Clinical Cases in Dermatology

Series Editor

Robert A. Norman, Tampa, USA

This series of concise practical guides is designed to facilitate the clinical decision-making process by reviewing a number of cases and defining the various diagnostic and management decisions open to clinicians.

Each title is illustrated and diverse in scope, enabling the reader to obtain relevant clinical information regarding both standard and unusual cases in a rapid, easy to digest format. Each focuses on one disease or patient group, and includes common cases to allow readers to know they are doing things right if they follow the case guidelines.

Nicholas Brownstone
Editor

Clinical Cases in Hidradenitis Suppurativa

Springer

Editor
Nicholas Brownstone
The Kimberly and Eric J. Waldman
Department of Dermatology at Mount Sinai
New York, NY, USA

ISSN 2730-6178 ISSN 2730-6186 (electronic)
Clinical Cases in Dermatology
ISBN 978-3-032-15199-5 ISBN 978-3-032-15200-8 (eBook)
https://doi.org/10.1007/978-3-032-15200-8

This Springer imprint is published by the registered company Springer Nature Switzerland AG
The registered company address is: Gewerbestrasse 11, 6330 Cham, Switzerland

To my family—thank you for your continued support and unconditional love

To AF, MC, AM, SH—I have wonderful memories that will last a lifetime

To my mentors from medical school, residency, fellowship, and beyond

To every patient suffering from HS

Foreword 1

Healthcare providers have the opportunity to change someone's life by learning more about recognizing and treating hidradenitis suppurativa (HS). This disease is not only overlooked but also commonly misdiagnosed. Consequently, a proper diagnosis takes an average of 7–10 years, leading to severe quality-of-life challenges for people living with HS.

Although new treatments are becoming available (and many more promising therapeutics are in clinical studies), these tools are only beneficial in the hands of knowledgeable providers. Educating dermatologists and other specialists about the diagnosis and treatment of HS is core to the mission of the HS Foundation—to improve the lives of people affected by HS.

We applaud Dr. Brownstone for writing this book and sharing vital knowledge with the dermatology community and beyond. We hope his efforts will meaningfully contribute to the rapidly evolving HS landscape, and above all, provide relief to those suffering from HS.

CEO, Hidradenitis Suppurativa Foundation
Apex, NC, USA
Brent Hazelett

Foreword 2

Hidradenitis suppurativa (HS) is a chronic skin condition characterized by recurrent painful nodules and abscesses that ultimately result in scars and tunnels and has a profound negative impact on quality of life. A mean delay in diagnosis of 7 years has hindered timely initiation of appropriate therapies for many patients with HS.

Fortunately, in recent years there have been revolutionary advancements in HS care, including a robust pipeline of therapeutics. A multimodal approach to care, utilizing both medical and procedural treatments, is often needed to optimize outcomes. The authors of this book, *Clinical Cases in Hidradenitis Suppurativa*, should be commended for presenting treatment principles in an accessible, easy-to-digest format. The cases in this book reflect patient scenarios that clinicians may encounter in a typical clinic day. Practical tips are also conveniently provided as key takeaway points at the end of every chapter.

In addition to covering therapies for HS in an up-to-date manner, chapters dedicated to patient populations that may require special treatment considerations such as women and children are included. A holistic approach to HS care is encouraged as can be seen by discussion of diet/lifestyle, complementary and alternative medicine, dressings, and wound care, along with patient resources and support groups. Topics including pain and itch management as well as HS comorbidities and complications are also addressed.

This book is a reflection of the immense progress that has been made in the HS field thus far and a window into further exciting advances to come. It is a wonderful companion text to have in clinic for the busy clinician!

Department of Dermatology
University of Southern California,
Los Angeles, CA, USA

Jennifer Hsiao

Preface

When we entered the profession of medicine, we all signed up to be "lifelong learners." The management of hidradenitis suppurativa (HS) illustrates this point beautifully. For many decades, our understanding of the pathophysiology of HS was limited and treatment was restricted to topical medications and oral antibiotics. In the last decade, a paradigm shift has occurred where we now have more clearly elucidated the immunopathogenic mechanisms of HS down to specific cell types and cytokines.

Within the last few years, there have been two new biologic agents approved for HS. Before 2015, there were no FDA-approved targeted therapies for HS, and from 2015 to 2023, there was only one. Furthermore, our understanding of the etiology, disease associations, and comorbidities of HS has expanded. Given this rapid change, new resources covering these topics are greatly needed.

This book seeks to address this need by covering the latest research on HS, including key chapters on the newest FDA-approved therapies, updates on comorbidities, special considerations in skin of color, the role of diet and environment, impact on quality of life, pipeline therapies, surgical/interventional management, a review of patient resources, and a chapter on the use of artificial intelligence in treating HS. I believe that practicing dermatologists, dermatology trainees, and medical students will all have something new to learn from this book. I also hope this book helps bridge the educational gap on HS for many other physicians who encounter this condition such as ER doctors, family medicine doctors, internal medicine doctors, OB/GYNs, pediatricians, and surgeons.

Many authors contributing to this book have outstanding expertise in the diagnosis and treatment of this disease. The topics they discuss will give the busy dermatology provider an excellent overview of the cutting-edge principles regarding the new therapies and concepts in the management of HS in a fun, case-based format. If the knowledge you gain from reading this book helps even just one patient, I view that as a success!

New York, NY, USA — Nicholas Brownstone

Contents

Chapter 1
Introduction to Hidradenitis Suppurativa (HS)

Elyse Mackenzie and Cindy Wassef

Case Title A 33-year-old female with recurring boils in the axilla and groin.

Case Presentation
A 33-year-old female with past medical history of obesity and metabolic syndrome presents to your clinic with recurrent painful nodules and abscesses primarily in the axillary and inguinal regions. These nodules have been recurrent over the past 5 years and intermittently drain purulent material with a notable foul odor and result in significant scarring. Symptoms worsen before menses. Previous treatments, mainly courses of antibiotics, have only offered transient relief. The patient notes a sibling with similar skin lesions. Her condition significantly affects her ability to perform daily tasks as a waitress, as friction from her uniform and repetitive movements while carrying food exacerbates the irritation. She has also begun experiencing sleep disturbances due to anxiety about how her pain is impacting her job performance.

Board Review Question
Which of the following is the most likely diagnosis in this patient?

A. Hidradenitis suppurativa
B. Cutaneous Crohn's disease
C. Furunculosis
D. Epidermoid cysts
E. Carbuncles

E. Mackenzie (✉) · C. Wassef
Rutgers Robert Wood Johnson Medical School, Piscataway, NJ, USA
e-mail: emm403@rwjms.rutgers.edu; wassefci@rutgers.edu

N. Brownstone (ed.), *Clinical Cases in Hidradenitis Suppurativa*, Clinical Cases in Dermatology, https://doi.org/10.1007/978-3-032-15200-8_1

Introduction to Hidradenitis Suppurativa (HS)

Definition and Epidemiology

Hidradenitis suppurativa (HS) is a chronic, relapsing inflammatory skin disease marked by recurrent painful nodules, abscesses, and draining sinus tracts in apocrine gland-rich, intertriginous regions. It primarily affects the axillae, groin, inframammary, and perianal areas. Onset typically occurs in the second to third decade of life, though pediatric and late-onset cases are reported. The global prevalence is approximately 1%, with estimates ranging from 0.1% in the United States to over 2% in parts of Europe and Africa depending on methodology and population studied [1]. The disease disproportionately affects women in Western countries, with a female-to-male ratio of 3:1, though this distribution may vary by region. In the United States, African American populations are particularly burdened [2].

Pathophysiology

The pathogenesis of HS is multifactorial, involving follicular occlusion, innate and adaptive immune dysregulation, microbial dysbiosis, and environmental and genetic contributors. It begins with follicular hyperkeratosis and infundibular occlusion leading to cyst formation and subsequent rupture, which initiates an exaggerated inflammatory response [3]. This response is characterized by neutrophil infiltration, cytokine release (notably TNF-α, IL-1β, and IL-17), bacterial dysbiosis, and the formation of sinus tracts and dermal fibrosis [4]. Obesity and smoking are well-established risk factors, and approximately one-third of patients report a family history, suggesting a genetic predisposition involving genes such as NCSTN [1].

Morphology and Clinical Presentation

HS lesions progress through a predictable morphological spectrum, beginning as painful, deep-seated nodules. These may evolve into abscesses, sinus tracts, and eventually extensive scarring. Common sites include the axillae, groin, perianal region, and inframammary folds. Patients often describe flares that worsen around menstruation, which may be attributed to cyclic sex hormone changes and peripheral androgen conversion [5]. The Hurley staging system, though limited in granularity, remains a widely used clinical tool, and is summarized by the following:

- *Stage I*: Isolated abscesses without sinus tracts or scarring.
- *Stage II*: Recurrent abscesses with isolated sinus tract formation and scarring.
- *Stage III*: Diffuse or near-complete area involvement with interconnected tracts and extensive scarring [1].

Despite its widespread use, the Hurley staging system does not allow for more nuanced evaluations of disease worsening or improvement. Emerging tools like the International Hidradenitis Suppurativa Severity Score System (IHS4) offer improved sensitivity for treatment response and disease monitoring [6]. Unlike the Hurley staging system, which categorizes disease into three broad stages and was primarily designed to guide surgical decision-making, the IHS4 is a dynamic and quantitative tool. It assigns numerical values to inflammatory nodules (×1), abscesses (×2), and draining tunnels (×4), allowing for a continuous measure of disease activity. This enables more precise monitoring of disease progression and treatment response, particularly in clinical trials and longitudinal care. The Dutch Hidradenitis Suppurativa Expert Group has also proposed a refinement of the Hurley staging system to address its limitations in assessing inflammation and disease extensiveness. Their updated model incorporates three components: the presence of sinus tracts, degree of inflammation, and anatomical distribution, providing a more nuanced stratification of disease severity and helping guide therapeutic decisions [7].

Histopathology of HS

Biopsies from HS lesions reveal a characteristic sequence of pathological changes beginning with follicular hyperkeratosis and epithelial hyperplasia, which lead to follicular occlusion and cystic dilation [1]. These changes are centered around terminal hair follicles in intertriginous areas, where the follicular unit includes associated sebaceous and apocrine glands. Dysregulated keratinization and accumulation of keratinous material within the follicular lumen, often influenced by environmental and metabolic factors such as obesity, smoking, and dysbiosis, contribute to early lesion formation [1]. Perilesional skin often shows psoriasiform hyperplasia, follicular plugging, and mild inflammatory cell infiltration, indicating subclinical activity [8]. As the disease progresses, follicular rupture occurs, releasing keratin debris and microbial components into the dermis and triggering a robust neutrophilic and histiocytic response. The subsequent inflammation promotes abscess formation and the development of sinus tracts lined with granulation tissue. Histologically, these tracts often appear as squamous epithelium-lined cysts or sinuses containing laminated keratin and hair shafts, suggesting origin from dilated and disrupted hair follicles rather than primary apocrine gland pathology [3]. In chronic lesions, dense aggregates of plasma cells, B-cells, and T-cells accumulate, sometimes forming tertiary lymphoid structures, while proliferating epithelial strands extend into the dermis and may contribute to tunnel formation and persistent disease [1, 8].

Treatment Options

Management of HS is multifaceted and depends on disease stage and severity. First-line interventions include lifestyle modifications such as smoking cessation and weight reduction, which may attenuate disease activity and reduce flare frequency [1]. Topical 1% clindamycin is recommended for mild disease, with intralesional triamcinolone injections used as an alternative treatment for symptomatic relief, especially during acute and painful flares [9]. Systemic antibiotics like doxycycline or combined rifampin-clindamycin are used for more extensive disease, with mono-therapy and combined treatments displaying clinically similar efficacy [10].

More recently, biologic therapies have revolutionized treatment for moderate-to-severe HS. Adalimumab, a TNF-alpha inhibitor, was the first FDA-approved biologic and has demonstrated efficacy in achieving HiSCR50 in over 40% of patients in clinical trials [11]. IL-17 inhibitors such as secukinumab and bimekizumab have since been FDA approved, with phase 3 trials showing superior efficacy compared to adalimumab, achieving HiSCR50 rates approaching or exceeding 50% [12]. These agents also show significant improvement in quality of life and reduction in lesion burden. Infliximab, another TNF-alpha inhibitor, while not FDA-approved for HS, is frequently used off-label in clinical practice for patients unresponsive to other therapies [1, 13]. Infliximab is an IV infusion medication while the other FDA approved biologics are subcutaneous injections. Infliximab may be dose adjusted based on the patient's weight. For refractory cases or those with extensive fibrotic changes, surgical options include incision and drainage, deroofing, or wide local excision. However, without targeting the underlying inflammatory process, surgical intervention alone is associated with high recurrence rate [1].

Differential Diagnosis of HS

Several dermatologic and systemic conditions can mimic HS, necessitating careful clinical differentiation (Table 1.1). Furunculosis presents as an acute, often solitary, painful nodule caused by *Staphylococcus aureus* infection. Unlike HS, it lacks chronicity and typically resolves without scarring [14]. Epidermoid cysts are benign, keratin-filled lesions with a central punctum and are generally non-inflammatory unless ruptured [15]. Carbuncles, which are clusters of furuncles, often occur in immunocompromised individuals and are localized to a single site, lacking the recurrent and scarring nature of HS [16]. Folliculitis in intertriginous areas may mimic HS, as this condition is also characterized by waxing and waning flares. However, folliculitis is characterized by pinpoint pustules on an erythematous base, which usually heals with hyperpigmented macules.

Cutaneous Crohn's disease may appear similarly to HS when affecting the perineal region, but is usually accompanied by systemic gastrointestinal symptoms,

Table 1.1 Differential diagnosis of hidradenitis suppurativa

Condition	Key clinical features	Differentiating points from HS
Furunculosis	Acute, tender, pus-filled nodule, often with central necrosis	Typically, a single lesion, short course; no sinus tracts, scarring; unlikely to be chronic and recurring
Carbuncles	Group of interconnected furuncles forming a painful nodule	Localized to a single site; bacterial etiology; not chronic or recurrent like HS
Epidermoid cysts	Firm, subcutaneous nodule with central punctum	Non-inflammatory unless ruptured; lacks sinus tracts and inflammatory flare pattern
Cutaneous Crohn's	Ulcerating plaques, nodules, or abscesses in perianal/perineal area with knife like ulcerations	Likely associated GI symptoms and systemic involvement; biopsy may reveal granulomatous inflammation
Acne conglobata	Nodulocystic acne with interconnected abscesses and comedones	Involves face, back, and chest; comedones are prominent; lacks sinus tracts in axilla/groin
SAPHO syndrome	Acne-like lesions with osteitis and joint pain	Presence of arthritis, hyperostosis, and systemic bone involvement distinguishes it from HS
Folliculitis	Pinpoint pustules on an erythematous base	Lesions are small and usually heal with hyperpigmented macules and do not form scarring or sinus tracts

including abdominal pain and diarrhea. However, in many cases of cutaneous Crohn's disease, the cutaneous symptoms precede the gastrointestinal symptoms. Biopsy, stool testing, and endoscopic evaluation help distinguish the two [17]. Referral to a gastroenterologist is important in suspected cases. A characteristic feature of cutaneous Crohn's disease is the presence of "knife-like" ulcerations in the skin. Acne conglobata involves cystic nodules and abscesses but predominantly affects the face, back, and chest, and is often comedone-rich [18]. SAPHO syndrome includes cutaneous pustulosis and is associated with osteitis and synovitis, which are not features of classic HS [19]. Recognizing these mimickers ensures timely and appropriate management and avoids unnecessary treatments.

Key Takeaways

- HS is a chronic inflammatory disorder marked by follicular occlusion, immune dysregulation, and recurrent painful lesions in intertriginous areas.
- The Hurley classification system and emerging tools like IHS4 are essential for staging and guiding therapy.
- Treatment ranges from lifestyle changes and topical therapies to biologics and surgical interventions.
- Mimickers such as furunculosis, cutaneous Crohn's disease, folliculitis, and epidermoid cysts must be differentiated carefully.
- Multidisciplinary care addressing comorbidities and psychosocial support is key to improving patient outcomes.

Board Review Question Explanation
Which of the following is the most likely diagnosis in this patient?

A. Hidradenitis suppurativa (Correct)
B. Cutaneous Crohn's disease
C. Furunculosis
D. Epidermoid cysts
E. Carbuncles

Answer Explanation The patient described displays hallmark features of HS: chronic, recurrent painful nodules in intertriginous regions, sinus tract formation, scarring, and a significant impact on quality of life.

The rationale for incorrect choices is as follows:

- B. Cutaneous Crohn's disease: Primarily affects the perianal area with concurrent GI symptoms
- C. Furunculosis: Presents as an acute, solitary bacterial abscess
- D. Epidermoid cysts: Non-inflammatory and identifiable by a central punctum
- E. Carbuncles: Localized bacterial infections lacking HS's chronic and relapsing course

References

1. Sabat R, Alavi A, Wolk K, Wortsman X, McGrath B, Garg A, Szepietowski JC. Hidradenitis suppurativa. Lancet. 2025;405(10476):420–38. https://doi.org/10.1016/S0140-6736(24)02475-9. Epub 2025 Jan 22. PMID: 39862870.
2. Garg A, Kirby JS, Lavian J, Lin G, Strunk A. Sex- and age-adjusted population analysis of prevalence estimates for hidradenitis suppurativa in the United States. JAMA Dermatol. 2017;153(8):760–4. https://doi.org/10.1001/jamadermatol.2017.0201. PMID: 28492923; PMCID: PMC5710402.
3. Yu CC, Cook MG. Hidradenitis suppurativa: a disease of follicular epithelium, rather than apocrine glands. Br J Dermatol. 1990;122(6):763–9. https://doi.org/10.1111/j.1365-2133.1990.tb06264.x. PMID: 2369556.
4. Krueger JG, Frew J, Jemec GBE, Kimball AB, Kirby B, Bechara FG, Navrazhina K, Prens E, Reich K, Cullen E, Wolk K. Hidradenitis suppurativa: new insights into disease mechanisms and an evolving treatment landscape. Br J Dermatol. 2024;190(2):149–62. https://doi.org/10.1093/bjd/ljad345. PMID: 37715694.
5. Karagiannidis I, Nikolakis G, Zouboulis CC. Endocrinologic aspects of hidradenitis suppurativa. Dermatol Clin. 2016;34(1):45–9. https://doi.org/10.1016/j.det.2015.08.005. PMID: 26617357.
6. Zouboulis CC, Tzellos T, Kyrgidis A, Jemec GBE, Bechara FG, Giamarellos-Bourboulis EJ, Ingram JR, Kanni T, Karagiannidis I, Martorell A, Matusiak Ł, Pinter A, Prens EP, Presser D, Schneider-Burrus S, von Stebut E, Szepietowski JC, van der Zee HH, Wilden SM, Sabat R, European Hidradenitis Suppurativa Foundation Investigator Group. Development and validation of the International Hidradenitis Suppurativa Severity Score System (IHS4), a novel dynamic scoring system to assess HS severity. Br J Dermatol. 2017;177(5):1401–9. https://doi.org/10.1111/bjd.15748. Epub 2017 Oct 30. PMID: 28636793.

7. Horváth B, Janse IC, Blok JL, Driessen RJ, Boer J, Mekkes JR, Prens EP, van der Zee HH. Hurley staging refined: a proposal by the Dutch Hidradenitis Suppurativa Expert Group. Acta Derm Venereol. 2017;97(3):412–3. https://doi.org/10.2340/00015555-2513. PMID: 27535129.
8. van der Zee HH, de Ruiter L, Boer J, van den Broecke DG, den Hollander JC, Laman JD, Prens EP. Alterations in leucocyte subsets and histomorphology in normal-appearing perilesional skin and early and chronic hidradenitis suppurativa lesions. Br J Dermatol. 2012;166(1):98–106. https://doi.org/10.1111/j.1365-2133.2011.10643.x. Epub 2011 Dec 5. PMID: 21929531.
9. Cuenca-Barrales C, Montero-Vílchez T, Sánchez-Díaz M, Martínez-López A, Rodríguez-Pozo JÁ, Díaz-Calvillo P, Arias-Santiago S, Molina-Leyva A. Intralesional treatments in hidradenitis suppurativa: a systematic review. Dermatology. 2022;238(6):1084–91. https://doi.org/10.1159/000524121. Epub 2022 Apr 27. PMID: 35477143.
10. van Straalen KR, Tzellos T, Guillem P, Benhadou F, Cuenca-Barrales C, Daxhelet M, Daoud M, Efthymiou O, Giamarellos-Bourboulis EJ, Jemec GBE, Katoulis AC, Koenig A, Lazaridou E, Marzano AV, Matusiak Ł, Molina-Leyva A, Moltrasio C, Pinter A, Potenza C, Romaní J, Saunte DM, Skroza N, Stergianou D, Szepietowski J, Trigoni A, Vilarrasa E, van der Zee HH. The efficacy and tolerability of tetracyclines and clindamycin plus rifampicin for the treatment of hidradenitis suppurativa: results of a prospective European cohort study. J Am Acad Dermatol. 2021;85(2):369–78. https://doi.org/10.1016/j.jaad.2020.12.089. Epub 2021 Jan 20. PMID: 33484766.
11. Kimball AB, Okun MM, Williams DA, Gottlieb AB, Papp KA, Zouboulis CC, Armstrong AW, Kerdel F, Gold MH, Forman SB, Korman NJ, Giamarellos-Bourboulis EJ, Crowley JJ, Lynde C, Reguiai Z, Prens EP, Alwawi E, Mostafa NM, Pinsky B, Sundaram M, Gu Y, Carlson DM, Jemec GB. Two phase 3 trials of adalimumab for hidradenitis suppurativa. N Engl J Med. 2016;375(5):422–34. https://doi.org/10.1056/NEJMoa1504370. PMID: 27518661.
12. Sabat R, Gudjonsson JE, Brembilla NC, van Straalen KR, Wolk K. Biology of Interleukin-17 and novel therapies for hidradenitis suppurativa. J Interf Cytokine Res. 2023;43(12):544–56. https://doi.org/10.1089/jir.2023.0105. Epub 2023 Oct 12. PMID: 37824200.
13. Ingram JR, Collier F, Brown D, Burton T, Burton J, Chin MF, Desai N, Goodacre TEE, Piguet V, Pink AE, Exton LS, Mohd Mustapa MF, Levell NJ, McHenry PM, Leslie TA, Wakelin S, Hunasehally RYP, Cork M, Johnston GA, Worsnop FS, Rakvit P, Salim A, McDonald B, Buckley D, Chua SL, Petrof G, Callachand N, Flavell T, Salad AA. British Association of Dermatologists guidelines for the management of hidradenitis suppurativa (acne inversa) 2018. Br J Dermatol. 2019;180(5):1009–17. https://doi.org/10.1111/bjd.17537.
14. Demos M, McLeod MP, Nouri K. Recurrent furunculosis: a review of the literature. Br J Dermatol. 2012;167(4):725–32. https://doi.org/10.1111/j.1365-2133.2012.11151.x. PMID: 22803835.
15. Zito PM, Scharf R. Epidermoid cyst [updated 2023 Aug 8]. In: StatPearls [Internet]. Treasure Island: StatPearls Publishing; 2025. Available from: https://www.ncbi.nlm.nih.gov/books/NBK499974/.
16. Troxell T, Hall CA. Carbuncle [updated 2023 July 3]. In: StatPearls [Internet]. Treasure Island: StatPearls Publishing; 2025. Available from: https://www.ncbi.nlm.nih.gov/books/NBK554459/.
17. Jørgensen AR, Thomsen SF, Karmisholt KE, Ring HC. Clinical, microbiological, immunological and imaging characteristics of tunnels and fistulas in hidradenitis suppurativa and Crohn's disease. Exp Dermatol. 2020;29(2):118–23. https://doi.org/10.1111/exd.14036. Epub 2019 Oct 1. PMID: 31519056.
18. Hafsi W, Arnold DL, Kassardjian M. Acne conglobata [2023 June 1]. In: StatPearls [Internet]. Treasure Island: StatPearls Publishing; 2025. PMID: 29083736.
19. Kahn MF, Khan MA. The SAPHO syndrome. Baillieres Clin Rheumatol. 1994;8(2):333–62. https://doi.org/10.1016/s0950-3579(94)80022-7. PMID: 8076391.

Chapter 2
HS in Skin of Color

Sidra Ibad and Victoria Farley

Case Title A 33-year-old African American female patient presents with foul-smelling axillary nodules and inguinal scarring

Case

A 33-year-old African American female patient presents with foul-smelling, draining nodules on her axillary vault. She also has significant inguinal scarring and notices a correlation between her menstrual cycles and the onset of symptoms. She has an 8-year smoking history and a BMI of 35. She has tried applying clindamycin to the affected areas and taken 100 mg doxycycline twice daily for the past 2–3 months without significant improvement.

Board Review Question

In the case presented above, which biologic is not FDA approved to treat the patient's disease?

A. Humira (adalimumab)
B. Cosentyx (secukinumab)
C. Bimzelx (bimekizumab)
D. Enbrel (etanercept)
E. None

S. Ibad
Department of Internal Medicine, HCA Sunrise/Mountainview Hospital, Las Vegas, NV, USA

V. Farley (✉)
Vivida Dermatology, Las Vegas, NV, USA
e-mail: vfarley@vivida.com

N. Brownstone (ed.), *Clinical Cases in Hidradenitis Suppurativa*, Clinical Cases in Dermatology, https://doi.org/10.1007/978-3-032-15200-8_2

The true incidence of hidradenitis suppurativa is unknown. HS has a prevalence of approximately 1.3% in African American populations, 0.75% in Caucasian populations, and 0.07% in Hispanic populations. HS develops due to a complex interplay between microbiome alteration, infundibular hyperkeratosis, and subclinical terminal hair follicle inflammation, leading to follicular plugging and eventual rupture. Following rupture, there is release of bacteria into the dermis, precipitating an inflammatory response and chronic inflammation. External factors that contribute to this disease process include genetics (gamma-secretase loss of function mutations) and the interplay between smoking and obesity [1]. This combination of factors leads to macrophage production of TNF alpha and IL-1beta, leading to dendritic production of IL-23. IL-23 production leads to Th17 polarization and culminates in the production of interleukins and increased autoinflammation. Some interleukins involved in the pathogenesis include IL-1, IL-12, IL-23, IL-17, and IL-36 (Fig. 2.1).

HS develops most often in intertriginous areas, such as the axilla, groin, buttocks, breast, inner thighs, and the waist. Manifestations include sinus tracts, nodules, abscesses, hypertrophic scarring, tunneling, pustules, and ulceration. The histopathology of HS includes hyperplasia of follicular epithelium, follicular occlusion and follicular hyperkeratosis [2]. The differential diagnosis for HS includes folliculitis, cutaneous Crohn's disease, intergluteal pilonidal cysts, carbuncles, and acne.

There are a limited number of controlled trials studying HS in skin of color patients, and HS remains underrepresented and underdiagnosed in skin of color patients. In the same vein, there are barriers to access for darker-skinned patients because they tend to have lower access to dermatologists, and therefore, difficulty

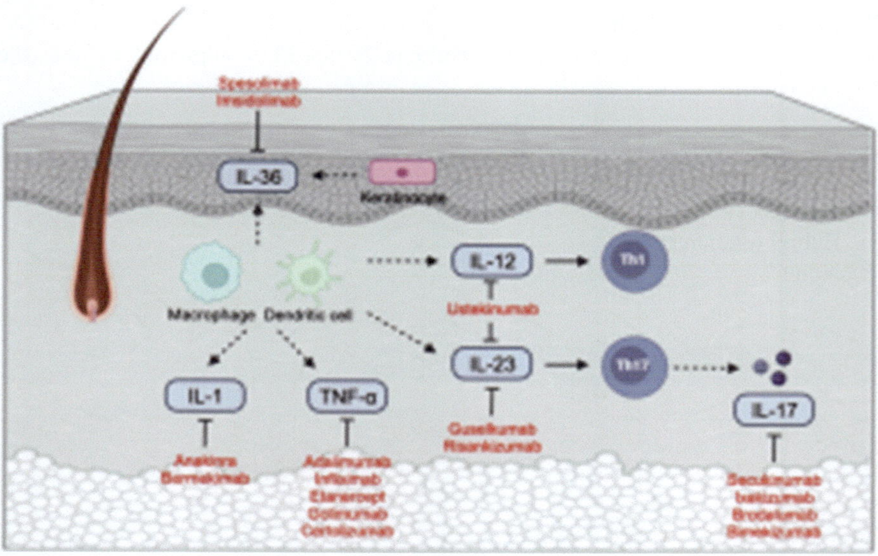

Fig. 2.1 Specific interleukins involved in the immunopathophysiology of HS. (Source: https://www.mdpi.com/2673-5601/4/1/4)

obtaining proper diagnosis. If left untreated, HS can lead to secondary infection, impaired lymph drainage, restrictions in movement, chronic pain, and detrimental psychological effects. Additionally, clinical trials between 2000 and 2019 included 68% Caucasian patients and a mere 14% African American patients, even though HS is significantly more common in patients with skin of color. It is unclear which factors, whether they be access to healthcare, lifestyle modifications, or distrust of the healthcare system contributed most to the limited involvement in clinical trials from skin of color patients.

One retrospective cohort study from Stanford University in 2021 studied access to care for HS patients with skin of color. The Hispanic patients in this study entered tertiary care centers at an earlier age (38.7 years of age for Caucasian patients and 30.8 years for Hispanics) but had increased symptom severity. Alternately, African American patients presented to tertiary care centers at a later age and with greater severity at the time of presentation. The African American and Hispanic patients included in this study were found to have significantly lower levels of incomes, which exacerbated healthcare disparities. This healthcare disparity is further exacerbated by the fact that patients with HS have increased unemployment, higher indirect costs, and slower income growth [3].African American patients were more likely to seek surgeons for complex excisions than their primary care providers and dermatologists, likely due to lack of health insurance. When these patients did pursue healthcare providers, they were given primarily pain-relief medications, including gabapentin and NSAIDs. Caucasian patients have shorter delays in diagnosis compared to their black counterparts [4]. Caucasian patients had approximately a 3.2-year delay in diagnosis when compared to their black and Hispanic counterparts who had a 4.8- and 4.7-year delay in diagnosis, respectively. The delay has been as much as 1.62 times that of Caucasian patients. For this reason, skin of color patients were found to have higher Hurley stages by the time of presentation. Similarly, African American patients with HS did not follow up as quickly after their initial diagnosis as compared to Caucasian patients. African American patients were approximately three times as likely to have an ED visit for their HS and to develop Hurley stage III. They were also approximately twice as likely to be hospitalized and require surgery when compared to their Caucasian counterparts. Black and Hispanic patients have poorer quality of life, with greater rates of depression, anxiety, and social isolation compared to their Caucasian counterparts at baseline [5].

Of the cases of the US National Library of Medicine, only 238 (13.7%) were African American patients and 20 (7.2%) were Hispanic patients, 14 (1.3%) were American Indian patients, and 26 (2.6%) were Asian patients [6]. Given the lack of racial heterogeneity in research databases, large population-based studies are required, and early interventions must be implemented to slow disease progression. Studies targeted at genetic factors, diet/lifestyle factors, and the response of skin of color to different therapies should be initiated. Reasons for underrepresentation of African American patients in HS trials include transportation difficulties, distrust with the healthcare system, difficulty finding time, and lack of awareness of trial opportunities. Hispanic patients may be underrepresented in trials due to language barriers.

Other necessary measures include increasing access to specialist HS clinics in areas that have high emergency room admission rates for HS. There should be increased resource distribution in communities of color. As for treatment approaches, it is important to develop less complex treatment strategies and cost-effective strategies. Education and training programs should be initiated to help recognize how HS appears different in darker skin tones, to develop provider directories of HS experts, and to incorporate skin of color images in existing continuing medical education and medical school courses. In addition, community outreach measures could be developed that include developing educational materials targeted to communities of color and hosting seminars and health care fairs at health clinics and churches. Other practical measures include developing culturally sensitive materials, providing financial assistance for patients with HS, translating materials into other languages, and creating partnerships with supporting organizations [7, 8].

Since many of these patients are unable to receive proper treatment in earlier stages of HS, their symptoms can deteriorate, and they may require Emergency Room care. African American and Hispanic patients have significantly higher rates of hospitalization and emergency department visits compared to their white counterparts. It is essential for clinicians to be made aware of how race and ethnicity play a factor in HS and be able to advocate for future clinical trials and cohort studies to investigate this role. Dermatologists must be willing to recognize race-based inequities for their patients and increase the availability of specialist hidradenitis suppurativa clinics where they are most needed.

Board Review Question Explanation
In the case presented above, which biologic is *not* FDA approved to treat the patient's disease?

A. Humira (adalimumab)
B. Cosentyx (secukinumab)
C. Bimzelx (bimekizumab)
D. Enbrel (etanercept) (Correct)
E. None

Correct Answer:
D. Enbrel (etanercept)

Humira (adalimumab) is a TNF-alpha inhibitor biologic used in patients 12 years and older with moderate to severe HS. Humira was the first FDA approved medication for HS. Cosentyx (secukinumab) is an IL-17A inhibitor biologic. Cosentyx received FDA approval in October of 2023. In November 2024, the FDA approved bimelkizumab (Bimzelx) for moderate to severe hidradenitis suppurativa. It is also a biologic and works via IL-17A and IL-17F inhibition. Potential risks of Il-17 inhibitors include exacerbation of inflammatory bowel disease, while adalimumab has been linked to cancers, including leukemia and lymphoma, multiple sclerosis, and new-onset heart failure. Although Enbrel is a TNF-alpha inhibitor like Humira, it has not been shown in clinical trials to improve hidradenitis suppurativa symptoms in the same way. Enbrel is not FDA approved to treat HS.

Key Takeaway Points

- There are a limited number of controlled trials studying HS in skin of color patients, and HS remains underrepresented and underdiagnosed in skin of color patients.
- African American patients are more likely to seek surgery, have greater delays in diagnosis, and be hospitalized for HS when compared to their white counterparts.
- African American and Hispanic patients with HS have poorer quality of life, with greater rates of depression, anxiety, and social isolation compared to their Caucasian counterparts.
- Given the lack of racial heterogeneity in research databases, large population-based studies are required, and early interventions must be implemented to slow disease progression.
- Necessary measures to address health disparities in HS include increasing access to specialist HS clinics, increased resource distribution, education and training programs, and community outreach measures.

References

1. Wolk K, Join-Lambert O, Sabat R. Aetiology and pathogenesis of hidradenitis suppurativa. Br J Dermatol. 2020;183(6):999–1010. https://doi.org/10.1111/bjd.19556.
2. Smith SDB, Okoye GA, Sokumbi O. Histopathology of hidradenitis suppurativa: a systematic review. Dermatopathology. 2022;9(3):251–7. https://doi.org/10.3390/dermatopathology9030029.
3. Kilgour JM, Li S, Sarin KY. Hidradenitis suppurativa in patients of color is associated with increased disease severity and healthcare utilization: a retrospective analysis of 2 U.S. cohorts [published correction appears in JAAD Int. 2021;3:88. doi: 10.1016/j.jdin.2021.03.006]. JAAD Int. 2021;3:42–52. https://doi.org/10.1016/j.jdin.2021.01.007.
4. Robinson I, Lee L, Cotton C. The impact of racial differences on treatment strategies in hidradenitis suppurativa: a retrospective review. J Drugs Dermatol. 2022;21(3):270–5. https://doi.org/10.36849/JDD.6446.
5. Serrano L, Ulschmid C, Szabo A, Roth G, Sokumbi O. Racial disparities of delay in diagnosis and dermatologic care for hidradenitis suppurativa. J Natl Med Assoc. 2022;114(6):613–6. https://doi.org/10.1016/j.jnma.2022.08.002.
6. Elhage KG, Davis MS, Hakimi M, et al. Ethnoracial representation in hidradenitis suppurativa clinical trials. Arch Dermatol Res. 2023;315(6):1793–6. https://doi.org/10.1007/s00403-022-02510-4.
7. Ulschmid C, Serrano L, Wu R, Roth GM, Sokumbi O. African American race is a risk factor for severe hidradenitis suppurativa. Int J Dermatol. 2023;62(5):657–63. https://doi.org/10.1111/ijd.16428.
8. Sachdeva M, Shah M, Alavi A. Race-specific prevalence of hidradenitis suppurativa. J Cutan Med Surg. 2021;25(2):177–87. https://doi.org/10.1177/1203475420972348.

Chapter 3
HS and Quality of Life

Madeline Tchack and Cindy Wassef

Case Title A 47-year-old female presents with recurrent, painful, malodorous nodules with evidence of multiple sinus tracts in the anogenital area.

Case

A 47-year-old female with a 15-year history of hidradenitis suppurativa presents with recurrent, painful, malodorous nodules and draining sinus tracts localized primarily to the anogenital region. She reports chronic fatigue and difficulty with ambulation due to persistent pain and swelling in the affected areas. She's been having trouble keeping a stable job and typically calls out from work 2–3 times/month from excessive pain or shame from drainage. She constantly worries about how she will be able to pay her medical bills and sometimes stays up all night worrying. She often avoids seeing friends and socializing and has not pursued a romantic relationship since the onset of disease. She has no suicidal ideation or prior suicide attempts. Vitals are within normal. On physical examination, the patient has an obese body habitus with multiple inflamed nodules, abscesses, and interconnected sinus tracts in the anogenital region with significant malodor and copious seropurulent drainage. There's evidence of extensive scarring, post-inflammatory hyperpigmentation, and areas of verrucous skin changes are present. PHQ-9 and GAD-7 scores are 12 and 10, respectively.

M. Tchack
Rutgers Robert Wood Johnson Medical School, Piscataway, NJ, USA

Rutgers Robert Wood Johnson, Department of Dermatology, Somerset, NJ, USA
e-mail: mst122@rwjms.rutgers.edu

C. Wassef (✉)
Premier Health Associates, Randolph, NJ, USA
e-mail: cindy.wassef@atlantichealth.org

N. Brownstone (ed.), *Clinical Cases in Hidradenitis Suppurativa*, Clinical Cases in Dermatology, https://doi.org/10.1007/978-3-032-15200-8_3

Board Review Question
A 36-year-old man with Hurley stage III hidradenitis suppurativa (HS) involving the axillae, groin, and perineum presents for evaluation. He reports significant pain, recurrent drainage, and social withdrawal due to embarrassment about odor and scarring. He has missed over 30 days of work in the past year and has recently been denied a promotion due to frequent absences. Which of the following statements best describes the economic and occupational burden associated with HS?

A. Financial burden is primarily driven by medication costs
B. Patients with HS are less likely to utilize emergency departments compared to patients with psoriasis
C. HS is associated with higher rates of work absenteeism, presenteeism, and unemployment compared to other dermatologic conditions
D. The financial burden of HS is largely mitigated by insurance coverage
E. Work function is generally preserved in patients with HS if disease severity is limited to Hurley stage I–II

Hidradenitis suppurativa (HS) is a chronic, recurrent, and debilitating inflammatory skin disease that profoundly impacts health-related quality of life (HRQoL) across physical, psychological, sexual, occupational, and financial domains. Although many dermatologic conditions are associated with impaired HRQoL, emerging evidence suggests that the burden of HS often exceeds that of other cutaneous conditions [1, 2]. Several studies have found that greater HS disease severity, assessed by Hurley stage, correlates with significantly worse Dermatology Life Quality Index (DLQI) scores [3, 4], with stronger positive relationships observed between DLQI scores and disease activity ($p < 0.0001$), the number of anatomical regions involved ($p = 0.045$), and anogenital localization ($p = 0.0051$) [3]. Early disease onset has also been identified as a key risk factor for more profound and enduring quality of life impairment in patients with HS [5], potentially contributing to the impaired development of social and romantic relationships as well impaired work function and decreased financial stability. A concise summary regarding the impact of quality of life on each health domain can be found in Table 3.1.

QoL and Other Dermatologic Skin Conditions

Psoriasis has been well documented to negatively impact HRQoL, comparable to serious systemic conditions like congestive heart failure, diabetes, and cancer [6], and emerging data suggests that HS may exert an even greater burden in key domains. In head-to-head comparisons, patients with moderate-to-severe HS reported greater pain, worse HRQoL, and more significant work impairment than patients with moderate-to-severe plaque psoriasis [7]. Financially, the burden appears similar, with annual out-of-pocket costs for HS patients approximating those seen in psoriasis ($2250 vs. $2528, respectively) [8].

Table 3.1 Summary of key findings in each quality-of-life domain

Domain	Key findings
Physical health	Pain, itching, burning, drainage, and bleeding arising from deep-seated nodules, abscesses, sinus tracts Restricted mobility; may interfere with activities of daily living Fatigue Impairment positively correlates with clinical severity, but even milder disease impairs physical function Early disease onset worsens impact Associated with many comorbidities
Mental health	Strongly associated with depression, anxiety, suicidality, substance use disorders, and other psychiatric conditions Distress from shame, low self-esteem, fear of stigmatization, social isolation, and lesion location Suicide completion is higher compared to general population Pediatric patients show mental health impairments comparable to the elderly Early disease onset worsens impact
Sexual health	Sexual dysfunction is highly prevalent; estimated to affect >50% of HS patients Physical symptoms in anogenital and perianal regions contribute to impaired sexual function Psychological factors strongly correlate with sexual dysfunction A stable romantic partner may mitigate sexual distress and improve outcomes Female HS patients experience greater sexual distress compared to male patients Both male and female patients score significantly lower on standardized sexual health measures compared to healthy controls
Work function	HS commonly emerges during the second and third decades of life and disrupts education and early workforce entry Patients miss substantial work time annually: ~26–47 days (absenteeism), ~63 days (presenteeism) Painful, malodorous lesions significantly impair work ability and mobility Psychological distress further contributes to presenteeism and reduced workplace performance Lower annual incomes, slower income growth, higher unemployment rates, and greater reliance on illness benefits compared to healthy individuals Increased risks of job dismissal, limited promotional opportunities, and higher rates of short- and long-term disability leave compared to healthy controls
Healthcare utilization	Higher direct healthcare costs than healthy controls—Increased ED, outpatient, and inpatient utilization Hospitalization accounts for over a third of total treatment expenses; over 40% of patients experience at least one hospitalization Pay an average of $2949.75 annually in direct costs, in addition to indirect costs from transportation, OTC products, and wound care supplies Noncurative surgeries contribute significantly to costs Medicaid and lower SES patients experience a disproportionate financial burden compared to commercially insured patients Treatment with anti-TNF agents (i.e., adalimumab) has demonstrated cost savings

Despite some similarities, important differences have been observed. When assessed using the 15D HRQoL questionnaire, both HS and psoriasis patients exhibited a similar pattern of impairment, but HS patients showed significantly worse outcomes in specific areas, particularly sexual activity ($p = 0.03$) [9]. Prior studies further revealed that sexual dysfunction scores were higher in HS patients than in those with psoriasis, even among psoriasis patients with genital involvement or comorbid depression [10–12]. Likewise, prevalence of sexual and erectile dysfunction appears to be slightly higher among individuals with HS compared to those with psoriasis [13]. Although psoriasis patients often experience high rates of anxiety, depression, low self-esteem, and social isolation [14, 15]—likely due to the highly visible nature of psoriatic lesions—HS patients face distressing, concealed symptoms such as deep nodules, malodor, and pain in sensitive areas, contributing profoundly to sexual dysfunction, social withdrawal, and psychological distress [9, 10, 13].

Social media sentiment analysis has reflected these nuances, with more frequent mentions of emotionally charged words like "crying" and aggressive language in tweets about HS compared to psoriasis and alopecia areata, possibly reflecting the higher prevalence of psychiatric comorbidities such as bipolar disorder and major depressive disorder in the HS population [16]. Furthermore, HS tends to present at a younger age than psoriasis, potentially magnifying its long-term HRQoL and economic consequences [1, 17]. In pediatric populations, the impact on quality of life was found to be more pronounced in HS, with Skindex-Teen scores more than twice as high as those of pediatric psoriasis patients (45.7 vs. 21.1) [18, 19].

Beyond psoriasis, HS has been shown to exert a worse quality of life burden than many other dermatologic and systemic diseases. Results of multiple studies have found great QoL impairment in HS patients compared to those with other dermatoses [2, 3, 10], including atopic dermatitis [20], acne vulgaris [21], alopecia [22], Darier disease, Hailey-Hailey [23], chronic urticaria [3], and skin cancer [24]. Patients with HS reported significantly poorer body image compared to patients with psoriasis, dermatitis, skin malignancies, and even systemic lupus erythematosus [25]. In comparisons with systemic diseases, HS patients reported worse quality of life scores than individuals suffering from inflammatory bowel disease, hepatitis C, lower limb amputation, major adverse cardiac events [26, 27], Crohn's disease, ulcerative colitis and rheumatoid arthritis [1, 15, 28]. Some findings suggest that the impact of HS on daily functioning and mental health may be comparable to that observed in conditions such as cardiovascular disease, COPD, diabetes mellitus, and cancer [24, 29, 30].

Healthcare utilization patterns further reflect the disease burden. Patients with HS require emergency department and inpatient care more frequently than those with other chronic inflammatory skin conditions [31, 32], and their healthcare costs exceed those for patients with breast, colorectal, or lung cancer [33]. During a 6-month period, 43.1% of HS patients reported missing work due to their illness, a much higher rate than those with psoriasis (17.7%) and atopic dermatitis (27.9%), and comparable to those with chronic urticaria (43.6%). HS patients were also more likely to require hospitalization (26.3%) compared to patients with psoriasis (8.1%), atopic dermatitis (5.8%), and chronic urticaria (13%) [34].

Pain, functional impairment, anxiety, depression, suicidal ideation, social stigmatization and isolation, low self-esteem, body image difficulties, and sexual dysfunction are key factors driving the heavy psychological burden seen across chronic skin diseases [35–37], but HS appears to disproportionately affect all domains of life. Kimball et al. explain that the cumulative life course impairment from HS, beginning early in life and the disease course and spanning decades, may prevent patients from achieving their full potential [38, 39].

Taken together, these findings demonstrate that while psoriasis and other chronic skin conditions such as atopic dermatitis, acne, and chronic urticaria significantly impact quality of life, HS is consistently associated with greater impairments across multiple realms. HS patients face a unique combination of physical pain, sexual dysfunction, psychological burden, and economic strain that may exceed the burden seen in many other dermatologic and systemic diseases.

Physical, Mental, and Sexual Health

Physical Health

Physical symptoms associated with HS, including pain, itching, burning, drainage, and bleeding arising from deep-seated nodules, abscesses, sinus tracts, and scar tissue have a profound impact on physical health [40]. In some studies, pain is the most frequently reported symptom [41, 42] and is often accompanied by high levels of irritation, itching, self-consciousness, embarrassment, and disability [4]. More than 75% of patients reported experiencing drainage, irritation, pain, itching, bleeding and odor, which significantly correlated with disease severity and functional limitations, including restricted arm movement and negative impacts on work, school, and personal relationships [4]. Even patients with mild-to-moderate HS experience reduced physical health status compared to the general population [39]. These physical limitations frequently interfere with activities of daily living and exercise, with 42.23% of patients reporting general activity impairment on Work Productivity and Activity Impairment scores [40], and many patients endorsing fatigue and having difficulty with basic tasks such as walking, climbing stairs, or lifting groceries [28].

Compared to healthy individuals, Hurley stage III HS patients report significantly worse physical functioning, increased bodily pain, reduced energy levels, and a more negative perception of general health [28]. These effects can begin early in life, as young adults with HS have reported physical health scores, daily living disabilities, and functional limitations similar in severity to individuals aged 65 years or older in the general population [39]. This dramatic physical toll may contribute to a phenomenon known as cumulative life course impairment, wherein chronic disease progressively limits a person's ability to achieve their "full life potential" or what life could have been without the disease [38, 39].

Furthermore, HS is often associated with a range of comorbid conditions such as obesity, smoking, Crohn's disease, and spondyloarthropathies, all of which exacerbate physical symptoms and increase systemic inflammation [43]. Components of metabolic syndrome, including hypertension, hyperlipidemia, diabetes, and anemia, are also more prevalent in HS patients, further exacerbating the overall physical burden these patients face [44]. Together, these findings underscore the substantial physical limitations imposed by HS, which reduce quality of life, restrict physical activity, and mimic the functional decline seen in much older populations.

Mental Health

Much like its effects on physical health, HS exerts a profound psychological toll on patients, contributing significantly to impaired quality of life and an increased risk of mental health disorders. Multiple studies have shown strong associations between HS and both psychological stressors such as, low self-esteem, fear of stigmatization, isolation, loneliness, and unemployment [24, 45–48] and a variety of mental health disorders, including depression, anxiety, schizophrenia, personality disorders, ADD/ADHD, substance use disorders, suicidality, and adjustment disorders [49]. One meta-analysis identified bipolar disorder and major depressive disorder as the most prevalent comorbidities in individuals with HS [50], while a recent US population-based study found that approximately 43% of people with HS had comorbid depression, a higher prevalence than in patients with other dermatologic conditions [24, 51].

Psychological distress in HS often stems from shame, low self-esteem, and social isolation, particularly when lesions are in exposed or anogenital regions [52–54]. Symptoms such as malodorous drainage, persistent discomfort, and unpredictable flares can significantly disrupt daily activities, impacting wardrobe choices and limiting participation in work, social, and sexual interactions, potentially leading to cycles of emotional withdrawal and avoidance behaviors [53, 55]. The mental health burden is further compounded by the disease's strong association with severe psychiatric outcomes; individuals with HS are up to twice as likely to die by suicide compared to the general population [48, 56], and a Finnish registry study reported that 4.4% of deaths in patients with HS were attributed to suicide [57]. In addition, a large cross-sectional study found that the prevalence of substance use disorder was two times higher in HS patients compared to the general population, especially involving alcohol, opioids, and marijuana [58].

The impact of HS on mental health begins early in the disease course. In pediatric HS patients, over 32% of patients screened positive for depression, more than double the rate in the general adolescent population [19]. Other studies have demonstrated that young patients with HS reported physical and mental health statuses comparable to elderly individuals from the general population, with the worst self-reported mental health seen in patients who had been suffering from the disease for at least a decade [39].

Despite the significant mental health burden, many patients likely do not receive appropriate psychiatric support. Integrating psychodermatology into HS care, such as routinely screening for depression and anxiety, discussing emotional and social challenges, and providing referrals to mental health professionals and support groups, has been recommended to improve outcomes. Studies suggest that topics like body image therapy, access to therapists specializing in skin disorders, insurance coverage for mental healthcare, HS-specific support groups, and increased funding for HS research may all help to mitigate psychological morbidity seen in HS patients [54].

Encouragingly, some studies suggest that effective management of HS symptoms can lead to improvements in mental health, offering a potential pathway for holistic treatment [49]. Given the multifactorial nature of mental distress in HS, a multidisciplinary approach addressing both dermatologic and psychological dimensions is critical to improving quality of life in this population.

Sexual Health

HS significantly affects sexual health and quality of life, particularly due to the physical, psychological, and social challenges associated with the disease. One study found that about 50% of the DLQI variance in HS patients was attributable to sexual dysfunction and distress [59]. In general, sexual dysfunction is highly prevalent in HS, with rates ranging from 51 to 62%, and erectile dysfunction reported in 52–60% of male patients [60]. Moreover, HS commonly involves intimate body areas, leading to discomfort, pain, and embarrassment that can severely disrupt sexual functioning [5, 28, 59, 61]. Patients with anogenital involvement and active painful lesions reported feeling ashamed of their lesions and scars, fearing that others, especially intimate partners, may find them unattractive or repulsive, negatively affecting both sexual health and social well-being [60–62].

Though the exact mechanisms by which sexual dysfunction occurs in HS patients is unclear, the cause is likely multifactorial and a combination of psychological factors and physical symptoms [55, 63]. Lesions in the groin, genital, and perianal areas may make sexual activity challenging [63], while systemic inflammation may alter hormone levels and vascular function, potentially leading to erectile dysfunction [5, 63, 64]. Psychological factors such as anxiety, depression, and body image disturbance also contribute significantly, with sexual dysfunction correlating strongly with depressive and anxiety symptoms in HS patients [65]. Having a stable romantic partner may help mitigate some of the emotional distress, leading to improved sexual confidence and reduced orgasm difficulty [63].

Multiple studies have found that, compared with healthy controls, both male and female HS patients scored significantly lower on standardized measures of sexual health [10, 66–68]. Nevertheless, women seem to experience greater sexual distress and impaired sexual function as compared to men, despite comparable disease severity [10, 60]. In one study by Kurek et al., all 44 participants with HS experienced some degree of sexual dysfunction, with worse impairment in women [10]. Strong correlations were observed in female HS patients between sexual function, distress, and quality of life, while in male HS patients, quality of life impairment did not correlate as significantly with sexual function. The authors also postulated that the impact on female patients may be attributed to their earlier age of disease onset (diagnosed approximately 6 years earlier in women), potentially leading to more profound disruptions to sexual development and self-image. Additionally, the authors suggested that higher impairment in sexual health in women may be a result of higher emotional and neuroendocrine responsiveness in females [10].

In sum, HS deeply impacts sexual health through a complex interplay of physical lesions, psychological distress, stigma, and systemic inflammation. This dimension of disease burden is often underrecognized, yet it plays a pivotal role in the overall quality of life for patients living with HS.

Work Function

HS poses a substantial burden on occupational functioning and economic productivity, particularly because it typically emerges during the critical years of education and workforce entry in the second or third decade of life [69, 70]. Patients with HS experience significant disruptions in work function, missing an average of 26 days annually and an additional 63 days from presenteeism, which is reduced productivity while present at work [71]. Other studies report similar findings: patients missed approximately 47 days annually for HS-related flares or medical visits [72], while 58% of employed patients cited HS as the cause of work absence, with a mean of 34 days missed per year [3, 73].

Workplace challenges are likely multifactorial for HS patients. The disease's physical manifestations often result in unavoidable absences [74], particularly when lesions are located in areas that limit mobility and make sitting difficult, such as the axillae, buttocks, or genitals [74, 75]. Presenteeism is also commonly reported and may stem from patients restricting movements to avoid exposing lesions or staining clothing due to malodorous discharge [74]. One pooled analysis found that patients with HS experienced a 10.17% rate of work time missed, with an additional 31.13% of time at work being impaired, culminating in a total work productivity impairment of 34.25% [40].

Beyond physical symptoms, HS also exerts a psychological toll that affects workplace performance. Patients with higher scores on the Hospital Anxiety and Depression Scale demonstrated greater impairment in work productivity [75, 76], while fear of stigmatization was also reported to contribute to mental distress and avoidance behaviors [36, 77].

Both physical and psychological effects appear to manifest in broader employment and financial trends. Compared to healthy individuals, patients with HS have significantly lower annual incomes, slower income growth, and increased risk of workforce exit [3, 73, 78]. A retrospective cohort study found that employed HS patients earned on average $7432.00 less annually and had $324.00 less income growth per year with higher risks of leaving the workforce compared to controls [73]. Similarly, 10% of patients reported being dismissed from work due to HS-related work impairments or absences, and 23.3% reported limited promotional opportunities [3]. In another cohort, only 60.6% of HS patients were employed, while 24% were unemployed and 15.2% received illness benefits despite having higher educational attainment than their parents and the general population [78]. One European study estimated that HS-related unemployment rates were twice that of the general population and resulted in a national loss of gross value totaling approximately 12.6 billion euros annually [76]. In the USA, it has also been found that patients with HS were more likely than matched controls to take short- and long-term disability leave and less likely to retire early, potentially due to financial constraints from ongoing medical costs and reduced earning capacity [73].

Collectively, these findings suggest that HS substantially impairs both work participation and advancement, compounding the disease's burden on individual quality of life and contributing to significant socioeconomic consequences at the population level.

Healthcare Costs

HS has been found to be associated with a significant economic burden that affects both individual patients and the healthcare system. Studies have found that HS patients incur substantially higher direct healthcare costs than those with psoriasis or the general population primarily due to the following factors: increased ED, outpatient and inpatient utilization, the cost of prescription medications and occupational difficulties [32, 36, 79]. Further, an estimated 69% of HS patients reported financial toxicity that was positively correlated with disease extent, number of affected body regions, procedures, and ED visits [80]. The chronic and relapsing nature of HS may contribute to its long-term financial toll [32] as patients frequently face catastrophic costs due to prolonged treatment needs, lost productivity, and extensive travel for care [72].

Multiple studies have demonstrated increased healthcare costs of HS patients compared to healthy controls. One study found that, compared to healthy controls, HS patients had estimated healthcare costs that were $6783.00 higher over a 7-year period [32], while another study estimated total costs to be nearly $7000.00 higher over a 3-year period [81, 82]. Another study revealed that HS patients pay an average of $2949.75/year in direct costs alone [72]. These direct expenses are likely further compounded by indirect costs, such as transportation, over-the-counter products, and out-of-pocket spending on dressings and analgesia [79].

Hospitalization represents a major driver of cost, accounting for an estimated 37.4% of overall treatment expenses [32]. Among HS patients, 43% experienced at least one hospitalization, far exceeding the national average of 0.12% [80], and

18.5% were hospitalized more than once [83]. Noncurative surgery alone was associated with a mean incremental cost of $4286.00 per patient, largely due to inpatient care [84].

These economic challenges appear to be especially pronounced in populations with lower socioeconomic status. Insurance coverage for medications and wound care supplies varies significantly, potentially adding another layer of financial uncertainty [85]. Medicaid and low socioeconomic status patients have shown an HS prevalence rate 3–3.5 times higher than those in Commercial/Medicare populations, likely influenced by racial disparities as HS is more common in Black individuals [86, 87]. Studied have demonstrated that, compared to their commercially insured counterparts, Medicaid HS patients are younger but suffer from more comorbidities and higher rates of ED visits, hospitalizations, and prescription pain medication use [44]. Further, lower income and educational attainment, more severe disease, and worse quality-of-life metrics all predict greater direct and indirect costs in HS patients [71].

Despite these challenges, targeted therapies may offer some cost-saving opportunities. Treatment with anti-TNF agents, such as adalimumab, has demonstrated cost reductions in both flare frequency and hospitalizations, resulting in overall lower annual costs per patient. These savings stem from decreased healthcare utilization and better disease control, highlighting the potential long-term economic value of appropriate medical management for patients with moderate-to-severe HS [88].

Board Review Question Explanation

A 36-year-old man with Hurley stage III hidradenitis suppurativa (HS) involving the axillae, groin, and perineum presents for evaluation. He reports significant pain, recurrent drainage, and social withdrawal due to embarrassment about odor and scarring. He has missed over 30 days of work in the past year and has recently been denied a promotion due to frequent absences. Which of the following statements best describes the economic and occupational burden associated with HS?

A. Financial burden is primarily driven by medication costs
B. Patients with HS are less likely to utilize emergency departments compared to patients with psoriasis
C. HS is associated with higher rates of work absenteeism, presenteeism, and unemployment compared to other dermatologic conditions (Correct)
D. The financial burden of HS is largely mitigated by insurance coverage
E. Work function is generally preserved in patients with HS if disease severity is limited to Hurley stage I–II

Answer Explanation

Patients with HS face substantial occupational and financial challenges. Studies show that HS is associated with higher rates of absenteeism, presenteeism, and workforce departure compared to patients with other skin conditions. In addition to direct medical costs, lost work productivity constitutes a major component of the overall economic burden. High reliance on emergency department visits and hospitalizations further exacerbates costs. Insurance coverage for wound care supplies, dressings, and medications is often inconsistent, contributing to significant out-of-pocket expenses and financial toxicity. Work impairment correlates strongly with disease severity, particularly in Hurley stage III disease, but still affects patients across all levels of severity level.

Key Takeaways

- HS profoundly impairs health-related quality of life, often exceeding the burden seen in other dermatologic and systemic diseases.
- Greater disease severity, earlier age of onset, and involvement of multiple anatomical regions are major risk factors for worsened quality of life outcomes in HS.
- HS negatively impacts physical health, mental health, sexual health, and work function, leading to substantial personal and socioeconomic consequences.
- Psychiatric comorbidities such as depression, anxiety, and suicidality are highly prevalent in HS and significantly contribute to overall disease burden.
- HS imposes a significant financial burden due to both direct healthcare costs and indirect losses from impaired work productivity and employment instability.

References

1. von der Werth JM, Jemec GB. Morbidity in patients with hidradenitis suppurativa. Br J Dermatol. 2001;144(4):809–13. https://doi.org/10.1046/j.1365-2133.2001.04137.x.
2. Wolkenstein P, Loundou A, Barrau K, Auquier P, Revuz J, Quality of Life Group of the French Society of Dermatology. Quality of life impairment in hidradenitis suppurativa: a study of 61 cases. J Am Acad Dermatol. 2007;56(4):621–3. https://doi.org/10.1016/j.jaad.2006.08.061.
3. Matusiak Ł, Bieniek A, Szepietowski JC. Hidradenitis suppurativa markedly decreases quality of life and professional activity. J Am Acad Dermatol. 2010;62(4):706–708.e1. https://doi.org/10.1016/j.jaad.2009.09.021.
4. McKenzie SA, Harview CL, Truong AK, et al. Physical symptoms and psychosocial problems associated with hidradenitis suppurativa: correlation with Hurley stage. Dermatol Online J. 2020;26(9):13030/qt4rm8w7kn.
5. Janse IC, Deckers IE, van der Maten AD, et al. Sexual health and quality of life are impaired in hidradenitis suppurativa: a multicentre cross-sectional study. Br J Dermatol. 2017;176(4):1042–7. https://doi.org/10.1111/bjd.14975.
6. Russo PA, Ilchef R, Cooper AJ. Psychiatric morbidity in psoriasis: a review. Australas J Dermatol. 2004;45(3):155–61. https://doi.org/10.1111/j.1440-0960.2004.00078.x.
7. Hamzavi IH, Sundaram M, Nicholson C, et al. Uncovering burden disparity: a comparative analysis of the impact of moderate-to-severe psoriasis and hidradenitis suppurativa. J Am Acad Dermatol. 2017;77(6):1038–46. https://doi.org/10.1016/j.jaad.2017.07.027.
8. Bhutani T, Wong JW, Bebo BF, Armstrong AW. Access to health care in patients with psoriasis and psoriatic arthritis: data from National Psoriasis Foundation survey panels. JAMA Dermatol. 2013;149(6):717–21. https://doi.org/10.1001/jamadermatol.2013.133.
9. Kluger N, Sintonen H, Ranta M, Serlachius M. Health-related quality of life of patients with hidradenitis suppurativa measured with the 15D instrument and comparison with the general population and patients with psoriasis. Skin Appendage Disord. 2018;4(3):131–5. https://doi.org/10.1159/000481117.

10. Kurek A, Peters EM, Chanwangpong A, Sabat R, Sterry W, Schneider-Burrus S. Profound disturbances of sexual health in patients with acne inversa. J Am Acad Dermatol. 2012;67(3):422–428.e1. https://doi.org/10.1016/j.jaad.2011.10.024.
11. Türel Ermertcan A, Temeltaş G, Deveci A, Dinç G, Güler HB, Oztürkcan S. Sexual dysfunction in patients with psoriasis. J Dermatol. 2006;33(11):772–8. https://doi.org/10.1111/j.1346-8138.2006.00179.x.
12. Meeuwis KA, de Hullu JA, van de Nieuwenhof HP, et al. Quality of life and sexual health in patients with genital psoriasis. Br J Dermatol. 2011;164(6):1247–55. https://doi.org/10.1111/j.1365-2133.2011.10249.x.
13. Molina-Leyva A, Salvador-Rodriguez L, Martinez-Lopez A, Ruiz-Carrascosa JC, Arias-Santiago S. Association between psoriasis and sexual and erectile dysfunction in epidemiologic studies: a systematic review. JAMA Dermatol. 2019;155(1):98–106. https://doi.org/10.1001/jamadermatol.2018.3442.
14. Bhosle MJ, Kulkarni A, Feldman SR, Balkrishnan R. Quality of life in patients with psoriasis. Health Qual Life Outcomes. 2006;4:35. https://doi.org/10.1186/1477-7525-4-35.
15. Kouris A, Platsidaki E, Efstathiou V, et al. Comparative study of quality of life and psychological aspects in patients with psoriasis and hidradenitis suppurativa. Acta Dermatovenerol Croat. 2021;29(4):203–10.
16. Lee IT, Juang SE, Chen ST, Ko C, Ma KS. Sentiment analysis of tweets on alopecia areata, hidradenitis suppurativa, and psoriasis: revealing the patient experience. Front Med. 2022;9:996378. https://doi.org/10.3389/fmed.2022.996378.
17. Villaseñor-Park J, Wheeler D, Grandinetti L. Psoriasis: evolving treatment for a complex disease. Cleve Clin J Med. 2012;79(6):413–23. https://doi.org/10.3949/ccjm.79a.11133.
18. Smidt AC, Lai JS, Cella D, Patel S, Mancini AJ, Chamlin SL. Development and validation of Skindex-Teen, a quality-of-life instrument for adolescents with skin disease. Arch Dermatol. 2010;146(8):865–9. https://doi.org/10.1001/archdermatol.2010.161.
19. McAndrew R, Lopes FCPS, Sebastian K, Diaz LZ. Quality of life in hidradenitis suppurativa: a cross-sectional study of a pediatric population. J Am Acad Dermatol. 2021;84(3):829–30. https://doi.org/10.1016/j.jaad.2020.09.072.
20. Ermertcan AT, Gencoglan G, Temeltas G, Horasan GD, Deveci A, Ozturk F. Sexual dysfunction in female patients with neurodermatitis. J Androl. 2011;32(2):165–9. https://doi.org/10.2164/jandrol.110.010959.
21. Klassen AF, Newton JN, Mallon E. Measuring quality of life in people referred for specialist care of acne: comparing generic and disease-specific measures. J Am Acad Dermatol. 2000;43(2 Pt 1):229–33. https://doi.org/10.1067/mjd.2000.105507.
22. Williamson D, Gonzalez M, Finlay AY. The effect of hair loss on quality of life. J Eur Acad Dermatol Venereol. 2001;15(2):137–9. https://doi.org/10.1046/j.1468-3083.2001.00229.x.
23. Harris A, Burge SM, Dykes PJ, Finlay AY. Handicap in Darier's disease and Hailey-Hailey disease. Br J Dermatol. 1996;135(6):959–63. https://doi.org/10.1046/j.1365-2133.1996.d01-1102.x.
24. Onderdijk AJ, van der Zee HH, Esmann S, et al. Depression in patients with hidradenitis suppurativa. J Eur Acad Dermatol Venereol. 2013;27(4):473–8. https://doi.org/10.1111/j.1468-3083.2012.04468.x.
25. Andersen PL, Nielsen RM, Sigsgaard V, Jemec GBE, Riis PT. Body image quality of life in patients with hidradenitis suppurativa compared with other dermatological disorders. Acta Derm Venereol. 2020;100(8):adv00107. https://doi.org/10.2340/00015555-3464.
26. Mortimore AM, Bullen A, McMeniman EK. The impact of hidradenitis suppurativa on quality of life is worse than inflammatory bowel disease and myocardial infarction. Australas J Dermatol. 2022;63(4):505–8. https://doi.org/10.1111/ajd.13910.
27. Vinding GR, Knudsen KM, Ellervik C, Olesen AB, Jemec GB. Self-reported skin morbidities and health-related quality of life: a population-based nested case-control study. Dermatology. 2014;228(3):261–8. https://doi.org/10.1159/000358009.

28. Alavi A, Anooshirvani N, Kim WB, Coutts P, Sibbald RG. Quality-of-life impairment in patients with hidradenitis suppurativa: a Canadian study. Am J Clin Dermatol. 2015;16(1):61–5. https://doi.org/10.1007/s40257-014-0105-5.
29. Matusiak Ł. Profound consequences of hidradenitis suppurativa: a review. Br J Dermatol. 2020;183(6):e171–7. https://doi.org/10.1111/bjd.16603.
30. Balieva F, Kupfer J, Lien L, et al. The burden of common skin diseases assessed with the EQ5D™: a European multicentre study in 13 countries. Br J Dermatol. 2017;176(5):1170–8. https://doi.org/10.1111/bjd.15280.
31. Khalsa A, Liu G, Kirby JS. Increased utilization of emergency department and inpatient care by patients with hidradenitis suppurativa. J Am Acad Dermatol. 2015;73(4):609–14. https://doi.org/10.1016/j.jaad.2015.06.053.
32. Kirby JS, Miller JJ, Adams DR, Leslie D. Health care utilization patterns and costs for patients with hidradenitis suppurativa. JAMA Dermatol. 2014;150(9):937–44. https://doi.org/10.1001/jamadermatol.2014.691.
33. Fu SJ, Rose L, Dawes AJ, Knowlton LM, Ruddy KJ, Morris AM. Out-of-pocket costs among patients with a new cancer diagnosis enrolled in high-deductible health plans vs traditional insurance. JAMA Netw Open. 2021;4(12):e2134282. https://doi.org/10.1001/jamanetworkopen.2021.34282.
34. Becherel PA, Reguiai Z, Fougerousse AC, et al. Compared burden of psoriasis, atopic dermatitis, hidradenitis suppurativa, and chronic urticaria: baseline characteristics of the patients included in the OMCCI cohort - a French, prospective Multicenter study of chronic inflammatory dermatoses. Dermatology. 2024;240(5-6):702–12. https://doi.org/10.1159/000540250.
35. Chernyshov PV. The evolution of quality of life assessment and use in dermatology. Dermatology. 2019;235(3):167–74. https://doi.org/10.1159/000496923.
36. Christensen RE, Jafferany M. Psychiatric and psychologic aspects of chronic skin diseases. Clin Dermatol. 2023;41(1):75–81. https://doi.org/10.1016/j.clindermatol.2023.03.006.
37. Balázs PG, Gáspár K, Gergely HL, et al. Comparison of health-related quality of life in atopic dermatitis, hidradenitis suppurativa, pemphigus and psoriasis. Arch Dermatol Res. 2025;317(1):291. https://doi.org/10.1007/s00403-024-03786-4.
38. Kimball AB, Gieler U, Linder D, Sampogna F, Warren RB, Augustin M. Psoriasis: is the impairment to a patient's life cumulative? J Eur Acad Dermatol Venereol. 2010;24(9):989–1004. https://doi.org/10.1111/j.1468-3083.2010.03705.x.
39. Sampogna F, Fania L, Mastroeni S, Ciccone D, Panebianco A, Abeni D. Age-specific physical and mental health status in Italian patients with hidradenitis suppurativa: a comparison with the general population. Arch Dermatol Res. 2021;313(1):41–7. https://doi.org/10.1007/s00403-020-02063-4.
40. Merchant SA, Shah SFH. The impact of hidradenitis suppurativa on work productivity and performance: a systematic review and meta-analysis. Clin Exp Dermatol. 2024;49(10):1156–63. https://doi.org/10.1093/ced/llae120.
41. Smith HS, Chao JD, Teitelbaum J. Painful hidradenitis suppurativa. Clin J Pain. 2010;26(5):435–44. https://doi.org/10.1097/AJP.0b013e3181ceb80c.
42. Garg A, Neuren E, Cha D, et al. Evaluating patients' unmet needs in hidradenitis suppurativa: results from the global survey of impact and healthcare needs (VOICE) project. J Am Acad Dermatol. 2020;82(2):366–76. https://doi.org/10.1016/j.jaad.2019.06.1301.
43. Deckers IE, van der Zee HH, Prens EP. Epidemiology of hidradenitis suppurativa: prevalence, pathogenesis, and factors associated with the development of HS. Curr Derm Rep. 2014;3:54–60. https://doi.org/10.1007/s13671-013-0064-8.
44. Marvel J, Vlahiotis A, Sainski-Nguyen A, Willson T, Kimball A. Disease burden and cost of hidradenitis suppurativa: a retrospective examination of US administrative claims data. BMJ Open. 2019;9(9):e030579. https://doi.org/10.1136/bmjopen-2019-030579.
45. Patel ZS, Hoffman LK, Buse DC, et al. Pain, psychological comorbidities, disability, and impaired quality of life in hidradenitis suppurativa [corrected] [published correction appears in Curr Pain Headache Rep. 2017;21(12):52. doi: 10.1007/s11916-017-0653-5.]. Curr Pain Headache Rep. 2017;21(12):49. https://doi.org/10.1007/s11916-017-0647-3.

46. Kouris A, Platsidaki E, Christodoulou C, et al. Quality of life and psychosocial implications in patients with hidradenitis suppurativa. Dermatology. 2016;232(6):687–91. https://doi.org/10.1159/000453355.
47. Kaaz K, Szepietowski JC, Matusiak Ł. Influence of itch and pain on sleep quality in patients with hidradenitis suppurativa. Acta Derm Venereol. 2018;98(8):757–61. https://doi.org/10.2340/00015555-2967.
48. Thorlacius L, Cohen AD, Gislason GH, Jemec GBE, Egeberg A. Increased suicide risk in patients with hidradenitis suppurativa. J Invest Dermatol. 2018;138(1):52–7. https://doi.org/10.1016/j.jid.2017.09.008.
49. Patel KR, Rastogi S, Singam V, Lee HH, Amin AZ, Silverberg JI. Association between hidradenitis suppurativa and hospitalization for psychiatric disorders: a cross-sectional analysis of the National Inpatient Sample. Br J Dermatol. 2019;181(2):275–81. https://doi.org/10.1111/bjd.17416.
50. Hedemann TL, Liu X, Kang CN, Husain MI. Associations between psoriasis and mental illness: an update for clinicians. Gen Hosp Psychiatry. 2022;75:30–7. https://doi.org/10.1016/j.genhosppsych.2022.01.006.
51. Vazquez BG, Alikhan A, Weaver AL, Wetter DA, Davis MD. Incidence of hidradenitis suppurativa and associated factors: a population-based study of Olmsted County, Minnesota. J Invest Dermatol. 2013;133(1):97–103. https://doi.org/10.1038/jid.2012.255.
52. Matusiak L, Bieniek A, Szepietowski JC. Psychophysical aspects of hidradenitis suppurativa. Acta Derm Venereol. 2010;90(3):264–8. https://doi.org/10.2340/00015555-0866.
53. Weigelt MA, Milrad SF, Kirby JRS, Lev-Tov H. Psychosocial impact of hidradenitis suppurativa: a practical guide for clinicians. J Dermatolog Treat. 2022;33(4):1861–8. https://doi.org/10.1080/09546634.2021.1937483.
54. Richards E, Joshi A. Psychosocial effects of hidradenitis suppurativa in the literature: a systematic review. Int J Psychiatry Med. 2025;60(1):97–110. https://doi.org/10.1177/00912174241249215.
55. Alavi A, Farzanfar D, Lee RK, Almutairi D. The contribution of malodour in quality of life of patients with hidradenitis suppurativa. J Cutan Med Surg. 2018;22(2):166–74. https://doi.org/10.1177/1203475417745826.
56. Garg A, Pomerantz H, Midura M, et al. 222 completed suicide in patients with hidradenitis suppurativa: a population analysis in the United States. J Invest Dermatol. 2017;137(5):S38. https://doi.org/10.1016/j.jid.2017.02.237.
57. Tiri H, Huilaja L, Jokelainen J, Timonen M, Tasanen K. Women with hidradenitis suppurativa have an elevated risk of suicide. J Invest Dermatol. 2018;138(12):2672–4. https://doi.org/10.1016/j.jid.2018.06.171.
58. Garg A, Papagermanos V, Midura M, Strunk A, Merson J. Opioid, alcohol, and cannabis misuse among patients with hidradenitis suppurativa: a population-based analysis in the United States. J Am Acad Dermatol. 2018;79(3):495–500.e1. https://doi.org/10.1016/j.jaad.2018.02.053.
59. Alavi A, Farzanfar D, Rogalska T, Lowes MA, Chavoshi S. Quality of life and sexual health in patients with hidradenitis suppurativa. Int J Womens Dermatol. 2018;4(2):74–9. https://doi.org/10.1016/j.ijwd.2017.10.007.
60. Cuenca-Barrales C, Montero-Vílchez T, Szepietowski JC, Matusiak L, Molina-Leyva A. Sexual impairment in patients with hidradenitis suppurativa: a systematic review. J Eur Acad Dermatol Venereol. 2021;35(2):345–52. https://doi.org/10.1111/jdv.16726.
61. Cuenca-Barrales C, Ruiz-Villaverde R, Molina-Leyva A. Sexual distress in patients with hidradenitis suppurativa: a cross-sectional study. J Clin Med. 2019;8(4):532. https://doi.org/10.3390/jcm8040532.
62. Deckers IE, Kimball AB. The handicap of hidradenitis suppurativa. Dermatol Clin. 2016;34(1):17–22. https://doi.org/10.1016/j.det.2015.07.003.
63. Cuenca-Barrales C, Molina-Leyva A. Risk factors of sexual dysfunction in patients with hidradenitis suppurativa: a cross-sectional study. Dermatology. 2020;236(1):37–45. https://doi.org/10.1159/000501905.

64. McCabe MP, Sharlip ID, Lewis R, et al. Risk factors for sexual dysfunction among women and men: a consensus statement from the fourth international consultation on sexual medicine 2015. J Sex Med. 2016;13(2):153–67. https://doi.org/10.1016/j.jsxm.2015.12.015.
65. Slyper M, Strunk A, Garg A. Incidence of sexual dysfunction among patients with hidradenitis suppurativa: a population-based retrospective analysis. Br J Dermatol. 2018;179(2):502–3. https://doi.org/10.1111/bjd.16483.
66. ter Kuile MM, Brauer M, Laan E. The female sexual function index (FSFI) and the female sexual distress scale (FSDS): psychometric properties within a Dutch population. J Sex Marital Ther. 2006;32(4):289–304. https://doi.org/10.1080/00926230600666261.
67. McGahuey CA, Gelenberg AJ, Laukes CA, et al. The Arizona sexual experience scale (ASEX): reliability and validity. J Sex Marital Ther. 2000;26(1):25–40. https://doi.org/10.1080/009262300278623.
68. Lim TO, Das A, Rampal S, et al. Cross-cultural adaptation and validation of the English version of the international index of erectile function (IIEF) for use in Malaysia. Int J Impot Res. 2003;15(5):329–36. https://doi.org/10.1038/sj.ijir.3901009.
69. Gulliver W, Alavi A, Wiseman MC, et al. Real-world moderate-to-severe hidradenitis suppurativa: decrease in disease burden with adalimumab. J Cutan Med Surg. 2022;26(4):361–70. https://doi.org/10.1177/12034754221088584.
70. McMillan K. Hidradenitis suppurativa: number of diagnosed patients, demographic characteristics, and treatment patterns in the United States. Am J Epidemiol. 2014;179(12):1477–83. https://doi.org/10.1093/aje/kwu078.
71. Gáspár K, Hunor Gergely L, Jenei B, et al. Resource utilization, work productivity and costs in patients with hidradenitis suppurativa: a cost-of-illness study. Expert Rev Pharmacoecon Outcomes Res. 2022;22(3):399–408. https://doi.org/10.1080/14737167.2021.1895753.
72. Feitosa MSC, Schulz DG, Pinzon APA, et al. Financial impact of hidradenitis suppurativa on family income and expenditures: a case-control study of out-of-pocket catastrophic costs. Int J Dermatol. 2024;63(12):e459–61. https://doi.org/10.1111/ijd.17488.
73. Tzellos T, Yang H, Mu F, Calimlim B, Signorovitch J. Impact of hidradenitis suppurativa on work loss, indirect costs and income. Br J Dermatol. 2019;181(1):147–54. https://doi.org/10.1111/bjd.17101.
74. Esmann S, Jemec GB. Psychosocial impact of hidradenitis suppurativa: a qualitative study. Acta Derm Venereol. 2011;91(3):328–32. https://doi.org/10.2340/00015555-1082.
75. Sandhu VK, Shah M, Piguet V, Alavi A. The impact of hidradenitis suppurativa on work productivity and activity impairment. Br J Dermatol. 2020;182(5):1288–90. https://doi.org/10.1111/bjd.18695.
76. Schneider-Burrus S, Kalus S, Fritz B, Wolk K, Gomis-Kleindienst S, Sabat R. The impact of hidradenitis suppurativa on professional life. Br J Dermatol. 2023;188(1):122–30. https://doi.org/10.1093/bjd/ljac027.
77. Ramasastry SS, Conklin WT, Granick MS, Futrell JW. Surgical management of massive perianal hidradenitis suppurativa. Ann Plast Surg. 1985;15(3):218–23. https://doi.org/10.1097/00000637-198509000-00005.
78. Kearney N, McCourt C, Hughes R, McGrath B, O'Kane D, Kirby B. High unemployment rate in patients with hidradenitis suppurativa despite high educational attainment. Dermatology. 2024;240(2):181–8. https://doi.org/10.1159/000533739.
79. Howard-James C, Tobin AM. An analysis of direct and indirect costs in hidradenitis suppurativa. Skin Health Dis. 2023;4(1):e306. https://doi.org/10.1002/ski2.306.
80. Towfighi P, Huffman SS, Bovill JD, et al. Financial toxicity of hidradenitis suppurativa: a single-center experience at an urban wound-care clinic. J Dermatol. 2023;50(10):1279–86. https://doi.org/10.1111/1346-8138.16868.
81. Zouboulis CC. The socioeconomic burden of hidradenitis suppurativa/acne inversa. Br J Dermatol. 2019;181(1):7–8. https://doi.org/10.1111/bjd.17396.

82. Hopson S, Gibbs LR, Syed S, Low R, McClung L, Beaty S. Treatment patterns and healthcare resource utilization among newly diagnosed psoriasis, psoriatic arthritis, axial spondyloarthritis, and hidradenitis suppurativa patients with past diagnosis of an inflammatory condition: a retrospective cohort analysis of claims data in the United States. Adv Ther. 2023;40(10):4358–76. https://doi.org/10.1007/s12325-023-02558-2.
83. Santos JV, Lisboa C, Lanna C, Costa-Pereira A, Freitas A. Hospitalisations with hidradenitis suppurativa: an increasing problem that deserves closer attention. Dermatology. 2016;232(5):613–8. https://doi.org/10.1159/000448515.
84. Jemec GB, Guérin A, Kaminsky M, Okun M, Sundaram M. What happens after a single surgical intervention for hidradenitis suppurativa? A retrospective claims-based analysis. J Med Econ. 2016;19(7):710–7. https://doi.org/10.3111/13696998.2016.1161636.
85. Carter MJ. Health economics information in wound care: the elephant in the room. Adv Wound Care. 2013;2(10):563–70. https://doi.org/10.1089/wound.2013.0479.
86. Reeder VJ, Mahan MG, Hamzavi IH. Ethnicity and hidradenitis suppurativa. J Invest Dermatol. 2014;134(11):2842–3. https://doi.org/10.1038/jid.2014.220.
87. Vlassova N, Kuhn D, Okoye GA. Hidradenitis suppurativa disproportionately affects African Americans: a single-center retrospective analysis. Acta Derm Venereol. 2015;95(8):990–1. https://doi.org/10.2340/00015555-2176.
88. Argyropoulou M, Kanni T, Kyprianou M, Melachroinopoulos N, Giamarellos-Bourboulis EJ. Cost-savings of adalimumab in hidradenitis suppurativa: a retrospective analysis of a real-world cohort. Br J Dermatol. 2019;180(5):1161–8. https://doi.org/10.1111/bjd.17151.

Chapter 4
HS, Diet and Lifestyle

Madeline Tchack, Meha Aggarwal, and Cindy Wassef

Case Title A 24-year-old female presents with a 2-year history of recurrent, painful nodules and abscesses in her bilateral axillae and the sub-pannus region.

Case

A 24-year-old female presents with a 2-year history of recurrent, painful nodules and abscesses in her bilateral axillae and the sub-pannus region. The patient reports occasional alcohol use and has smoked 1 pack of cigarettes/day for the past 6 years. Her diet primarily consists of fast food. The patient has a body mass index (BMI) of 39.41 kg/m^2. Vitals are within normal limits. Physical exam shows inflamed, tender nodules, with draining sinus tracts in the bilateral axillae and sub-pannus with evidence of post-inflammatory hyperpigmentation. Laboratory studies identify mild leukocytosis (12.5 L/cells), non-fasting hyperglycemia (212 mg/dL), elevated hemoglobin A1c (9.3%), elevated C-reactive protein (14.3 mg/dL), low zinc (59 mcg/dL), and low vitamin D (16 ng/mL). She presents today with questions regarding any lifestyle factors that she can adjust to improve her disease.

M. Tchack · M. Aggarwal
Rutgers Robert Wood Johnson Medical School, Piscataway, NJ, USA

Rutgers Robert Wood Johnson, Department of Dermatology, Somerset, NJ, USA

C. Wassef (✉)
Premier Health Associates, Randolph, NJ, USA
e-mail: cindy.wassef@atlantichealth.org

N. Brownstone (ed.), *Clinical Cases in Hidradenitis Suppurativa*, Clinical Cases in Dermatology, https://doi.org/10.1007/978-3-032-15200-8_4

Board Review Question
Which of the following interventions is most effective for improving disease severity?

A. Ketogenic diet
B. Wearing tight polyester fabrics
C. Vitamin E supplementation
D. Smoking cessation
E. Sitz baths

Obesity in HS

A subclinical proinflammatory state is characteristic of both HS and obesity; both conditions are thus intricately linked at the molecular level [1]. Obesity is marked by increased adipose tissue, which acts as an endocrine organ by secreting proinflammatory adipokines and cytokines, such as leptin and resistin, and TNF-α, IL-1β, and IL-6, respectively [2, 3]. Obesity shares an adipokine and cytokine profile with HS [4]. At the clinical level, this association is significant; development of HS is associated with weight gain and severity of HS correlates with BMI [5]. Elevated childhood BMI is significantly associated with adulthood HS development, although this risk can be reduced to normal levels by returning to normal weight [6]. Elevated BMI can also hinder treatment efforts; obesity is associated with poor treatment response, increases the likelihood of postoperative axillary recurrence, and is an independent marker of severe, recalcitrant HS [4].

Weight reduction is thus a first-line recommendation for HS, with lifestyle modifications and bariatric surgery both associated with HS regression [7]. Bariatric surgery for obese patients reduces their risk of developing de novo HS and may even have a mild protective effect on HS recurrence in patients with HS and obesity, who undergo bariatric surgery [8]. Recently, glucagon-like-peptide-1 (GLP-1) receptor agonists such as semaglutide and liraglutide, which are FDA-approved for weight loss in patients with obesity, have been hypothesized to exert anti-inflammatory effects through modulation of adipose milieu and cytokine production [9]. Semaglutide therapy has been shown to improve HS patients' Dermatology Life Quality Index (DLQI) scores [10]. In a study of semaglutide's effect on HS improvement, males, active smokers, and patients taking higher doses of semaglutide showed significant symptom improvement [11]. Liraglutide may also be used, having shown a significant reduction in DLQI scores and Hurley stage in a small-scale study [12].

Diet

Dietary factors have been found to play a significant role in HS, influencing both disease severity and progression. Some studies found that dairy products, refined carbohydrates, and high-fat and high-sugar diets may have similar effects on HS lesions as they do on acne vulgaris, promoting anabolic and pro-inflammatory signaling cascades [13] and increasing inflammatory cytokines (e.g., TNF-α, IL-1β and IL-17) [14, 15]. The Western diet, characterized by high-glycemic index foods, red meat, dairy, and egg protein, has been associated with acne vulgaris, and, thus, may negatively impact HS [16].

Several studies have investigated the benefits of eliminating foods or adapting certain diets. Eliminating dairy, gluten [14, 15, 17–20], and brewer's yeast [20] from the diet have all shown to lead to HS symptom improvement or even resolution, sometimes independently of weight loss [20], suggesting not only that specific dietary components may influence HS severity [21], but also food quality may be more important than mere caloric restriction [22]. Adherence to anti-inflammatory diets that emphasize the consumption of healthy fats while discouraging refined grain and carbohydrate intake, such as low-glycemic, ketogenic [14, 23, 24], paleo [25], and Mediterranean diets, have all been associated with reduced HS severity [18, 19, 26–28]. Intermittent fasting has also been explored, with patients reporting significant improvements in HS severity despite minimal weight changes [29], emphasizing that dietary modifications may exert effects beyond simple weight loss. Though the effects of alcohol remain inconclusive, some studies suggest that decreasing alcohol consumption may improve symptom severity [30, 31].

Patient-reported data further underscore these dietary connections. In one study, 75.8% of HS patients made dietary alterations that excluded gluten, dairy, refined sugars, tomatoes, and alcohol, with 30.9% of patients reporting significant symptom improvement [15]. In another large study, nearly one-third of HS patients identified sweets, bread, pasta, dairy, and high-fat foods as triggering agents [14]. One small study even noted that 83% of their patients reported improvement on a dairy-free diet while none had worsening symptoms [32].

Nutritional deficiencies may also contribute to HS pathogenesis. Observational studies have reported correlations between low levels of zinc and vitamin D and increased numbers of HS lesions [33, 34]. Moreover, lower serum levels of zinc [33] and vitamin D [34–36] have been consistently observed in HS patients compared to healthy controls. Additionally, zinc, crucial for immune regulation and wound healing, and vitamin D, which significantly contributes to innate immunity and keratinocyte function, have both been suggested to facilitate disease onset when deficiencies exist [25, 37], and may reduce lesion severity with supplementation [33, 34, 38]. Emerging evidence also suggests a role for vitamin B12 in mitigating inflammation in HS, particularly in patients with comorbid inflammatory bowel disease [39].

Based on the evidence described herein, dietary interventions, addressing nutritional deficiencies, and eliminating specific trigger foods (Table 4.1) may be lifestyle changes that can serve as potential therapeutic strategies in HS treatment. While further research is needed to solidify these recommendations and clarify their long-term benefits, dietary modifications may be a cost-effective adjunct to medical management [25].

Table 4.1 Diet and supplement recommendations aimed at improving HS symptoms with associated evidence

	Diet/food/supplement	Examples/doses	Effects/benefits
Eliminations	Brewer's yeast	Baked goods (brownies, cakes, cookies, donuts), beer, bread, cider, wine	Studies reported improved HS lesions, symptoms, and fewer flare-ups following a yeast-free diet for 3–12 months [20]
	Alcohol	Beer, cider, liquor (gin, tequila, vodka, whiskey), wine	30.9% of HS patients who had made dietary alterations excluding gluten, dairy, refined sugars, tomatoes, and alcohol reported significant improvement [15] Dairy was the most likely food item to exacerbate symptoms, followed by high-glycemic index foods and red meat [25] 83% of patients improved under a dairy free diet and none worsened [32] 32.6% of patients identified sweets, bread, pasta, dairy, and high-fat foods as triggers [14] Elimination diets excluding gluten and dairy showed positive outcomes in individual cases [14, 15, 17–20, 25] Some studies suggest that high-fat and high-sugar diets may exacerbate symptoms by increasing inflammatory cytokines [14, 15]
	Dairy	Butter, cream, cheese, ice cream, milk, yogurt	
	Gluten	Baked goods, beer, bread, cereal, pasta, whiskey	
	High-sugar/glycemic foods	Baked goods, cereal, fast food, pineapple, refined grains (white bread/pasta/rice), snacks (candy, chips, pretzels) starchy vegetables (potatoes), sugar-sweetened beverages (fruit juice, soda, sports drink, sweet tea), watermelon	
	Western diet	Baked goods, dairy, fried foods, processed/prepackaged foods, red meat, refined grains, sugar-sweetened beverages	Western diet has been associated with worsening acne vulgaris, and is suggested to have a potential negative impact on HS [14, 16, 24, 32]

Beneficial diets	Dairy-free diet	Eliminating dairy; see "dairy" above	
	Gluten-free diet	Eliminating gluten; see "gluten" above	
	Intermittent fasting	"Ramadan fasting" (only allowed to eat or drink from sunset until dawn)	Though patients did not report any significant weight changes, they did report significant improvement in HS severity [29]
	Ketogenic diet (high fat and protein, low carbohydrates)	Avocados, eggs, fish, meat, non-starchy vegetables (broccoli, carrots, peppers, zucchini), nuts, olives, poultry, unsweetened dairy	Ketogenic diet showed potential benefits in reducing HS severity markers and inflammation [19, 28] Low-glycemic and ketogenic diets have been observed to improve HS severity [14, 24, 25, 32]
	Low-sugar/glycemic foods	Fruits, garlic, legumes, low-fat/unsweetened dairy, non-starchy vegetables, nuts, whole grains	
	Mediterranean diet	Extra virgin olive oil, fish/seafood, fruits, legumes (beans, lentils, peanuts, peas), nuts, seeds, vegetables, whole grains (brown rice, oats, quinoa, whole wheat bread/pasta)	Adherence to a Mediterranean diet could potentially be a supportive factor in managing HS and reducing its clinical severity [27] Mediterranean diet has been associated with reduced HS severity, likely due to its inflammatory properties [18, 26, 27]
	Paleo diet	Fruits, vegetables, lean meats (chicken/turkey breast, pork tenderloin, filet mignon), nuts, seeds	The most significant improvements occurred following the paleo and anti-inflammatory diet (e.g., Mediterranean diet) [25]
Nutrient supplementation	Vitamin B12	1000 mcg IM for every 4–6 weeks [39]	Vitamin B12 supplementation showed promise in managing HS in patients with comorbid IBD [39]
	Vitamin D	3–6 months supplementation recommended depending on baseline deficiency [35, 40]	Multiple studies have consistently reported lower vitamin D levels in HS patients compared to healthy controls [34–36]
	Zinc	90 mg of zinc gluconate daily for 3 months [38, 41, 42]	3-month duration of zinc supplementation boosted the expression of innate immunity markers [41] 90 mg zinc supplementation was suggested to reduce the severity and induce remission in Hurley grade I–II HS patients [38, 42]

Smoking in HS

The differentiation pathway of T helper (Th) 17 cells and regulatory T (Treg) cells has been studied in relation to HS due to its dysregulation in multiple proinflammatory states such as obesity, smoking, and autoimmunity. HS is characterized by increased Th17/Treg ratio, with Th17 being proinflammatory and Treg being immunosuppressive. The impact of smoking on the Th17/Treg axis is multi-factorial. Smoking is independently associated with increased Th17 expression as well as impaired Treg function and quantity. Additionally, smoking has been associated with the downregulation of the Notch signaling pathway, which lies upstream of the Th17/Treg axis and is likely also affected by familial HS mutations. Cigarette smoke also contains aryl hydrocarbon receptor (AhR) agonists, which independently upregulate Th17 cells. Moreover, cigarette smoke fumes contain benzopyrene, which strengthens AhR's effects on Th17 [43, 44]. There is strong evidence to suggest that smoking dysregulates immunological pathways and contributes to HS development.

This association can be seen at the clinical level. Literature suggests a strong association between smoking status and HS, with one meta-analysis finding that patients with HS are 4 times more likely to be smokers [45]. Among HS patients, never-smokers had significantly lower HS Sartorius scores than smokers, suggesting that smoking status is associated with disease severity [46]. A later study found that any smoking history is associated with significantly greater disease severity [47]. Smoking not only predisposes patients to HS, but also worsens their disease severity in comparison with non-smoking HS patients and even blunts disease response to treatment; smoking status is associated with significantly lower odds of improvement in response to treatment, regardless of pack-year history [48]. Smoking cessation and remaining abstinent is associated with reduced risk of new-onset HS development compared to that of active smokers. Those who quit smoking saw their risk of HS development fall to that of never-smokers around 3 years after quitting [49].

Environment and Physical Irritants

Environmental factors, particularly heat and humidity, seem to play a significant role in the exacerbation of HS. Heat is thought to exacerbate HS through multiple mechanisms, including heightened sweat production and retention, which can promote friction, hyperkeratosis, follicular plugging, and subsequent inflammation [50, 51]. Additionally, excessive heat and perspiration may alter skin microbiota, encouraging the proliferation of pathogenic bacteria that may contribute to dysbiosis within intertriginous areas [51]. High humidity likely amplifies these effects by impairing the evaporation of sweat, leading to prolonged skin exposure to moisture and heat, which can damage eccrine structures and induce inflammation [52]. As

HS frequently impacts apocrine sweat gland-bearing skin, persistent exposure to sweat and humidity in these regions often exacerbates HS lesions [53].

Studies that investigated seasonal patterns of HS flares noted a higher frequency of flares, measured by national Emergency Department visits, in the summer months (July and August) and October while observing a decrease in flares in the winter [52, 54]. In qualitative surveys, heat, sweating, and mechanical stress were among the most frequently cited factors exacerbating HS, with 32% of patients reporting worsening symptoms during the summer months [17]. As global temperatures continue to rise from climate change, it is possible that the burden of HS incidence and severity may likewise progressively increase worldwide [55].

Mechanical stress is also well-documented in the literature as both an inciting event in the pathogenesis of HS and a potential trigger for HS flares [56, 57]. In response to mechanical stress, follicular epithelium may become hypoplastic [58] or promote keratinocyte differentiation and proliferation [59], leading to retention of hair follicle debris, subsequent follicle occlusion, and eventual cyst formation [58, 59]. Furthermore, formed cysts that have continuous exposure to mechanical stress are more likely to rupture, inciting an inflammatory response that's seen with HS [56].

Intertriginous areas, where heat retention, sweating, and mechanical stress are common, are areas of the body where HS lesions most frequently form. Moreover, behavioral factors that increase heat, moisture, or mechanical friction may also contribute to increased flares. Undergarments and tightly fitted clothing that hugs the body in these areas can drastically exacerbate the degree of inflammation, discomfort, pain, and pruritus associated with these lesions [59]. Shaving and the regrowing of hair shafts may also lead to irritation and folliculitis, especially in skin folds, and may be responsible for initiating the inflammatory cascade seen in HS [59]. Some studies have also found an association between shaving intertriginous areas and earlier disease onset [60, 61]. Additionally, aluminum salt-containing deodorants have been found to be irritative and were noted as an HS trigger by 13% of patients [60].

Certain lifestyle modifications may play a key role in the management of HS and may complement medical therapies to reduce disease flares and symptoms and improve quality of life. To mitigate irritation and inflammation, patients should avoid aluminum salt-containing deodorants and shaving while practicing good skin hygiene as much as possible [17]. Laser-assisted hair removal in intertriginous areas has shown promise, particularly in the early stages of HS, and may even help to prevent the onset of the disease as HS inflammation is believed to start at the hair follicle [17].

Clothing and undergarment selections are also critical yet often overlooked aspects of HS management. The goal of appropriate undergarment selection in HS management is to minimize mechanical stress, heat, humidity, and microbial colonization [56]. Breathable, absorbent, and antimicrobial fabrics, such as bamboo, cellulose-derived rayon [62, 63], or silver-containing materials, can reduce sweat retention, microbial colonization, and odor [56]. These materials deflect water and sweat away from the skin rather than absorbing them, which optimizes evaporation to heat and moisture dissipation [64]. For patients unable to access these specialized fabrics, 100% cotton offers a more affordable and practical alternative. In general, undergarments should minimize mechanical stress and sheering forces with loose-fitting designs [56].

For women, bra designs like sports bras or camisole tanks with built-in wireless support can offload pressure and prevent irritation [56]. Women 's underwear that may help reduce friction in the sub-pannus include "boy shorts," briefs (low- or high-cut), "cheeky" underwear, or seamless or laser-cut underwear that lack elastic bands. Undergarments with elastic bands or bras with thin, tight straps or metal wires should be avoided because they can exert significant pressure that may lead to inflammation [56]. Men should opt for loose boxers or trunks over tight briefs, though snug-fitting clothing may sometimes reduce tissue movement and associated friction in some situations. Practical additions, such as abdominal or bra liners and breast pads, can reduce friction and absorb sweat and discharge in patients with actively draining lesions or a large pannus [56]. These strategies, alongside patient education on proper skincare and sweat management, should be considered in comprehensive HS management guidelines [55].

Stress Management and Mitigation

HS can have profound psychological and social consequences, significantly impacting patients' quality of life. Compared to individuals without the condition, those with HS report higher levels of depression, anxiety, loneliness, and social isolation [65, 66]. Many patients describe feelings of shame stemming from self-perceived disgust and fear of judgment by others, compounded by the physical pain that leaves them feeling powerless over their bodies [66, 67]. Patients also associate HS with shame, isolation, irritation, unpleasant odors, scarring, itching, and chronic pain [68, 69], with the disease's burden exceeding that of other skin conditions like psoriasis, atopic dermatitis, chronic urticaria, and neurofibromatosis-1 [69, 70].

HS, regardless of severity, often disrupts everyday social activities, including hobbies, public outings, family gatherings, and even intimate relationships [66, 71]. Numerous studies have found that HS patients, especially women, commonly report sexual dysfunction [66, 72]. While coping mechanisms vary among individuals, positive strategies that include seeking social support from peers or support groups and using humor may help to manage the often debilitating psychologic distress. In contrast, maladaptive responses such as social withdrawal, concealing symptoms, and avoiding discussions about their condition can exacerbate psychological struggles [57, 66]. The deeply distressing nature of HS, often described by patients as "miserable" or "evil," [69] underscores the critical need for holistic care addressing both physical and mental health.

Board Review Question Explanation
Which of the following interventions is most effective for improving disease severity?

A. Ketogenic diet
B. Wearing tight polyester fabrics
C. Vitamin E supplementation
D. Smoking cessation (Correct)
E. Sitz baths

Answer Explanation Smoking cessation is associated with reduced risk of HS onset and improved treatment response in patients with existing HS [44]. There is no evidence to suggest that a ketogenic diet improves disease severity. Wearing tight polyester fabrics can irritate HS lesions, could be painful and uncomfortable, and do not improve disease severity. There is no evidence to suggest that vitamin E supplementation improves disease severity. While Sitz baths can temporarily provide pain relief for extensive HS lesions, they are not associated with improved disease severity.

Key Takeaways

- Obesity is associated with a greater risk of developing HS and poorer treatment response. While diet and exercise changes are first-line treatments for losing weight, bariatric surgery and GLP-1RAs can facilitate the weight loss process.
- Eliminating trigger foods like dairy and high-glycemic-index items, adopting anti-inflammatory diets, and supplementing with zinc and vitamin D may improve HS symptoms by reducing systemic inflammation.
- Smoking creates a pro-inflammatory state, driving HS development. Smoking cessation can reduce de novo HS risk and improve treatment response.
- Heat, humidity, tight clothing, and mechanical stress intensify HS symptoms by promoting sweat retention, friction, and microbial imbalances, particularly in intertriginous areas.
- HS is associated with profound psychological burdens, including depression, anxiety, and social isolation. Stress management strategies and addressing the mental health impacts of HS are essential components of holistic care.

References

1. Frew JW. Hidradenitis suppurativa is an autoinflammatory keratinization disease: a review of the clinical, histologic, and molecular evidence. JAAD Int. 2020;1(1):62–72.
2. Nowak-Liduk A, Kitala D, Ochała-Gierek G, Łabuś W, Bergler-Czop B, Pietrauszka K, et al. Hidradenitis suppurativa: an interdisciplinary problem in dermatology, gynecology, and surgery-pathogenesis, comorbidities, and current treatments. Life. 2023;13(9):1895. https://doi.org/10.3390/life13091895.

3. Krajewski PK, Matusiak Ł, Szepietowski JC. Adipokines as an important link between hidradenitis suppurativa and obesity: a narrative review. Br J Dermatol. 2023;188(3):320–7.
4. Mintoff D, Agius R, Benhadou F, Das A, Frew JW, Pace NP. Obesity and hidradenitis suppurativa: targeting meta-inflammation for therapeutic gain. Clin Exp Dermatol. 2023;48(9):984–90.
5. Boer J. Should hidradenitis suppurativa be included in dermatoses showing koebnerization? Is it friction or fiction? Dermatology. 2017;233(1):47–52.
6. Jørgensen AHR, Aarestrup J, Baker JL, Thomsen SF. Association of birth weight, childhood body mass index, and height with risk of hidradenitis suppurativa. JAMA Dermatol. 2020;156(7):746–53.
7. Sivanand A, Gulliver WP, Josan CK, Alhusayen R, Fleming PJ. Weight loss and dietary interventions for hidradenitis suppurativa: a systematic review. J Cutan Med Surg. 2020;24(1):64–72.
8. Chierici A, Bulsei J, Alromayan M, Alamri A, Pavone G, Fontas E, et al. Bariatric surgery reduces the incidence of hidradenitis suppurativa in individuals with obesity: results of a nationwide administrative data study in France. Surg Obes Relat Dis. 2024;20(10):947–52.
9. Bendotti G, Montefusco L, Lunati ME, Usuelli V, Pastore I, Lazzaroni E, et al. The anti-inflammatory and immunological properties of GLP-1 receptor agonists. Pharmacol Res. 2022;182:106320.
10. Lyons D, Louly Nathan A, Pender E, Murray G, Smith C, Kirby B, et al. Semaglutide for weight loss in people with obesity as an adjunctive treatment for hidradenitis suppurativa: its impact on disease control and quality of life. Br J Dermatol. 2024;191(4):631–3.
11. Posada Posada MI, Alora MB, Lima XTV. Impact of semaglutide use in obese and diabetic patients with hidradenitis suppurativa. J Eur Acad Dermatol Venereol. 2025;39(8):e662–4. https://doi.org/10.1111/jdv.20392.
12. Nicolau J, Nadal A, Sanchís P, Pujol A, Masmiquel L, Nadal C. Liraglutide for the treatment of obesity among patients with hidradenitis suppurativa. Med Clin (Barc). 2024;162(3):118–22.
13. Melnik BC. Linking diet to acne metabolomics, inflammation, and comedogenesis: an update. Clin Cosmet Investig Dermatol. 2015;8:371–88.
14. Fernandez JM, Marr KD, Hendricks AJ, Price KN, Ludwig CM, Maarouf M, et al. Alleviating and exacerbating foods in hidradenitis suppurativa. Dermatol Ther. 2020;33(6):e14246.
15. Dempsey A, Butt M, Kirby JS. Prevalence and impact of dietary avoidance among individuals with hidradenitis suppurativa. Dermatology. 2020;236(4):289–95.
16. Maarouf M, Platto JF, Shi VY. The role of nutrition in inflammatory pilosebaceous disorders: implication of the skin-gut axis. Australas J Dermatol. 2019;60(2):e90–8.
17. Kurzen H, Kurzen M. Secondary prevention of hidradenitis suppurativa. Dermatol Rep. 2019;11(2):8243.
18. Lorite-Fuentes I, Montero-Vilchez T, Arias-Santiago S, Molina-Leyva A. Potential benefits of the Mediterranean diet and physical activity in patients with hidradenitis suppurativa: a cross-sectional study in a Spanish population. Nutrients. 2022;14(3):551. https://doi.org/10.3390/nu14030551.
19. Macklis PC, Tyler K, Kaffenberger J, Kwatra S, Kaffenberger BH. Lifestyle modifications associated with symptom improvement in hidradenitis suppurativa patients. Arch Dermatol Res. 2022;314(3):293–300.
20. Cannistrà C, Finocchi V, Trivisonno A, Tambasco D. New perspectives in the treatment of hidradenitis suppurativa: surgery and brewer's yeast-exclusion diet. Surgery. 2013;154(5):1126–30.
21. Haddad NR. The role of diet in managing hidradenitis suppurativa: a review of current evidence and future directions. Arch Dermatol Res. 2024;316(8):508.
22. Boer J. Resolution of hidradenitis suppurativa after weight loss by dietary measures, especially on frictional locations. J Eur Acad Dermatol Venereol. 2016;30(5):895–6.
23. Roster K, Xie L, Nguyen T, Lipner SR. Impact of ketogenic and low-glycemic diets on inflammatory skin conditions. Cutis. 2024;113(2):75–80.
24. Yamanaka-Takaichi M, Revankar R, Shih T, Gall M, Hsiao JL, Shi VY, et al. Expert consensus on priority research gaps in dietary and lifestyle factors in hidradenitis suppurativa: a Delphi consensus study. Arch Dermatol Res. 2023;315(7):2129–36.

25. Vural S, Baskurt D, Yıldırıcı Ş, Rasulova G, Danacı S, Botsalı A. Evaluating dietary considerations in hidradenitis suppurativa: a critical examination of existing knowledge. Int J Dermatol. 2024;63(8):987–98.
26. Velluzzi F, Anedda J, Pisanu S, Dell'Antonia M, Deledda A, Boi A, et al. Mediterranean diet, lifestyle and quality of life in Sardinian patients affected with hidradenitis suppurativa. J Public Health Res. 2021;11(2):jphr-2021. https://doi.org/10.4081/jphr.2021.2706.
27. Barrea L, Fabbrocini G, Annunziata G, Muscogiuri G, Donnarumma M, Marasca C, et al. Role of nutrition and adherence to the Mediterranean diet in the multidisciplinary approach of hidradenitis suppurativa: evaluation of nutritional status and its association with severity of disease. Nutrients. 2018;11(1):57. https://doi.org/10.3390/nu11010057.
28. Verde L, Cacciapuoti S, Caiazzo G, Megna M, Martora F, Cavaliere A, et al. Very low-calorie ketogenic diet (VLCKD) in the management of hidradenitis suppurativa (Acne Inversa): an effective and safe tool for improvement of the clinical severity of disease. Results of a pilot study. J Transl Med. 2024;22(1):149.
29. Damiani G, Mahroum N, Pigatto PDM, Pacifico A, Malagoli P, Tiodorovic D, et al. The safety and impact of a model of intermittent, time-restricted circadian fasting ("Ramadan fasting") on hidradenitis suppurativa: insights from a multicenter, observational, cross-over, pilot, exploratory study. Nutrients. 2019;11(8):1781. https://doi.org/10.3390/nu11081781.
30. Shlyankevich J, Chen AJ, Kim GE, Kimball AB. Hidradenitis suppurativa is a systemic disease with substantial comorbidity burden: a chart-verified case-control analysis. J Am Acad Dermatol. 2014;71(6):1144–50.
31. Walter AC, Meissner M, Kaufmann R, Valesky E, Pinter A. Hidradenitis suppurativa after radical surgery-long-term follow-up for recurrences and associated factors. Dermatol Surg. 2018;44(10):1323–31.
32. Danby FW. Diet in the prevention of hidradenitis suppurativa (acne inversa). J Am Acad Dermatol. 2015;73(5 Suppl 1):S52–4.
33. Poveda I, Vilarrasa E, Martorell A, García-Martínez FJ, Segura JM, Hispán P, et al. Serum zinc levels in hidradenitis suppurativa: a case-control study. Am J Clin Dermatol. 2018;19(5):771–7.
34. Kelly G, Sweeney CM, Fitzgerald R, O'Keane MP, Kilbane M, Lally A, et al. Vitamin D status in hidradenitis suppurativa. Br J Dermatol. 2014;170(6):1379–80.
35. Fabbrocini G, Marasca C, Luciano MA, Guarino M, Poggi S, Fontanella G, et al. Vitamin D deficiency and hidradenitis suppurativa: the impact on clinical severity and therapeutic responsivity. J DermatolTreat. 2021;32(7):843–4.
36. Moltrasio C, Tricarico PM, Genovese G, Gratton R, Marzano AV, Crovella S. 25-Hydroxyvitamin D serum levels inversely correlate to disease severity and serum C-reactive protein levels in patients with hidradenitis suppurativa. J Dermatol. 2021;48(5):715–7.
37. Cervantes J, Eber AE, Perper M, Nascimento VM, Nouri K, Keri JE. The role of zinc in the treatment of acne: a review of the literature. Dermatol Ther. 2018;31(1):e12576. https://doi.org/10.1111/dth.12576.
38. Brocard A, Knol AC, Khammari A, Dréno B. Hidradenitis suppurativa and zinc: a new therapeutic approach. A pilot study. Dermatology. 2007;214(4):325–7.
39. Mortimore M, Florin THJ. A role for B_{12} in inflammatory bowel disease patients with suppurative dermatoses? An experience with high dose vitamin B_{12} therapy. J Crohns Colitis. 2010;4(4):466–70.
40. Guillet A, Brocard A, Bach Ngohou K, et al. Verneuil's disease, innate immunity and vitamin D: a pilot study. J Eur Acad Dermatol Venereol. 2015;29(7):1347–53.
41. Dréno B, Khammari A, Brocard A, et al. Hidradenitis suppurativa: the role of deficient cutaneous innate immunity. Arch Dermatol. 2012;148(2):182–6.
42. Hessam S, Sand M, Meier NM, Gambichler T, Scholl L, Bechara FG. Combination of oral zinc gluconate and topical triclosan: an anti-inflammatory treatment modality for initial hidradenitis suppurativa. J Dermatol Sci. 2016;84(2):197–202.

43. Melnik BC, John SM, Chen W, Plewig G. T helper 17 cell/regulatory T-cell imbalance in hidradenitis suppurativa/acne inversa: the link to hair follicle dissection, obesity, smoking and autoimmune comorbidities. Br J Dermatol. 2018;179(2):260–72.
44. Bukvić Mokos Z, Miše J, Balić A, Marinović B. Understanding the relationship between smoking and hidradenitis suppurativa. Acta Dermatovenerol Croat. 2020;28(1):9–13.
45. Acharya P, Mathur M. Hidradenitis suppurativa and smoking: a systematic review and meta-analysis. J Am Acad Dermatol. 2020;82(4):1006–11.
46. Sartorius K, Emtestam L, Jemec GBE, Lapins J. Objective scoring of hidradenitis suppurativa reflecting the role of tobacco smoking and obesity. Br J Dermatol. 2009;161(4):831–9.
47. Chu CB, Li WL, Lin SH, Hsu CK, Yang CC, Tsai SJ. The influence of gender and smoking on hidradenitis suppurativa. Dermatol Sin. 2021;39(3):125–31.
48. Denny G, Anadkat MJ. The effect of smoking and age on the response to first-line therapy of hidradenitis suppurativa: an institutional retrospective cohort study. J Am Acad Dermatol. 2017;76(1):54–9.
49. Kim SR, Choi YG, Jo SJ. Smoking cessation and risk of hidradenitis suppurativa development. JAMA Dermatol. 2024;160(10):1056–65.
50. de Winter K, van der Zee HH, Prens EP. Is mechanical stress an important pathogenic factor in hidradenitis suppurativa? Exp Dermatol. 2012;21(3):176–7.
51. von Laffert M, Helmbold P, Wohlrab J, Fiedler E, Stadie V, Marsch WC. Hidradenitis suppurativa (acne inversa): early inflammatory events at terminal follicles and at interfollicular epidermis. Exp Dermatol. 2010;19(6):533–7.
52. Atluri S, Masson R, Tran K, Hsiao JL, Shi VY. Managing seasonal flares in hidradenitis suppurativa. J Am Acad Dermatol. 2024;90(1):e23–4.
53. Matusiak Ł, Szczęch J, Kaaz K, Lelonek E, Szepietowski JC. Clinical characteristics of pruritus and pain in patients with hidradenitis suppurativa. Acta Derm Venereol. 2018;98(2):191–4.
54. Tripathi R, Korman NJ, Ezaldein HH. Seasonal burden of National Emergency Department visits due to hidradenitis suppurativa. J Am Acad Dermatol. 2022;86(6):1362–5.
55. Singh R, Fathy R, Kassamali B, Noe MH, Barbieri JS, LaChance A, et al. Increased ambient outdoor temperatures are associated with increased disease flaring in hidradenitis suppurativa. Arch Derm Res. 2023;316(1):49.
56. Loh TY, Hendricks AJ, Hsiao JL, Shi VY. Undergarment and fabric selection in the management of hidradenitis suppurativa. Dermatology. 2021;237(1):119–24.
57. Thompson AM, Fernandez JM, Rick J, Hendricks AJ, Maarouf M, Mata EM, et al. Identifying triggers for hidradenitis suppurativa flare: a patient survey. Br J Dermatol. 2021;185(1):225–6.
58. Kelly G, Prens EP. Inflammatory mechanisms in hidradenitis suppurativa. Dermatol Clin. 2016;34(1):51–8.
59. Boer J, Nazary M, Riis PT. The role of mechanical stress in hidradenitis suppurativa. Dermatol Clin. 2016;34(1):37–43.
60. von der Werth JM, Williams HC. The natural history of hidradenitis suppurativa. J Eur Acad Dermatol Venereol. 2000;14(5):389–92.
61. Morgan WP. The role of depilation and deodorants in hidradenitis suppurativa. Arch Dermatol. 1982;118(2):101.
62. Frazer L. New spin on an old fiber. Environ Health Perspect. 2004;112(13):A754–7.
63. Woodings CR. The development of advanced cellulosic fibres. Int J Biol Macromol. 1995;17(6):305–9.
64. Dai XQ, Imamura R, Liu GL, Zhou FP. Effect of moisture transport on microclimate under T-shirts. Eur J Appl Physiol. 2008;104(2):337–40.
65. Kouris A, Platsidaki E, Christodoulou C, Efstathiou V, Dessinioti C, Tzanetakou V, et al. Quality of life and psychosocial implications in patients with hidradenitis suppurativa. Dermatology. 2016;232(6):687–91.
66. Christensen RE, Jafferany M. Psychiatric and psychologic aspects of chronic skin diseases. Clin Dermatol. 2023;41(1):75–81.

67. Keary E, Hevey D, Tobin AM. A qualitative analysis of psychological distress in hidradenitis suppurativa. Br J Dermatol. 2020;182(2):342–7.
68. Esmann S, Jemec GBE. Psychosocial impact of hidradenitis suppurativa: a qualitative study. Acta Derm Venereol. 2011;91(3):328–32.
69. Gooderham M, Papp K. The psychosocial impact of hidradenitis suppurativa. J Am Acad Dermatol. 2015;73(5 Suppl 1):S19–22.
70. Wolkenstein P, Loundou A, Barrau K, Auquier P, Revuz J, Quality of Life Group of the French Society of Dermatology. Quality of life impairment in hidradenitis suppurativa: a study of 61 cases. J Am Acad Dermatol. 2007;56(4):621–3.
71. Perche PO, Singh R, Senthilnathan A, Feldman SR, Pichardo RO. Hidradenitis suppurativa's impact on social activities: an observational study. Cureus. 2022;14(5):e25292.
72. Seetan K, Al-Zubi M, Al-Omari R. Sexual dysfunction in patients with hidradenitis suppurativa: a systematic review and meta-analysis. J Clin Aesthet Dermatol. 2021;14(8):61–5.

Chapter 5
Treatment of HS with Complementary and Alternative Medicine

Theresa Tran

Case Title A 28-year-old female presents with a history of hidradenitis suppurativa (HS).

Case
A 28-year-old female presents with a history of hidradenitis suppurativa (HS). The patient has tried multiple different treatments. However, she has some residual nodules that are somewhat painful. She is disappointed with results from the conventional medicinal therapies and tells you she is working on prioritizing her health and inquires about natural remedies. Furthermore, she asks about changes she can make in her daily life, as well as alternative therapies to help her disease improve. What do you tell her?

Board Review Question
A 28-year-old woman with Hurley stage I hidradenitis suppurativa (HS) presents to clinic seeking non-pharmacologic options to supplement her current treatment. Laboratory evaluation reveals a zinc deficiency. Which of the following is the most appropriate next step in management?

A. Initiate zinc picolinate 50 mg daily and vitamin B12 injections
B. Begin turmeric supplementation and recommend bleach baths
C. Prescribe zinc gluconate 90 mg daily and counsel on potential side effects
D. Recommend routine vitamin D supplementation regardless of levels
E. Start oral cannabinoids for systemic symptom control

T. Tran (✉)
Department of Dermatology, Temple University Hospital, Philadelphia, PA, USA
e-mail: Theresa.Tran@tuhs.temple.edu

N. Brownstone (ed.), *Clinical Cases in Hidradenitis Suppurativa*, Clinical Cases in Dermatology, https://doi.org/10.1007/978-3-032-15200-8_5

Table 5.1 A summary of complementary and alternative medicines

Therapy	Target symptom/effect	Clinical studies available
Zinc supplementation	Inflammation, lesion resolution	Yes—small studies, partial/complete remission observed
Vitamin D supplementation	Immune modulation, nodule reduction	Yes—limited studies in deficient patients
Vitamin B12	Skin healing, support with other micronutrients	Limited—anecdotal and case-based evidence
Turmeric (curcumin)	Inflammation, antimicrobial effects	Limited—studies in related conditions (e.g., psoriasis)
Cannabinoids (topical/systemic)	Pain relief, inflammation, wound healing	No RCTs—survey and anecdotal data only
Magnesium (oral)	Pain relief	No—theoretical benefits, not HS-specific
Bleach baths (sodium hypochlorite)	Antimicrobial, anti-inflammatory	No—recommended antibacterial alternatives preferred
Epsom salt baths (magnesium sulfate)	Pain, inflammation, stress relief	No—anecdotal support, lack of evidence
Balneotherapy	Skin inflammation, flare reduction	Limited—studied in other dermatologic conditions
Acupuncture/acupressure	Pain, itch, inflammation	No—theoretical benefit, minimal HS-specific evidence
Dietary modifications	Disease modulation, inflammation	Limited—most patients self-report, minimal objective evidence

Many patients with recalcitrant chronic diseases that do not improve with conventional medication regimens explore complementary and alternative medicines. Adjuncts to standard therapeutics such as dietary modifications and alternative remedies have been increasingly investigated in recent years. However, the strength of evidence for non-pharmacologic therapies is limited by small study sizes and lack of randomized controlled trials. If a dermatology provider chooses not to recommend or prescribe any of these complementary and alternative medicines, it is still beneficial to be aware of these options as patients may inquire about them during their office visit. Table 5.1 provides a summary of complementary and alternative medicines discussed in this chapter.

Complementary and Alternative Medicines

Zinc

Zinc is an essential micronutrient for cellular processes including cell proliferation, differentiation, apoptosis, and a part of both innate and adaptive immune functions. Zinc exhibits anti-inflammatory effects by suppressing development of IL-17 producing cells and downregulating toll-like receptor response. The relationship between zinc deficiency and HS has been demonstrated particularly in patients with new-onset HS, or with worsening HS following bariatric surgery and weight loss. The efficacy of zinc supplementation has been studied, with the preferred formulation of zinc gluconate (zinc picolinate has better absorption but is more expensive) at a dose of 90 mg daily, citing complete or partial remission of HS in patients. Zinc supplementation is recommended for patients with Hurley stage I or II disease, if deficient. Common side effects include nausea, vomiting, and loss of appetite which can be mitigated by adhering to the recommended dose. Patients who chronically receive prolonged zinc supplementation are also recommended to take copper supplementation to avoid copper deficiency. Symptoms of copper deficiency include hair loss, diarrhea, cutaneous and ophthalmic sores, and loss of appetite. When supplementing copper, the ratio of zinc:copper is 10:1 [1–6].

Vitamin D

The exact relationship between vitamin D and HS is continuing to be studied. Current research shows that vitamin D helps to modulate immune function within the folliculo-pilosebaceous subunit and increases synthesis of antimicrobial peptides, which reduces secondary infections and skin inflammation. HS patients were found to have a higher prevalence of vitamin D deficiency compared to those without HS, and supplementation with vitamin D in HS patients could theoretically help normalize keratinocyte proliferation and differentiation. However, current guidelines indicate insufficient evidence to recommend routine Vitamin D supplementation for HS patients. There are some studies which have demonstrated a reduction in inflammatory nodules with vitamin D supplementation in vitamin D deficient HS patients [7–10].

Vitamin B12 (Cobalamin)

The relationship between vitamin B12 and HS is not extensively documented, but there are some insights from the medical literature that suggest potential benefits of vitamin B12 supplementation in certain contexts, such as in conjunction with other micronutrients like zinc and vitamin D, leading to partial or complete lesion resolution in HS patients. Also, there was a noted improvement with vitamin B12 supplementation in patients with irritable bowel disease who also had suppurative dermatoses [11, 12].

Turmeric

Curcumin, the active compound in turmeric, has been theorized to help HS due to its anti-inflammatory and antimicrobial properties by disrupting bacterial membranes, inhibiting bacterial replication, and disrupting microbial biofilms. The concomitant use of both oral curcumin and topical curcumin has shown improvement in other inflammatory conditions such as psoriasis and atopic dermatitis; however, the evidence regarding its use is limited in HS patients. Side effects at higher doses include diarrhea, headache, yellow stool, rash, and nausea [13–15].

Cannabinoids

There are three classes of cannabinoids: phytocannabinoids (plant-derived) that include delta-9-tetrahydrocannabinol (THC) and cannabidiols (CBD), endogenous cannabinoids, and synthetic cannabinoids. In general, oral cannabinoids have been shown to target systemic symptoms such as anorexia, nausea, and pain. Topical cannabinoids decrease pain perception and can therefore aid in pain relief by targeting localized pain and inflammation. It can also assist in wound healing through its promotion of apoptosis of both keratinocytes and sebocytes. Cannabinoids are not currently established as a treatment for HS. However, there is increased quantity, frequency, and proportion of cannabis use in patients with HS in comparison to those with other painful and pruritic chronic skin conditions. In a survey, the primary motivation for use was recreation, with pain and stress relief as other motivations. Topical cannabis or cannabinoid creams/oils were also favored, with anecdotal reports of improvement in their skin conditions. Notable side effects of systemic cannabinoid use include tachycardia (acute), bradycardia (chronic), decreased systemic vascular resistance, nystagmus, conjunctival injection, lethargy, decreased concentration, and generalized psychomotor impairment. Side effects of topical CBD use include dryness and pain at the application site [16, 17].

Magnesium

Magnesium has been shown to be an effective complimentary therapy for reducing pain, and therefore may be beneficial in alleviating pain in HS patients. In patients with renal disease or increased magnesium intake, hypermagnesemia can occur with notable symptoms including weakness, nausea, dizziness, and confusion. Serious adverse effects include cardiovascular complications, flaccid paralysis, lethargy, and coma [18].

Bathing Regimens

Bathing can be considered as an alternative to antiseptic and medicated washes used in the shower. Generally, the act of bathing can reduce stress, pain, and fatigue. It is important to note that not every patient may have access to a bathtub to implement these techniques. The different bathing additives discussed are associated with anti-inflammatory, reparative, and antioxidative properties [6].

Sodium Hypochlorite (Bleach) Baths

Bleach is best known for its antimicrobial properties, creating superoxide radicals to destroy bacteria, spores, viruses, and fungi. In addition, it demonstrates anti-inflammatory properties through decreasing inflammatory cytokine levels. There are no direct studies in the efficacy of bleach baths for HS, and the current guidelines recommend other antibacterial agents such as chlorhexidine washes [6].

Magnesium Sulfate (Epsom Salt) Baths

Epsom salt baths have been favored for those seeking non-pharmacologic treatments, with anecdotal experiences citing healing of illnesses, reducing bodily aches and pains, and reducing inflammation. There are no studies which have been able to provide further data on these benefits or elucidate a mechanism of action. Patients can continue these regimens if they desire, however first-line recommendation of this practice is not preferred, and counseling on other disease-modifying interventions should be offered [6].

Balneotherapy

This method of bathing in mineral water, often with elevated levels of magnesium, sodium, potassium, calcium, chloride, sulfate, and carbonate. Side effects are rare, but can include itch and skin irritation. Balneotherapy has been studied to show improvement of flares in patients with atopic dermatitis, psoriasis, and acne. However, more research is required for HS patients [18].

Acupuncture and Acupressure

Acupuncture is based on traditional Chinese medicine, where the body's meridian lines are stimulated via insertion of thin needles through the skin. The mechanism is not completely understood; however, the practice helps reduce inflammation, pain, and itch potentially due to stimulation of inhibitory nerve fibers, therefore educing signals to the central nervous system or reducing neurotransmitter modulation. For those with a fear of needles, acupressure can be used which consists of applying external pressure to similarly designated acupoints. Acupuncture and acupressure may be beneficial for patients with HS, especially for pain management during acute flares. However, further research is needed to investigate whether there are notable improvements for patients with HS. Side effects reported with acupuncture related techniques include fever, pain, and dizziness. Side effects reported with acupressure include bruising, soreness, and pruritus [18].

Dietary Management

There are several diets that have been studied in relation to hidradenitis suppurativa, including low carbohydrate diets, low dairy diets, and Mediterranean diets. Most HS patients alter their diet; however, only a small portion report significant improvement [7]. The current clinical guidelines acknowledge the potential role of dietary modifications, though evidence continues to remain limited. Please see the chapter on HS, Diet and Lifestyle for further information.

Board Review Question Explanation

A 28-year-old woman with Hurley stage I hidradenitis suppurativa (HS) presents to clinic seeking non-pharmacologic options to supplement her current treatment. Laboratory evaluation reveals a zinc deficiency. Which of the following is the most appropriate next step in management?

A. Initiate zinc picolinate 50 mg daily and vitamin B12 injections
B. Begin turmeric supplementation and recommend bleach baths
C. Prescribe zinc gluconate 90 mg daily and counsel on potential side effects (Correct)
D. Recommend routine vitamin D supplementation regardless of levels
E. Start oral cannabinoids for systemic symptom control

Answer Explanation

Zinc gluconate at 90 mg daily is the preferred formulation and dose for zinc supplementation in HS patients with documented deficiency, especially in Hurley stage I or II disease. Side effects such as nausea and appetite loss can be mitigated by following dosing guidelines. While zinc picolinate may have better absorption, it is more expensive and not typically first-line. Vitamin D and B12 should only be supplemented if deficient. Turmeric and cannabinoids have limited evidence, and bleach baths are not established for HS treatment.

Key Takeaway Points

- Many patients with HS seek complementary and alternative medicine (CAM) to manage symptoms alongside conventional treatments. If a dermatology provider chooses not to recommend or prescribe any of these complementary and alternative medicines, it is still beneficial to be aware of these options as patients may inquire about them during their office visit.
- Zinc supplementation, especially in deficient patients, shows the strongest evidence among CAM therapies for improving HS lesions.
- Vitamin D may modulate immune function and reduce inflammation, but routine supplementation is not currently recommended without deficiency.
- Evidence for turmeric (curcumin), vitamin B12, and cannabinoids is limited to anecdotal reports or small studies, though theoretical benefits exist.
- Bathing regimens, including bleach baths, Epsom salt, and balneotherapy, may provide symptom relief but lack strong clinical data in HS.
- Acupuncture and acupressure may help reduce pain and inflammation during HS flares, but more research is needed.
- Magnesium, both oral and in bathing forms, may help with pain but requires caution due to potential toxicity in certain patients.
- Dietary modifications are commonly attempted by patients, but current evidence is insufficient to support specific diets as effective interventions.

References

1. Hessam S, Sand M, Meier NM, Gambichler T, Scholl L, Bechara FG. Combination of oral zinc gluconate and topical triclosan: an anti-inflammatory treatment modality for initial hidradenitis suppurativa. J Dermatol Sci. 2016;84(2):197–202. https://doi.org/10.1016/j.jdermsci.2016.08.010. Epub 2016 Aug 10. PMID: 27554338.
2. Weir SA, Roman B, Jiminez V, Burns M, Sanyi A, Elewski B, Mayo T. Hidradenitis suppurativa and five key vitamins and minerals. Skin Appendage Disord. 2023;9(3):153–9. https://doi.org/10.1159/000528122. Epub 2023 Mar 23. PMID: 37325281; PMCID: PMC10264908.
3. Serra-García L, Morgado-Carrasco D. RF—usefulness of zinc gluconate and other nondrug treatments for managing hidradenitis suppurativa. Actas Dermosifiliogr. 2022;113(6):627–31. https://doi.org/10.1016/j.ad.2020.08.027. Epub 2021 Nov 16. PMID: 35728916 (English, Spanish).
4. Brocard A, Knol AC, Khammari A, Dréno B. Hidradenitis suppurativa and zinc: a new therapeutic approach. A pilot study. Dermatology. 2007;214(4):325–7. https://doi.org/10.1159/000100883. PMID: 17460404.
5. Brocard A, Dréno B. Innate immunity: a crucial target for zinc in the treatment of inflammatory dermatosis. J Eur Acad Dermatol Venereol. 2011;25(10):1146–52. https://doi.org/10.1111/j.1468-3083.2010.03934.x. Epub 2011 Jan 24. PMID: 21261748.
6. Buechler CR, Daveluy SD. 15 – Topical therapeutics. In: Shi VY, Hsiao JL, Lowes MA, Hamzavi IH, editors. A comprehensive guide to hidradenitis suppurativa. Elsevier; 2022. p. 145–54. ISBN 9780323777247.

7. Alikhan A, Sayed C, Alavi A, Alhusayen R, Brassard A, Burkhart C, Crowell K, Eisen DB, Gottlieb AB, Hamzavi I, Hazen PG, Jaleel T, Kimball AB, Kirby J, Lowes MA, Micheletti R, Miller A, Naik HB, Orgill D, Poulin Y. North American clinical management guidelines for hidradenitis suppurativa: a publication from the United States and Canadian hidradenitis suppurativa foundations: part I: diagnosis, evaluation, and the use of complementary and procedural management. J Am Acad Dermatol. 2019;81(1):76–90. https://doi.org/10.1016/j.jaad.2019.02.067. Epub 2019 Mar 11. PMID: 30872156; PMCID: PMC9131894.
8. Lackner L, Zyriax BC, Stephan B. To what extent does vitamin D and its serum levels influence the severity of hidradenitis suppurativa: a literature review. Acta Derm Venereol. 2024;104:adv40321. https://doi.org/10.2340/actadv.v104.40321. PMID: 39254290; PMCID: PMC11407108.
9. Seetan K, Eldos B, Saraireh M, et al. Prevalence of low vitamin D levels in patients with hidradenitis suppurativa in Jordan: a comparative cross-sectional study. PLoS One. 2022;17(3):e0265672. https://doi.org/10.1371/journal.pone.0265672.
10. Kelly G, Sweeney CM, Fitzgerald R, et al. Vitamin D status in hidradenitis suppurativa. Br J Dermatol. 2014;170(6):1379–80. https://doi.org/10.1111/bjd.12900.
11. Choi F, Lehmer L, Ekelem C, Mesinkovska NA. Dietary and metabolic factors in the pathogenesis of hidradenitis suppurativa: a systematic review. Int J Dermatol. 2020;59(2):143–53. https://doi.org/10.1111/ijd.14691. Epub 2019 Oct 25. PMID: 31651051.
12. Mortimore M, Florin TH. A role for B_{12} in inflammatory bowel disease patients with suppurative dermatoses? An experience with high dose vitamin B_{12} therapy. J Crohns Colitis. 2010;4(4):466–70. https://doi.org/10.1016/j.crohns.2010.02.007. Epub 2010 Mar 21. PMID: 21122544.
13. Savage KT, Singh V, Patel ZS, Yannuzzi CA, McKenzie-Brown AM, Lowes MA, Orenstein LAV. Pain management in hidradenitis suppurativa and a proposed treatment algorithm. J Am Acad Dermatol. 2021;85(1):187–99. https://doi.org/10.1016/j.jaad.2020.09.039. Epub 2020 Sept 17. PMID: 32950543; PMCID: PMC8176324.
14. Witte K, Wolk K, Witte-Händel E, Krause T, Kokolakis G, Sabat R. Targeting metabolic syndrome in hidradenitis suppurativa by phytochemicals as a potential complementary therapeutic strategy. Nutrients. 2023;15(17):3797. https://doi.org/10.3390/nu15173797. PMID: 37686829; PMCID: PMC10490062.
15. Witte K, Sabat R, Witte-Händel E, Ghoreschi K, Wolk K. Phytotherapeuthics affecting the IL-1/IL-17/G-CSF Axis: a complementary treatment option for hidradenitis suppurativa? Int J Mol Sci. 2022;23(16):9057. https://doi.org/10.3390/ijms23169057. PMID: 36012322; PMCID: PMC9408811.
16. Metko D, Mehta S, Piguet V. Cannabis usage among patients with hidradenitis suppurativa: a scoping review. J Cutan Med Surg. 2024;28(3):307–8. https://doi.org/10.1177/12034754241238719. Epub 2024 Mar 10. PMID: 38462895; PMCID: PMC11141092.
17. Fernandez JM, Thompson AM, Borgstrom M, Orenstein LAV, Hsiao JL, Shi VY. Pain management modalities for hidradenitis suppurativa: a patient survey. J Dermatolog Treat. 2022;33(3):1742–5. https://doi.org/10.1080/09546634.2020.1822501. Epub 2020 Sep 20. PMID: 32914659.
18. Price KN, Thompson AM, Shi VY. 28 – Complementary and alternative medicine. In: Shi VY, Hsiao JL, Lowes MA, Hamzavi IH, editors. A comprehensive guide to hidradenitis suppurativa. Elsevier; 2022. p. 273–82. https://doi.org/10.1016/B978-0-323-77724-7.00028-0. ISBN 9780323777247.

Chapter 6
Dressings and Wound Care for HS Patients

Erin R. Pomerantz, Romina Garakani, and Emily Correia

Case Title A 35-year-old female with persistent boils and open wounds in the axilla region.

Case

A 35-year-old female with a 10-year history of hidradenitis suppurativa presents to your office during the summer with complaints of intermittent lesions in her axilla that have become inflamed, red, and painful without drainage. She says this has affected her quality of life and has made her feel self-conscious, especially when she goes to the beach. She states that she has been doing a lot of research on the internet to find something that would help these "red bumps." She has come across different dressings and is overwhelmed by her choices. She is unsure which one is the best and is hopeful that you could give her a recommendation.

Board Review Question

Which of the following wound dressing types would you recommend for the above patient?

A. Silver Iodine Dressing
B. Hydrocolloid Dressing

E. R. Pomerantz (✉)
Lewis Katz School of Medicine at Temple University, Philadelphia, PA, USA
e-mail: erin.pomerantz@temple.edu

R. Garakani
Drexel University College of Medicine, Philadelphia, PA, USA
e-mail: rag338@drexel.edu

E. Correia
The Department of Dermatology and Cutaneous Biology at the Sidney Kimmel Medical College, Thomas Jefferson University Hospital, Philadelphia, PA, USA
e-mail: exc203@jefferson.edu

N. Brownstone (ed.), *Clinical Cases in Hidradenitis Suppurativa*, Clinical Cases in Dermatology, https://doi.org/10.1007/978-3-032-15200-8_6

C. Alginate Dressing
D. Chlorhexidine Dressing
E. Benzoyl Peroxide Dressing

Introduction

Hidradenitis suppurativa (HS) is a chronic, inflammatory skin condition that predominantly affects the hair follicles, leading to painful lesions [1]. These lesions typically manifest as nodules, abscesses, and sinus tracts that often arise in intertriginous areas of the body, making wound care a challenge. The recurrent and debilitating nature of this disease significantly impacts a patient's emotional wellbeing. Furthermore, infected lesions can worsen symptoms and complicate treatment, making effective wound care essential. Proper wound care not only alleviates pain and reduces the risk of further flare-ups but also promotes healing, prevents infections, and minimizes the likelihood of scarring.

Proper wound care should focus on patient comfort, accessibility, and the quality of lesions. Ideal wound dressings should facilitate an optimal healing environment, support tissue regeneration, and reduce the risk of secondary bacterial infections [2]. Dressings act as a protective barrier, absorb exudate from draining lesions, and help maintain the moisture balance needed for healing. These qualities can also be therapeutic when managing HS lesions.

While a variety of wound dressings are available, many patients with HS continue to rely on over-the-counter options like gauze and absorbent pads [3]. These dressings are accessible and cost-effective, which is important considering that HS lesions may require frequent dressing changes [4]. However, while gauze and similar products provide some protection, they do not offer the advanced features to manage HS lesions effectively. Specifically, these dressings lack the moisture-retentive and antimicrobial properties found in newer, more specialized dressings [2]. Advanced dressings such as hydrocolloids, alginates, negative pressure wound therapy (NPWT), and those with bactericidal properties, are preferable in managing exudate, promoting a moist healing environment, and reducing the risk of infection. These options can also conform to the shape of the wound, enhancing comfort and minimizing irritation. Unfortunately, they are often more expensive and less accessible for many patients, presenting a barrier to their widespread use.

This chapter will explore the role of wound dressings in the management of HS, focusing on the importance of selecting the right dressing to optimize patient outcomes. A range of available dressings will be reviewed to provide a comprehensive overview of their benefits and limitations. This chapter aims to equip healthcare providers with the knowledge needed to enhance wound healing, improve patient comfort, and minimize complications.

Antimicrobial Dressings

Silver and Iodine

Silver antimicrobial dressings are widely used in wound care due to the bactericidal properties of silver ions, which are released into the wound bed and reduce bacterial growth. A study by Lin et al. showed that silver-containing dressings were more effective in reducing bacterial contamination and growth than standard gauze dressings [5]. These silver dressings not only prevent bacterial entry into the wound but also trap bacteria within the dressing, thereby protecting the wound from potential infection [5]. Similarly, iodine-based antimicrobial dressings have been shown to support wound healing through the release of iodine and its antimicrobial effects. However, a study by Jiang et al. found that silver dressings led to a greater reduction in healing time compared to iodine dressings [6]. Further research has highlighted additional benefits of silver ions in wound healing. Silver ions have been shown to stimulate the production of vascular endothelial growth factor (VEGF), promoting angiogenesis, skin contraction, and tissue remodeling [7]. Moreover, silver dressings are more effective at absorbing wound exudate and conforming to the shape of the wound, enhancing patient comfort by reducing dressing movement and irritation [8]. Overall, while more research is needed to establish the role of silver dressings in specific conditions like HS, their broad antimicrobial properties and ability to promote wound healing make them a promising option in wound care management.

Honey

Honey is another effective antimicrobial agent used in wound dressings. Its antimicrobial activity stems from several factors, including the production of hydrogen peroxide, its natural acidity, and the presence of bioactive compounds such as methylglyoxal in Manuka honey [9]. Additionally, honey's high viscosity creates a protective barrier over the wound, helping to prevent contamination [9]. Beyond its antimicrobial effects, honey also supports tissue regeneration in wound healing. Its moisture content, high sugar concentration, and the generation of reactive oxygen species (ROS) contribute to the promotion of cell growth and tissue repair [10]. Together, these properties make honey a valuable adjunct in wound care, particularly for its ability to both protect against infection and enhance the healing process.

Topical Antiseptics

Chlorhexidine

Chlorhexidine gluconate is a topical antiseptic frequently recommended for treating lesions of HS due to its antimicrobial properties. Studies by Cheong et al. using both ex vivo human skin models and in vivo xenograft mouse models have shown its strong antimicrobial activity [11]. However, chlorhexidine also has significant cytotoxic effects, causing cellular damage across the epidermis and dermis, which can hinder wound healing [11]. After an initial 24-h treatment, its ability to reduce bacterial growth was not sustained, with bacterial levels rebounding after 48 h, highlighting its transient effect [11]. These findings underscore the importance of carefully considering alternative antiseptics when managing HS lesions.

Benzoyl Peroxide

Benzoyl peroxide is a highly effective antiseptic often recommended for managing HS lesions. As an alternative to chlorhexidine in clinical practice, it provides both anti-inflammatory and antibacterial benefits. Benzoyl peroxide is degraded to benzoic acid to generate free radicals, causing damage to bacterial cell walls and inducing cell death. Its bactericidal properties help reduce the bacterial load of microorganisms frequently associated with cutaneous infections [12]. Additionally, this agent has keratolytic properties, which help reduce the follicular occlusion that occurs in HS lesions. Its anti-inflammatory, microbicidal, and keratolytic properties optimize its effectiveness in managing HS.

Zinc Pyrithione

Zinc pyrithione is a commonly used antifungal for treating seborrheic dermatitis, offering superior antibacterial effects over chlorhexidine gluconate, with enhanced bacterial suppression at 72 hours [13, 14]. Its antiproliferative, anti-inflammatory, and anti-androgenic properties effectively promote wound healing [15]. More cost-effective and accessible than chlorhexidine, its prolonged antimicrobial action is attributed to its strong adhesion to hair follicles and the stratum corneum, ensuring effectiveness even after thorough rinsing [14].

Alginates

Alginate dressings, derived from brown algae or bacteria, are recognized for their high absorption capacity [16]. Their hydrophilic properties allow the absorption of large volumes of fluid while maintaining a moist environment in the wound bed, preventing both dehydration and maceration of surrounding tissue [17]. Additionally, alginate-based hydrogels are gentle on the wound bed and cause minimal disruption when removed, which makes them a suitable choice for wounds that require frequent dressing changes [16]. Alginate dressings are particularly beneficial for managing wounds with significant levels of exudate, such as those lesions commonly associated with HS. The high absorbency of alginate dressings helps manage wounds with heavy exudate, maintaining a controlled moist environment that promotes healing.

Hydrocolloids

The term "hydrocolloid" describes a type of dressing in which the semisolid form of a hydrophilic mass is applied to a flexible semipermeable carrier [18]. Later on, this term began to also include an amorphous hydrogel dressing and a fibrous dressing made of carboxymethyl cellulose [18]. Hydrocolloid dressings are preferably used as postoperative dressings or for secondary retention purposes as they are less permeable than alginates or hydrogels [18]. In addition, these dressings have more commonly been used for the treatment of chronic wounds, like pressure ulcers [18]. However, they are still effective for acute wounds as they can absorb excess fluid, provide a barrier to infection, and facilitate debridement [18]. In the case of HS, one study investigated the use of hydrocolloid dressings for patients who had undergone wide excision of perianal HS lesions and were healing by granulation [19]. On the third post-operative day, hydrocolloid dressings were applied daily to the excision sites [19]. They found that this type of dressing minimized patient discomfort, allowed faster patient mobilization, and allowed the area to remain dry for longer periods [19]. Therefore, these types of dressings may be most useful after HS procedures, such as deroofing.

Negative Pressure Wound Therapy

Negative pressure wound therapy (NPWT) promotes wound healing that occurs through the use of sub-atmospheric pressure [20]. This method works by reducing inflammatory exudate and promoting granulation tissue [20]. In general, NPWT is commonly used when a wound is complex, non-healing, or at great risk of not healing [20]. For acute wounds, NPWT is indicated when the wound cannot be closed by primary intention due to active or increased risk of infection, skin tension, or swelling [20]. This type of wound therapy can also be utilized for acute or chronic dehisced wounds [20]. In the case of HS management, NPWT creates a symmetrical physical pressure layer of lesions, reducing wound contamination and promoting granulation [21]. Parrado et al. presented a case in which NPWT created a sterile environment to open HS wounds in the perineal regions after debridement. The report found that NPWT helped the healing process in addition to providing better results after skin grafting procedures [21].

Biodegradable Temporizing Matrix (BTM)

The application of NovoSorb BTM (Biodegradable Temporizing Matrix) in the management of post-surgical wounds in patients with HS offers a promising strategy for enhancing healing outcomes. Post-surgical wound care in HS is particularly challenging due to extensive excisional lesions and the heightened risk of infection. NovoSorb BTM serves as a temporary, synthetic dermal matrix that promotes cellular infiltration and tissue regeneration within the wound bed [22]. Acting as both a scaffold for new tissue growth and a protective barrier against bacteria, BTM has been shown to facilitate more effective healing. Recent studies underscore its advantages as a cost-effective intervention that minimizes the need for intensive wound care while reducing the risks of infection, graft rejection, and skin contractures [23]. Furthermore, a retrospective analysis demonstrated that BTM use was associated with fewer hospitalizations and contributed to the restoration of a full range of motion following wound closure, highlighting its potential to improve both functional and clinical outcomes [24].

Gauze Dressings for Post-Surgical Wounds

Gauze, abdominal pads, and adhesive bandages are commonly used over-the-counter dressing options for managing HS lesions [25]. The North American Clinical Management Guidelines for Hidradenitis Suppurativa emphasize the importance of selecting a dressing with strong absorption capabilities to effectively manage the exudate associated with these lesions [26]. While gauze is a widely available and cost-effective option, it has several limitations. It can adhere to the wound bed, making removal painful and potentially causing further tissue damage. Additionally, gauze lacks the moisture-retentive properties of more refined dressings, which are important in creating an optimal healing environment [4]. As a result, although gauze may be an affordable short-term solution, it is less effective for long-term wound care in HS lesions, particularly when compared to alternative dressings that better support healing and reduce discomfort.

Conclusions

Selecting the correct type of dressing can be overwhelming to both patients and providers as there are a wide array of choices available. Proper wound care is complex due to the fluctuating nature of HS. Furthermore, there is no single dressing that can address the needs of HS patients at different stages of their lives and disease. Another compounding factor is the cost of dressings and insurance coverage. Such factors can hinder accessibility to proper wound care, exacerbating the already difficult management of this disease.

In this chapter, the authors have provided an overview of the different types of dressings that are available. While data does exist on these dressings, the literature is lacking in regard to dressings in the setting of HS. It is important that our field continues to add to the literature to increase knowledge and facilitate better wound care management of HS patients. Table 6.1 summarizes the types of dressings that may be used for HS, along with their mechanism of action, benefits, and limitations.

Board Review Question Explanation

Which of the following wound dressing types would you recommend for the above patient?

A. Silver Iodine Dressing
B. Hydrocolloid Dressing
C. Alginate Dressing
D. Chlorhexidine Dressing
E. Benzoyl Peroxide Dressing (Correct)

Answer Explanation

Correct Answer: E. Benzoyl Peroxide Dressing.

Explanation: This patient is presenting with inflamed lesions in her axillary regions and is hoping to mitigate the pain and frequency of these lesions. A dressing that would be best suited for her situation is benzoyl peroxide dressing. This type of dressing is preferred for the management of active lesions that are inflamed as it has both antibacterial and anti-inflammatory effects. Additionally, it may reduce future lesions due to these effects along with its keratolytic properties.

Key Takeaways

- Proper wound care and an understanding of the different types of wound dressings available is important knowledge, especially when caring for HS patients. Such care can optimize healing, decrease infection risk, and improve patient quality of life.
- Antimicrobial dressings, including silver and iodine dressings as well as honey, are promising for wound healing as they facilitate environments with less bacterial entry and provide protection against wound infection.
- Chlorhexidine, benzoyl peroxide, and zinc pyrithione are available dressing options that are anti-septic.

Table 6.1 Summary of dressings. This table summarizes the types of dressings that may be used for HS, along with their mechanism of action, benefits, and limitations

Dressing type	Mechanism	Benefits	Limitations	Best use
Silver-based dressings	Silver ions reduce bacterial growth and prevent infection	Bactericidal; promotes healing and conforms to the wound	Expensive; potential for allergic reactions	High-risk or infected wounds; chronic HS lesions
Iodine-based dressings	Releases iodine for antimicrobial effects and healing support	Bactericidal; accelerates healing, and reduces infection risk	Can irritate the skin; staining risk; needs careful application	Infected or high-bacterial load wounds
Honey (Manuka)	Antimicrobial from hydrogen peroxide, acidity, and methylglyoxal. Creates a protective barrier	Antibacterial; promotes tissue regeneration and maintains moisture	Risk of an allergic reaction. Can be messy and not convenient to use	Chronic or infected wounds; ulcers
Chlorhexidine	Disrupts bacterial cell walls to prevent infection	Strong antimicrobial; effective for short-term use; reduces potential antibiotic resistance	Cytotoxic; inhibits healing; effectiveness wanes over time	Acute infections; HS lesion prevention
Zinc pyrithione	Antibacterial, antifungal, and anti-inflammatory	Prolonged antimicrobial action, anti-inflammatory, cost-effective, and reduces potential antibiotic resistance	May not be as effective for deep or chronic wounds	Mild to moderate HS, seborrheic dermatitis
Benzoyl peroxide	Antiseptic with antibacterial and anti-inflammatory effects	Reduces bacterial load; controls and reduces potential antibiotic resistance and inflammation	Can dry out or irritate the skin; fabric bleaching	Inflammatory or acne-related HS lesions
Alginate dressings	Absorbs exudate and forms a gel to maintain moisture	High absorbency, minimal disruption during removal, reduces maceration	Not suitable for dry wounds; may require frequent changes	Wounds with heavy exudate (e.g., HS flare-ups)
Hydrocolloid dressings	Maintains a moist environment and barrier to infection	Absorbs exudate, promotes healing, and reduces discomfort	Not for highly exudative wounds; can cause maceration if not changed	Post-surgical, chronic wounds, minor HS

(continued)

Table 6.1 (continued)

Dressing type	Mechanism	Benefits	Limitations	Best use
Negative pressure wound therapy (NPWT)	Uses sub-atmospheric pressure to reduce exudate and stimulate tissue growth	Promotes granulation tissue, reduces swelling and infection risk	Requires specialized equipment; expensive, uncomfortable	Complex, non-healing, or deep HS lesions
Biodegradable temporizing matrix (BTM)	Synthetic dermal matrix that supports tissue regeneration and protects against infection	Enhances healing, reduces infection risk, and minimizes contractures	Requires careful application; not widely available	Post-surgical HS wounds, tissue regeneration
Gauze dressings	Absorbs exudate and act as a barrier	Economical; widely available	Adheres to wounds, painful removal, lacks moisture balance, and has antimicrobial effects	Simple, short-term wound care or minor lesions. Lesions requiring frequent dressing changes

- Alginate and hydrocolloid dressings provide moist environments while providing barrier protection to wounds.
- Gauze dressings are economical and are a good choice for simple, short-term wound care.

References

1. Bukvić Mokos Z, Markota Čagalj A, Marinović B. Epidemiology of hidradenitis suppurativa. Clin Dermatol. 2023;41(5):564–75. https://doi.org/10.1016/j.clindermatol.2023.08.020.
2. Vowden K, Vowden P. Wound dressings: principles and practice. Surgery (Oxford). 2014;32(9):462–7. https://doi.org/10.1016/j.mpsur.2014.07.001.
3. Poondru S, Scott K, Riley JM. Patient perspectives of wound care management in hidradenitis suppurativa. Arch Dermatol Res. 2023;315(6):1847–50. https://doi.org/10.1007/s00403-023-02576-8.
4. Jones VJ. The use of gauze: will it ever change? Int Wound J. 2006;3(2):79–86. https://doi.org/10.1111/j.1742-4801.2006.00215.x.
5. Lin YH, Hsu WS, Chung WY, Ko TH, Lin JH. Silver-based wound dressings reduce bacterial burden and promote wound healing. Int Wound J. 2016;13(4):505–11. https://doi.org/10.1111/iwj.12467.
6. Jiang Y, Zhang Q, Wang H, Välimäki M, Zhou Q, Dai W, Guo J. Effectiveness of silver and iodine dressings on wound healing: a systematic review and meta-analysis. BMJ Open. 2024;14(8):e077902. https://doi.org/10.1136/bmjopen-2023-077902.
7. Bourdillon KA, Delury CP, Cullen BM. Biofilms and delayed healing – an in vitro evaluation of silver- and iodine-containing dressings and their effect on bacterial and human cells. Int Wound J. 2017;14(6):1066–75. https://doi.org/10.1111/iwj.12761.

8. Alimov V, Lovecchio F, Sinha M, Foster KN, Drachman D. Use of a silver-containing hydrofiber dressing for filling abscess cavity following incision and drainage in the emergency department: a randomized controlled trial. Adv Skin Wound Care. 2013;26(1):20–5. https://doi.org/10.1097/01.ASW.0000425936.94874.9a.
9. Yupanqui Mieles J, Vyas C, Aslan E, Humphreys G, Diver C, Bartolo P. Honey: an advanced antimicrobial and wound healing biomaterial for tissue engineering applications. Pharmaceutics. 2022;14(8):1663. https://doi.org/10.3390/pharmaceutics14081663.
10. Dunnill C, Patton T, Brennan J, Barrett J, Dryden M, Cooke J, Leaper D, Georgopoulos NT. Reactive oxygen species (ROS) and wound healing: the functional role of ROS and emerging ROS-modulating technologies for augmentation of the healing process. Int Wound J. 2017;14(1):89–96. https://doi.org/10.1111/iwj.12557.
11. Cheong JZA, Liu A, Rust CJ, et al. Robbing Peter to Pay Paul: Chlorhexidine gluconate demonstrates short-term efficacy and long-term cytotoxicity. Wound Rep Reg. 2022;30(5):573–84. https://doi.org/10.1111/wrr.13044.
12. Okamoto K, Kanayama S, Ikeda F, et al. Broad spectrum in vitro microbicidal activity of benzoyl peroxide against microorganisms related to cutaneous diseases. J Dermatol. 2021;48(4):551–5. https://doi.org/10.1111/1346-8138.15739.
13. Danesh MJ, et al. Pyrithione zinc as a general management strategy for hidradenitis suppurativa. J Am Acad Dermatol. 2015;73(5):e175.
14. Guthery E, Seal LA, Anderson EL. Zinc pyrithione in alcohol-based products for skin antisepsis: persistence of antimicrobial effects. Am J Infect Control. 2005;33(1):15–22.
15. Gupta M, et al. Zinc therapy in dermatology: a review. Dermatol Res Pract. 2014;2014(1):709152.
16. Zhang M, Zhao X. Alginate hydrogel dressings for advanced wound management. Int J Biol Macromol. 2020;162:1414–28. https://doi.org/10.1016/j.ijbiomac.2020.07.311.
17. Varaprasad K, Jayaramudu T, Kanikireddy V, Toro C, Sadiku ER. Alginate-based composite materials for wound dressing application: a mini review. Carbohydr Polym. 2020;236:116025. https://doi.org/10.1016/j.carbpol.2020.116025.
18. Thomas S. Hydrocolloid dressings in the management of acute wounds: a review of the literature. Int Wound J. 2008;5(5):602–13. https://doi.org/10.1111/j.1742-481X.2008.00541.x.
19. Michel L. Use of hydrocolloid dressing following wide excision of perianal hidradenitis suppurativa. Proc R Soc Med. 1985;88:144–8.
20. Zaver V, Kankanalu P. Negative Pressure Wound Therapy. In: StatPearls [Internet]. Treasure Island (FL): StatPearls Publishing; 2024. [Updated 2023 Sep 4]. Available from: https://www.ncbi.nlm.nih.gov/books/NBK576388/.
21. Parrado R, Cadena M, Vergara A, Cadena D, Chalela JG. The role of negative pressure wound therapy in the management of hidradenitis suppurativa: a case report and literature review. Int Wound J. 2017;14:35–9. https://doi.org/10.1111/iwj.12544.
22. NovoSorb® BTM | Biodegradable Synthetic Dermal Substitute. (n.d.). United States. https://polynovo.com/novosorb-btm/.
23. Aldin Malkoc, Wong DT, Woodward B. Single staged treatment of a complex full thickness debridement for hidradenitis suppurativa using NovoSorb Biodegradable Temporizing MatrixTM. Burns Open. 2022;6(3):125–8. https://doi.org/10.1016/j.burnso.2022.05.001.
24. Smith HG. Treatment of hidradenitis with synthetic biodegradable matrix eliminated post-surgical hospitalization. J Am Coll Surg. 2019;229(4):e46–7. https://doi.org/10.1016/j.jamcollsurg.2019.08.793.
25. Poondru S, et al. Patient perspectives of wound care management in hidradenitis suppurativa. Arch Dermatol Res. 2023;315(6):1847–50. https://doi.org/10.1007/s00403-023-02576-8.
26. Alikhan A, et al. North American clinical management guidelines for hidradenitis suppurativa: a publication from the United States and Canadian Hidradenitis Suppurativa Foundations: Part I: diagnosis, evaluation, and the use of complementary and procedural management. J Am Acad Dermatol. 2019;81(1):76–90. https://doi.org/10.1016/j.jaad.2019.02.067.

Chapter 7
Pain and Itch Control in HS (Clinical Cases in HS)

Jason Kauper, Sidney M. Leno, and Sarah K. Whitley

Case Title A 23-year-old male with HS presents with acute-on-chronic pain in his right axilla.

Case

Today a patient with Hurley stage II HS presents for an urgent visit to address severe pain in his right axilla. His current treatment regimen includes clindamycin gel, benzoyl peroxide solution, and adalimumab 40 mg weekly. Since starting these medications, he has noticed fewer new nodules and less pain and drainage from existing HS lesions. However, he endorses chronic pruritus in HS-affected body sites. Three days ago, he noted acute worsening of pain and drainage from an established lesion in his right axilla. On clinical exam, you note a tender 5 × 2 cm erythematous fluctuant and firm plaque that is spontaneously draining purulent material. Also, hyperpigmented firm nodules and plaques are present at other intertriginous sites. Your assessment is that this patient is experiencing a localized disease flare. The patient asks what treatment(s) you can recommend for this exacerbation in HS pain.

Jason Kauper and Sidney M. Leno contributed equally with all other contributors.

J. Kauper
T.H. Chan School of Medicine, University of Massachusetts, Worcester, MA, USA

S. M. Leno
Department of Dermatology, University of Massachusetts, Worcester, MA, USA

S. K. Whitley (✉)
T.H. Chan School of Medicine, University of Massachusetts, Worcester, MA, USA

Department of Dermatology, University of Massachusetts, Worcester, MA, USA

Autoimmune Therapeutics Institute, University of Massachusetts, Worcester, MA, USA
e-mail: Sarah.Whitley@umassmed.edu

N. Brownstone (ed.), *Clinical Cases in Hidradenitis Suppurativa*, Clinical Cases in Dermatology, https://doi.org/10.1007/978-3-032-15200-8_7

Board Review Question
A patient with hidradenitis suppurativa and peptic ulcer disease has already been prescribed disease-directed therapies for treatment of his HS. To target severe pain associated with an acute HS abscess, which of the following would be first-line therapy?

A. Acetaminophen 325 mg every 4–8 h PRN
B. Oxycodone 5 mg every 4–6 h PRN
C. Tramadol 50 mg every 4–6 h PRN
D. Ibuprofen 200 mg every 4–8 h PRN
E. Incision and drainage

Introduction

Patients with hidradenitis suppurativa (HS) experience debilitating symptoms related to chronic inflammation [3, 5, 8]. Chief among these symptoms is pain. Most HS patients report pain severe enough to limit function and activities of daily living [1, 4, 9, 10]. In a global survey including more than 1900 patients with HS, 61.4% rated their pain as moderate to high and 4.5% described it as the worst pain possible [11]. In another study of 103 patients with HS, 35.0% reported moderate to severe pain and 60.4% reported moderate to severe pruritus [4]. Notably, 59.5% of HS patients experienced both pain and itch at the same anatomical site, underscoring the need to address both symptoms [4, 12].

Despite the central role of pain and itch in disease-related quality of life (QoL) burden, lack of prospective studies to evaluate pain management strategies in HS has yielded guidelines that rely solely on expert opinion [6, 7, 9]. Because pain and itch arise from overlapping yet distinct somatosensory pathways, they require targeted assessment and intervention. Accordingly, this chapter will examine mechanisms of pain processing in HS, review current concepts of itch pathogenesis, and describe approaches for clinical assessment and treatment of both symptoms.

Pain and Itch Mechanisms in HS

Pain may be classified according to physiologic mechanism—nociceptive (arising from tissue injury), neuropathic (resulting from nerve injury), or nociplastic (reflecting a sensitized nervous system) [6, 9, 11]. Pain may also be categorized by pain duration (acute, chronic, or episodic), anatomic location, and etiology (cancer-associated or non-cancer-associated) [13]. Clinically, HS-related pain most commonly presents as acute nociceptive pain arising from active inflammation or as chronic pain with neuropathic features [2, 5, 11]. A foundational study by Alsouhibani et al. [14] used quantitative sensory testing (QST) to objectively characterize pain mechanism in HS. QST applies precisely controlled thermal, mechanical, or pressure stimuli to HS and control skin, then measures perceptual responses. In this way, QST functions as a "stress test" for the nervous system, revealing how sensory nerves detect and process stimuli. In HS lesions, QST uncovered patterns of sensory gain and loss, establishing that nociceptive, neuropathic, and nociplastic pathways all shape HS patients' experience of pain [14]. Though QST is not practical for routine use in dermatologic practice, it is a tool that can be used in conjunction with patient reported outcomes, nerve conduction studies, histology, and neuroimaging (e.g., functional magnetic resonance imaging or positron emission tomography) to delineate pain contributions in HS.

Inflammatory mediators can directly sensitize peripheral pain-sensing nerves (e.g. nociceptors) by lowering nerve action potential thresholds and increasing nerve responsiveness to mechanical stimuli to produce hyperalgesia [15–18]. Sustained inflammation increases central nervous system responsiveness to painful stimuli, causing altered and amplified pain perception termed central sensitization [14, 19]. This involves a cascade of structural, functional, and neurochemical changes in the central nervous system that amplify ascending (excitatory/pain) signaling while reducing descending (inhibitory/downregulatory) signaling. Central sensitization strongly associates with psychological comorbidities, particularly depression [11, 19, 20]. Central sensitization is significantly more common among HS patients with a prior diagnosis of depression (odds ratio 6.16; 95% CI, 2.81–13.54), underscoring close interplay between mood disorders and central pain processing [19, 20]. This relationship is likely bidirectional. The psychological burden of HS—social isolation, reduced quality of life, and disease-related stigma—may exacerbate central sensitization through stress-mediated neuroplastic changes [8, 21, 22]. In advanced HS, chronic inflammation causes damage to cutaneous nerve fibers [14]. This impairs transduction of both innocuous and noxious thermal and mechanical stimuli, producing QST findings suggestive of neuropathy [5, 14]. Taken together, available evidence indicates that HS pain arises from overlapping nociceptive, neuropathic, and nociplastic mechanisms driven by neuroimmune interactions within affected skin, with multiple pain processes often coexisting in individual patients [2, 6, 9, 11, 23].

The pathogenesis of itch in HS is poorly defined, and there are currently no HS-specific therapeutic guidelines for its management [4, 5, 12, 24, 25]. The quality-of-life impact of HS-associated itch is likely underestimated, with studies reporting that up to 82.6% of patients experience mild to moderate pruritus [4, 12, 24]. Patients frequently describe HS-associated itch as burning or stinging, and itch commonly co-localizes with pain at affected anatomic sites [25]. HS-associated itch exhibits specific temporal features, commonly occurring in brief episodic flares lasting up to 10 min, most frequently during the evening and nighttime [4]. Pruritus in HS appears closely linked to disease activity, correlating with lesion presence and severity, and is most pronounced in patients with Hurley stage III disease [7, 12, 24].

Type 2 cytokines (IL-4/IL-13) and IL-31 activate downstream JAK/STAT signals to transduce chronic idiopathic pruritus and atopic dermatitis-related itch [26, 27]. IL-4/-13/-31 have not been reported to be enriched in HS skin; thus, it is likely that

HS-related itch occurs through distinct mechanisms. Despite a reported link between HS and asthma [28], currently there is no evidence that mast cell release of histamine or proteases contributes to HS-associated pruritus.

Common to itch and pain perception is sensitization of peripheral small-diameter sensory neurons (Aδ and C-fiber afferents) [15, 17]. Both nociceptors and itch-sensing nerves (e.g., pruriceptors) are activated by inflammatory cytokines, mast cell mediators, and microbial products [16, 26]. The HS-associated cytokine TNF-α enhances both pain and itch by sensitizing peripheral sensory nerves through TNFR1 and downstream p38, ERK, and NK-κB signaling [29]. IL-6 and IL-1β are well-established contributors to nociceptive and neuropathic pain in other diseases and organ systems and may promote itch indirectly through amplification of inflammatory circuits and central sensitization [30, 31]. The mammalian target of rapamycin (mTOR) represents a shared molecular substrate for chronic itch and pain [32]. TNF-α, IL-6, IL-31, and the protease-activated receptor PAR2 have been shown to induce mTOR expression, and Karagianni et al. [33] reported elevated mTOR levels in both lesional and nonlesional HS skin that correlated with disease severity. These data suggest that mTOR dysregulation contributes to heightened sensory neuron excitability in HS, and that mTOR-targeting therapies such as metformin may attenuate both itch and pain. These findings highlight neuroimmune crosstalk as a central driver of HS-associated itch and pain and establish it as a rational target for therapeutic intervention.

Assessment of HS Itch and Pain

A structured approach to evaluating pain and itch in HS supports both day-to-day clinical decision-making and standardized measurement of treatment response in clinical trials. In routine clinical practice, pain and itch are commonly assessed using the numeric rating scale (NRS) or visual analog scale (VAS), which quantify symptom intensity in a simple and reproducible manner on a 0–10 scale [34, 35]. The Dermatology Life Quality Index (DLQI) [36] and the Hidradenitis Suppurativa Quality of Life (HiSQOL) [37] instruments can be used alongside these measures to provide a broader assessment of disease impact on daily functioning. These validated tools are practical to administer, well accepted by patients, and position the clinician to factor health-related quality of life and symptomology into clinical care decisions. (Table 7.1).

Among available pain measures, the NRS (0–10 scale) is often preferred due to its simplicity, reliability, and low rate of incomplete responses [34]. Both the NRS and VAS are sensitive to changes in pain intensity and correlate with disease severity and quality of life [2, 34]. In HS, pain is typically assessed as maximum or average intensity over a defined period, such as the preceding 24 h or 7 days. An NRS score of ≥3 is generally considered clinically significant [34]. When used in combination patient-reported quality of life (QoL) outcome measures such as the DLQI or HiSQOL, these tools can inform the impact of HS itch and pain on daily functioning.

Table 7.1 Patient Reported Outcome Tools for Assessment of Pain and Itch in HS

Setting	Instrument	Notes
Pain or itch severity	Pain Numeric Rating Scale (NRS)	Simple 0–10 scale; high patient acceptability; sensitive to change; commonly used to assess average or maximum pain over 24 hr maximum and 7 day average
	Pain Visual Analog Scale (VAS)	Continuous measure of pain intensity; responsive to treatment effects; used clinical and research settings
	Brief Pain Inventory	9 items that measure pain severity and interference with daily life over 24 h and 1 week
	Hidradenitis Suppurativa Symptom Daily Diary (HSSDD)	11-point NRS capturing worst skin pain over the preceding 24 h
	Itchy Quant	0–10 rating NRS scale for itch
Pain categorization	PainDETECT	9 item screening tool for neuropathic pain
	Central sensitization inventory (CSI)	25 item screening tool for centrally sensitized, e.g., nociplastic pain
Quality of life	Dermatology Life Quality Index (DLQI)	Consists of 3 domains: symptoms, psychosocial impacts, and activities/adaptations; 17 items with a 7-day recall period scored 0 (not at all) to 4 (extremely); total score ranges from 0–68 with higher scores indicating worse QoL
	Hidradenitis Suppurativa Quality of Life (HiSQOL)	Consists of 3 domains: symptoms, psychosocial impacts, and activities/adaptations; 17 items with a 7-day recall period scored 0 (not at all) to 4 (extremely); total score ranges from 0 to 68 with higher scores indicating worse QoL
Treatment response	Hidradenitis Suppurativa Impact Assessment (HSIA)	HS-specific patient-reported outcome; assesses disease impact and functional impairment
	Hidradenitis Suppurativa Symptom Assessment (HSSA)	HS-specific patient-reported outcome; captures symptom burden and treatment-related change
Anxiety and depression	GAD-7	Generalized anxiety assessment
	PHQ-9	Screen for presence and severity of depression

Abbreviations: *HS* hidradenitis suppurativa, *NRS* numeric rating scale, *VAS* visual analog scale, *DLQI* Dermatology Life Quality Index, *HiSCR* Hidradenitis Suppurativa Clinical Response, *HS-PGA/HS-PhGA* Hidradenitis Suppurativa Physician Global Assessment, *HSSA* Hidradenitis Suppurativa Symptom Assessment, *HSIA* Hidradenitis Suppurativa Impact Assessment, *HASI-R* Hidradenitis Suppurativa Area and Severity Index-Revised, *HS-IGA* Hidradenitis Suppurativa Investigator Global Assessment, *IHS4* International Hidradenitis Suppurativa Severity Score System, *HiSQoL* Hidradenitis Suppurativa Quality of Life

In research settings, additional survey tools are used to assess response to treatment and to supplement the clinician's physical exam. HS-specific instruments such as the Hidradenitis Suppurativa Impact Assessment (HSIA) and the Hidradenitis Suppurativa Symptom Assessment (HSSA) are designed to capture treatment-related changes in symptom burden and functional impact that may not be fully reflected by generic quality-of-life metrics [2, 5, 9]. Achievement of a 30% reduction in NRS pain score (NRS30) and a four-point reduction in DLQI score (range 0–30; 30 = max QoL burden) have been cited as minimal clinically important differences [38]. Of note, efforts are underway to standardize a core outcomes set for use in interventional clinical trials for HS [39].

Assessment of itch in HS is less standardized than pain, and validated disease-specific tools for itch are lacking. However, exploratory evaluation of itch using NRS or VAS measures may be of clinical utility, given its high prevalence and contribution to QoL burden.

HS Pain and Itch-Directed Therapies

Existing therapeutic guidelines focus on disease modifying therapies; however, the high morbidity burden of HS pain has prompted development of additional pain-focused guidelines [2, 6, 9, 23]. Current HS pain management guidelines are based on expert opinion. These consensus guidelines endorse a multimodal approach to pain management that encompasses disease-directed therapies, analgesics, non-pharmacologic pain management including physical therapy, wound care, or cognitive behavior therapy, and neuromodulators for treatment of comorbid psychological conditions [6, 13]. Management strategies are tailored according to disease severity and the presence of comorbid conditions (Table 7.2). National and international guidelines emphasize routine assessment of pain severity and control of underlying inflammation as pillars of HS pain management [6, 38]. Accordingly, disease-directed therapy should be implemented before escalation to adjunctive pain treatments.

Current FDA-approved biologic therapies for HS offer limited relief of pain and itch. TNF-α inhibition with adalimumab 40 mg weekly reduces average HS pain severity by 0.4 points to achieve a final NRS pain score of 4 out of 10 [40]. The SUNSHINE and SUNRISE phase 3 trials demonstrated that IL-17A inhibition with secukinumab diminishes "worst skin pain" as early as week 4; this is sustained through week 52 [41]. Pain reduction was consistent across patient subgroups and was observed in placebo-treated patients who transitioned to secukinumab, supporting a direct treatment effect. However, the number of patients achieving a 30% reduction in pain severity score (NRS30) at week 16 was only modestly higher in patients treated with secukinumab (37%) versus placebo (23%) [41]. The dual IL-17A/F inhibitor bimekizumab demonstrates the most rapid and clinically meaningful improvements in HS-related pain amongst FDA-approved treatments for HS. The BE HEARD I and II trials revealed a 1.2-point reduction ($p = 0.0022$) in

Table 7.2 Summary of existing guidelines and recommendations for pain management in HS [1, 6, 26]

	Therapy	Mechanism of action	Adverse effects and special population considerations
Acute HS pain management	Disease-directed therapy	Reduces acute inflammatory burden driving pain	Foundational step for all acute pain
	Warm compresses	Vasodilation improves perfusion and promotes drainage	N/A
	Intralesional triamcinolone	Local corticosteroid effect reduces inflammation and nociceptor sensitization	Mixed efficacy data; limited data in pregnancy; consider tolerance in pediatrics
	Incision and drainage	Decompresses abscesses and relieves pressure	Procedural pain; recurrence without disease control
	Resorcinol 15% cream	Keratolytic and antiseptic effects reduce abscess duration	Irritant contact dermatitis common
	Lidocaine, menthol, pramoxine	Local sodium channel blockade or counter-irritation	Minimal systemic risk
	COX-2 nonselective NSAIDs (ibuprofen, ketorolac, naproxen)	Reduce prostaglandin synthesis thereby impairing gastric mucosal protection and platelet function	Avoid with prior CABG, aspirin-exacerbated asthma, or GI bleeding; use caution in CV or liver disease, uncontrolled hypertension, age >65, or bleeding risk. Higher GI bleed risk than COX-2-selective NSAIDs—consider PPI co-therapy.
	COX 2 selective NSAIDs (celecoxib, diclofenac, etodolac, meloxicam)	Reduces prostaglandins while sparing GI lining and platelet function	GI bleeding, renal risk; naproxen preferred with CV risk
	Short-acting opioids for breakthrough pain (e.g., tramadol, oxycodone)	Central μ-opioid receptor activation	Sedation, respiratory depression; limit duration and quantity
Chronic HS pain management	Optimization of medical therapy	Reduces persistent inflammatory drivers of pain	Inadequate control limits analgesic response

(continued)

Table 7.2 (continued)

	Therapy	Mechanism of action	Adverse effects and special population considerations
Nociceptive pain throbbing, aching, sharp	NSAIDs (first-line nociceptive pain)	Peripheral anti-inflammatory effect	Avoid long-term use in renal/GI disease
Nociplastic pain Widespread and diffuse aching with extreme sensitivity to touch	SNRIs, TCAs (second-line nociceptive pain) 1st line: Duloxetine 2nd line: Venlafaxine 3rd line: Amitriptyline, Nortriptyline	Central pain modulation	QTc prolongation (venlafaxine); anticholinergic effects (TCAs)
Neuropathic pain burning, stabbing, shooting, "pins and needles"	Anticonvulsants, SNRIs (neuropathic pain) 1st line: Gabapentin 2nd line: Pregabalin	Reduce neuronal hyperexcitability and enhance descending inhibition	Sedation, dizziness; avoid serotonergic combinations; may be safely combined with SNRIs
	Pain specialist referral	Advanced pharmacologic or interventional options	Indicated after failure of ≥2 therapies or chronic opioid use
Psychological treatments	Cognitive behavioral therapy (CBT)	Reframes maladaptive pain cognitions; improves coping	First-line psychosocial therapy
	Acceptance and commitment therapy (ACT)	Enhances psychological flexibility and pain acceptance	Useful when physical impairment limits CBT
Wound care optimization	Appropriate dressings, drainage management	Reduces mechanical irritation and secondary inflammation	Individualize by lesion location
Physical therapy	Targeted mobility and strengthening	Reduces musculoskeletal contributors to pain	Tailor to disease severity

Hidradenitis Suppurativa Symptom Daily Diary (HSSDD) worst skin pain and a 5-point improvement in DLQI score ($p = 0.0005$) from baseline in patients treated with bimekizumab relative to placebo [42].

For acute HS pain, intralesional triamcinolone, incision and drainage procedures, nonsteroidal anti-inflammatory drugs (NSAIDs), and acetaminophen are recommended first-line treatments [6, 38]. Tramadol or other short-acting opioids are second-line acute pain therapies, appropriate for recalcitrant or breakthrough pain [9]. Daily NSAIDs, anticonvulsants (gabapentin or pregabalin), serotonin and norepinephrine reuptake inhibitors (duloxetine, venlafaxine, or nortriptyline), and tricyclic antidepressants comprise the pharmacologic armamentarium for chronic HS pain [2, 6, 9]. These drugs can be used when disease-directed therapies fail to relieve

HS pain, and/or pain character is suggestive of neuropathic or centrally sensitized pain. A meta-analysis of randomized controlled trials comparing pharmacologic agents for the treatment of chronic noncancer pain reported that opioids performed similarly to NSAIDs, tricyclic antidepressants, and anticonvulsants in alleviating pain and improving physical function [13]. These data suggest that current pain management practices do not adequately control HS-related pain, and some types of pain are not opioid responsive. Notably, reduction in pain scores correlate strongly with improvement in DLQI but do not consistently correlate with inflammatory lesion burden or biomarkers of inflammation, e.g., erythrocyte sedimentation rate (ESR) and C-reactive protein (CRP), highlighting a discordance between HS pain and inflammation that warrants further investigation [11, 23, 43].

Depressive symptoms are frequently observed in patients with HS and strongly correlate with heightened pain experiences [20, 44]. Evidence-based psychological treatments for chronic pain include cognitive behavioral therapy (CBT) and acceptance and commitment therapy (ACT). Among these, CBT is regarded as the first-line psychosocial treatment for chronic pain [45, 46]. CBT addresses pain and emotional distress through structured problem-solving strategies, with an emphasis on the connection of pain perceptions to cognitive processes, emotional responses, and behavioral patterns [46]. Maladaptive, pain-related, catastrophizing thoughts such as "this pain may last forever" contribute to negative affect and increase behaviors that intensify pain, such as "pushing through" or self-isolation. Core components of CBT that can help HS patients with chronic pain include reframing unhelpful thought patterns, relaxation techniques, and activity pacing, which involves completing large tasks in smaller segments with planned breaks [47, 48].

Acceptance and commitment therapy (ACT) is a psychological intervention for chronic pain that aims to impart psychological flexibility through six interrelated processes: acceptance, cognitive defusion, present-moment awareness, self-as-context, values clarification, and committed action [49]. Although ACT has demonstrated benefit in other chronic pain populations, it has not yet been specifically studied in patients with HS experiencing comorbid pain and depression. Still, this approach is deemed to have value in supporting psychological health [47].

Evidence supporting cannabinoids (e.g., tetrahydrocannabinol (THC), cannabidiol (CBD), and synthetic derivatives (nabilone) for chronic pain demonstrates, at best, small reductions in pain severity, with benefit primarily observed for products containing comparable ratios of THC to CBD (e.g., nabiximols) or select synthetic cannabinoids [6, 9]. High-THC formulations may provide modest analgesia, whereas low-THC or CBD-ratio products appear ineffective. The American College of Physicians advises caution, noting that for many patients the potential harms, particularly cognitive impairment, sedation, dizziness, and psychiatric effects, outweigh the limited analgesic benefit. In dermatology, cannabinoids have been shown to improve inflammatory pruritus in allergic contact dermatitis [50], and topical endocannabinoids have demonstrated benefit in reducing uremic pruritus [51].

Cannabis use is common among patients with HS, though available data suggest use often precedes onset of HS and may not be primarily driven by pain symptoms [6, 11, 52]. Of note, adolescents and young adults may be at increased risk for cognitive impairment and psychotic symptoms with long-term cannabis use which is important to elucidate upon patient interview. Additionally, most cannabinoid products are not regulated by U.S. Food and Drug Administration, complicating safe dosing [52].

Acupuncture has moderate-strength evidence supporting benefit in nociceptive pain diseases like osteoarthritis, chronic headache, and low back pain. In neuropathic pain, evidence remains inconsistent, with meta-analyses showing either no benefit or small effect sizes based on low-quality data [53]. Limited studies in dermatologic disease suggest possible improvements in sleep but not disease severity or pruritus. Adverse events are uncommon but include granuloma formation, localized argyria, and sclerosing lipogranulomatosis [6, 23, 53]. At present, a role for acupuncture in HS pain management is uncertain and warrants further study.

Although some studies show that Alpha-lipoic acid (ALA) improves symptoms of diabetic peripheral neuropathy (DPN), tendon reflex, and nerve conduction velocity, its efficacy in DPN evidence remains mixed [54–58]. ALA (300–600 mg/day) administered intravenously offered maximal relief though ALA 600 mg/day orally improved burning and stinging [54, 55]. ALA is thought to exert its effects through antioxidant mechanisms, including free radical scavenging, metal chelation, regeneration of endogenous antioxidants (glutathione, vitamins C and E), and reduction of oxidative stress [57]. It also suppresses proinflammatory cytokines such as IL-6 and may improve microcirculation, thereby enhancing nerve perfusion and conduction. ALA is generally well tolerated, though patients may experience nausea at higher doses (600 mg/day). Because ALA can interfere with thyroid hormone metabolism, thyroid-stimulating hormone should be monitored in patients receiving levothyroxine [55]. Rare but important safety concerns include insulin autoimmune syndrome. Given its safety profile, ALA may be considered a low-risk adjunct in neuropathic pain, though evidence of efficacy in HS is limited [57, 58].

Curcumin demonstrates strong evidence for pain reduction and functional improvement in osteoarthritis at doses of 1000–1500 mg/day, with efficacy comparable to NSAIDs and fewer cardiovascular adverse events [59, 60]. Curcumin, the main anti-inflammatory molecule in turmeric, exerts its effect through inhibition of TNF-α, IL-1, IL-6, and COX-2, pathways relevant to HS pathophysiology [60]. Although direct evidence in HS-related pain is limited, curcumin's favorable safety profile and systemic anti-inflammatory effects make it a reasonable adjunctive option [6].

Surapaneni et al. [23] proposed tiered management recommendations based on pain refractoriness, while Li et al. [2] base their recommendations on established pharmacologic approaches for other painful conditions. A summary of the North American HS clinical management guidelines for treating HS pain [6, 38] is provided in Table 7.2 and summarized as follows: begin pain management with disease control; incorporate topical analgesics, oral acetaminophen, and oral NSAIDs as needed for acute pain; consider addition of short-acting opioid analgesics for refractory acute pain; collaborate with multidisciplinary teams such as psychiatry or pain specialists when necessary; manage chronic pain according to the World Health Organization (WHO) pain ladder. The WHO pain ladder advises use of non-opioid analgesics (acetaminophen, NSAIDs) ± non-pharmacological methods for *mild* chronic pain, weak opioids (codeine, tramadol, hydrocodone) plus non-opioids adjuncts for *moderate* chronic pain, and strong opioids (morphine, oxycodone, fentanyl, methadone) plus non-opioids adjuncts for *severe* chronic pain [16, 17].

HS-associated itch is underrecognized and lacks disease-specific management guidelines [4, 25]. Table 7.3 summarizes emerging strategies for itch modulation. IL-17A blockade with brodalumab reduced itch, pain, and depression in patients with HS observed over a 24-week period [61, 62]. JAK inhibition produces dose-dependent improvements in HS quality-of-life scores and has proven off-label success in treating chronic pruritus associated with other dermatologic conditions [27, 63]. Statins have also been shown to reduce itch intensity [64–66]. Finally, metformin has potential efficacy in treatment of HS-associated itch related to its activation of the 5′ AMP-activated protein kinase (AMPK) pathway and subsequent inhibition of mTOR [32, 67]. In contrast, oral antihistamines demonstrate limited efficacy in HS-associated pruritus, and there is currently no evidence to support their routine use in this context [9].

In summary, despite the substantial burden of HS-associated pain and itch on quality of life, there are no prospective, mechanism-driven studies specifically investigating their management. Current treatment approaches are largely extrapolated from other inflammatory dermatoses and focus on reducing HS inflammation rather than targeting the neuroimmune pathways that underlie pain and pruritus, highlighting a critical need for targeted, evidence-based therapeutic development.

Board Review Question Explanation

A patient with hidradenitis suppurativa and peptic ulcer disease has already been prescribed disease-directed therapies for treatment of his HS. To target severe pain associated with an acute HS abscess, which of the following would be first-line therapy?

A. Acetaminophen 325 mg every 4–8 h PRN
B. Oxycodone 5 mg every 4–6 h PRN
C. Tramadol 50 mg every 4–6 h PRN
D. Ibuprofen 200 mg every 4–8 h PRN
E. Incision and drainage (correct)

Answer Explanation

- After employing disease-directed immunomodulatory therapy (e.g., TNF-α or IL-17A/F inhibition) to address the underlying inflammatory process, a patient with HS who presents with severe pain due to an acute abscess should receive incision and drainage (I&D) as first-line therapy (answer choice E). This is consistent with the most up-to-date recommendations [16].
- Although incision and drainage is first-line for acute, tense, painful abscesses, intralesional steroid injection (range 5–40 mg/mL), topical lidocaine, oral acetaminophen (answer choice A), and oral NSAIDs (answer choice D) are also suitable treatments for acute HS pain.

Table 7.3 Summary of recommendations for management of HS itch

Medication	Suggested adult dosing	Mechanism/target	Risks/cautions
Topical therapies *Menthol*	4% ointment or cream: 4 times max daily Menthol 1%–3% OTC Max: up to 16%	Activation of TRPM8 (transient receptor potential melastatin-8) channels	Hypersensitivity reaction Avoid contact with eyes, mucous membranes, open wounds, damaged or irritated skin, sensitive skin Avoid use under occlusion or with heating pads Common adverse effects: erythema, glazing, peeling
Lidocaine	4%–5% Cream: Every 3–4 h (6× daily) 4% or Patch: Every 12 h, max of 3 patches 2.5% Lidocaine with 2.5% prilocaine (EMLA): Max 20 g over 200 cm^2 area for <4 h	Blocks voltage-gated sodium channels, preventing depolarization and thereby blocking pain signal transmission	Application site reaction (erythema, edema) Avoid application to large open wounds to reduce risk of systemic absorption and toxicity Use extreme caution in those with G6PD deficiency, elderly, acutely ill, infants
Ketamine-Amitriptyline-Lidocaine compound cream	5% to 10% ketamine/5% amitriptyline/5% lidocaine compounded in Lipo derm cream 3–4 times daily	Blocking N-methyl-D-aspartate receptors and sodium channels, reducing sensitivity of peripheral nerve fibers	Application site burning, erythema
Corticosteroids	Class I (super-high potency): Clobetasol propionate 0.05%, halobetasol 0.05%, betamethasone dipropionate 0.05% Class II (High potency): Fluocinonide 0.05%, betamethasone dipropionate 0.05%, Class III (Upper mid-potency): Triamcinolone acetonide 0.5%, fluticasone propionate 0.005% Class IV (Mid-potency): Triamcinolone acetonide 0.1%, mometasone furoate 0.1% Class V (Lower mid-potency): Fluticasone propionate 0.05%, hydrocortisone valerate 0.2% Class VI (Low potency): Desonide 0.05%, alclometasone dipropionate 0.05% Class VII (Least potent): Hydrocortisone 1–2.5%	Induction of phospholipase A_2 inhibitory proteins (lipocortins), which suppress the biosynthesis of inflammatory mediators such as prostaglandins and leukotrienes by inhibiting the release of arachidonic acid from membrane phospholipids Targeting immune cells and suppressing proinflammatory cytokines	Skin atrophy, pigment alteration, acne, petechiae, telangiectasia

(continued)

Systemic therapies *Statins*	precise mechanism of any antipruritic effect has not been definitively characterized	Inhibition of HMG-CoA reductase Suppression of dendritic cell-mediated Th2 responses Activate temperature-gated TRP channels (TRPA1, TRPV1, TRPM8) expressed on nociceptive sensory neurons Decrease expression of proinflammatory neuropeptides calcitonin gene-related peptide (CGRP) and substance P in sensory neurons	Contraindication in liver disease; baseline liver and kidney function should be checked before initiation; intermittent monitoring for hyperkalemia and acute kidney injury
Anticonvulsants	*Gabapentin* *300 mg BID on day 2* *300 mg TID on day 3* *Subsequent dose increases* may be made as tolerated *Taper gradually over 1 week* when discontinuing *Pregabalin* Initial does: 150 mg/day (divided BID or TID) After 1 wk can increase to 300 mg/day Max dose: 600 mg/day (divided by BID or TID) Taper gradually in >1 week	Binds with high affinity to the $\alpha 2\delta$ subunit of voltage-activated calcium channels leading to both analgesic and antiepileptic effects Neuropathic pain agents	*Gabapentin* *First-line anticonvulsant* due to a favorable risk–benefit profile *Avoid combination with other antiepileptics* to reduce additive toxicity *Potential adverse effects:* tremors, altered mental status, respiratory depression, dizziness, fatigue, and visual disturbances *Renal considerations:* obtain baseline creatinine and creatinine clearance for appropriate dose adjustment in patients with kidney disease *Pregabalin* *Second-line anticonvulsant* *Crosses the blood–brain barrier*, may cause euphoria *Avoid combination with other antiepileptics* *Renal considerations:* check baseline creatinine and creatinine clearance; use with caution in patients with renal failure *Controlled substance*

(continued)

Table 7.3 (continued)

Medication	Suggested adult dosing	Mechanism/target	Risks/cautions
Antidepressants	*Duloxetine (1st line)* *Initial dose:* 30 mg/day *After 1 week:* increase to 60 mg/day *Further titration:* may increase up to 120 mg/day *Maximum dose:* 120 mg/day (no established benefit typically observed above 60 mg/day) *Tapering:* reduce dose by 50% in week 1, then an additional 50% in week 2 *Venlafaxine (2nd line)* *Initial dose 37.5 mg/day* *After 1 wk increase to 75 mg/day* *Then, may increase by 75 mg every 7 days up to 225 mg/day* *Taper by 75 mg/week to discontinue*	Serotonin-norepinephrine reuptake inhibitors (SNRIs) Enhance descending inhibitory pathways in the spinal cord via increased noradrenergic transmission action on α-adrenoceptors, with serotonin contributing via activation of specific 5-HT receptor subtypes (particularly $5\text{-}HT_3$, $5\text{-}HT_7$, $5\text{-}HT_4$, and $5\text{-}HT_6$)	*Duloxetine* *First-line SNRI* due to a favorable risk profile *Serotonergic effects:* headache, fatigue, nausea, sexual dysfunction *Noradrenergic effects:* night sweats, xerostomia *Risk of serotonin syndrome:* avoid concurrent use with MAOIs, SSRIs, TCAs, linezolid, and methylene blue *Renal and hepatic considerations:* use with caution in patients with renal or hepatic impairment *Additional benefit:* may also be used for management of pruritus *Venlafaxine* *QTc prolongation risk*, in addition to risks associated with duloxetine *Renal considerations:* check baseline creatinine and creatinine clearance; use with caution in patients with renal impairment
Aprepitant	80 mg daily for 1–4 weeks	Selective NK_1 receptor antagonist blocking substance P signaling Modulates pain/itch pathways Minimal activity at $5\text{-}HT_3$ or dopamine receptors; reduces substance P-mediated pruritus	Fatigue, diarrhea, constipation, abdominal pain, decrease blood cell count, hypotension Inhibits CYP3A4 and may increase plasma concentrations of drugs that are metabolized through this liver enzyme
Other Therapies *Cognitive behavioral therapy*	Patient dependent	Address scratching, stress, and dysfunctional illness perceptions Habit reversal training to reduce scratching, relaxation techniques to alleviate stress and cognitive restructuring to modify negative beliefs	–

- Oxycodone (immediate-release) and tramadol (answer choices B, C) are both short-acting opioids which should be reserved for acute pain refractory to acetaminophen, NSAIDs, intralesional steroid injection, and disease modifying therapies [17].

Key Take Home Points

- Pain and itch are central symptoms of hidradenitis suppurativa that substantially impair daily functioning and quality of life.
- Pain in HS arises from the convergence of nociceptive, neuropathic, and nociplastic mechanisms, driven by chronic inflammation, recurrent tissue injury, and altered peripheral and central neuronal excitability.
- Itch in HS is comparatively understudied and is likely mediated by cytokine dysregulation and aberrant cutaneous neuroimmune signaling, through mechanisms that are distinct from—and not fully explained by—pain pathways.
- Dysregulated mTOR signaling may contribute to HS-associated itch by promoting neuroimmune activation, representing a promising therapeutic target.
- Nociceptive pain should be managed by prioritizing disease-directed therapy and anti-inflammatory analgesics (e.g., topical agents, NSAIDs, COX-2-selective inhibitors) for acute flares, with escalation to systemic or adjunctive therapies when pain becomes persistent or refractory.
- Neuropathic and nociplastic pain require early recognition and sustained, mechanism-targeted management using neuromodulators such as gabapentin, SNRIs, and TCAs.
- There are currently no formal guidelines or FDA-approved therapies specifically targeting HS-associated itch, underscoring the need for individualized, patient-centered management.
- Integrated management of pain and itch in HS remains an active area of investigation, and future mechanistic and clinical studies are needed to develop targeted strategies that improve patient outcomes.

References

1. Patel ZS, Hoffman LK, Buse DC, Grinberg AS, Afifi L, Cohen SR, Lowes MA, Seng EK. Pain, psychological comorbidities, disability, and impaired qualify of life in Hidradenitis Suppurativa. Curr Pain Headache Rep. 2017;21:49. https://doi.org/10.1007/s11916-017-0647-3.
2. Li YH, Williams MN, Jedrzejczak MJ, Orenstein LAV, Singh V. A practical, comprehensive guide to pain management hidradenitis suppurativa. Dermatol Rev. 2022;3:137–49. https://doi.org/10.1002/der2.122.
3. Wolk K, Join-Lambert O, Sabat R. Aetiology and pathogenesis of hidradenitis suppurativa. Br J Dermatol. 2020;183:999–1010. https://doi.org/10.1111/bjd.19556.
4. Matusiak Ł, Szczęch J, Kaaz K, Lelonek E, Szepietowski JC. Clinical characteristics of Pruritus and pain in patients with Hidradenitis Suppurativa. Acta Derm Venereol. 2018;98:191–4. https://doi.org/10.2340/00015555-2815.

5. Orenstein LAV, Salame N, Siira MR, Urbanski M, Flowers NI, Echuri H, Garg A, McKenzie-Brown AM, Curseen KA, Patzer RE, et al. Pain experiences among those living with hidradenitis suppurativa: a qualitative study. Br J Dermatol. 2022;188:41–51. https://doi.org/10.1093/bjd/ljac018.
6. Savage KT, Singh V, Patel ZS, Yannuzzi CA, McKenzie-Brown AM, Lowes MA, Orenstein LAV. Pain management in hidradenitis suppurativa and a proposed treatment algorithm. J Am Acad Dermatol. 2021;85:187–99. https://doi.org/10.1016/j.jaad.2020.09.039.
7. Molina-Leyva A, Cuenca-Barrales C. Pruritus and Malodour in patients with Hidradenitis Suppurativa: impact on quality of life and clinical features associated with symptom severity. Dermatology. 2020;236:59–65. https://doi.org/10.1159/000502139.
8. Matusiak Ł, Bieniek A, Szepietowski J. Psychophysical aspects of Hidradenitis Suppurativa. Acta Derm Venereol. 2010;90:264–8. https://doi.org/10.2340/00015555-0866.
9. Pulminskas A, Hojjatie R, Karatas TB, Li YH, Orenstein LAV. Hidradenitis Suppurativa symptom relief pain and itch. Dermatol Clin. 2025;43:247–60. https://doi.org/10.1016/j.det.2024.12.009.
10. Deckers IE, Kimball AB. The handicap of Hidradenitis Suppurativa. Dermatol Clin. 2016;34:17–22. https://doi.org/10.1016/j.det.2015.07.003.
11. Reddy S, Orenstein LAV, Strunk A, Garg A. Incidence of long-term opioid use among opioid-naive patients with Hidradenitis Suppurativa in the United States. JAMA Dermatol. 2019;155:1284–90. https://doi.org/10.1001/jamadermatol.2019.2610.
12. Vossen ARJV, Schoenmakers A, van Straalen KR, Prens EP, van der Zee HH. Assessing Pruritus in Hidradenitis Suppurativa: a cross-sectional study. Am J Clin Dermatol. 2017;18:687–95. https://doi.org/10.1007/s40257-017-0280-2.
13. Whitley SK. Elucidation of pain mechanisms in Hidradenitis Suppurativa. JAMA Dermatol. 2023;159:1047–9. https://doi.org/10.1001/jamadermatol.2023.3264.
14. Alsouhibani A, Speck P, Cole EF, Mustin DE, Li Y, Barron JR, Orenstein LAV, Harper DE. Quantitative sensory testing to characterize sensory changes in Hidradenitis Suppurativa skin lesions. JAMA Dermatol. 2023;159:1102–11. https://doi.org/10.1001/jamadermatol.2023.3243.
15. Chu C, Artis D, Chiu IM. Neuro-immune interactions in the tissues. Immunity. 2020;52:464–74. https://doi.org/10.1016/j.immuni.2020.02.017.
16. Chiu IM, Sokol CL. Neuroimmune recognition of allergens. Curr Opin Immunol. 2024;90:102458. https://doi.org/10.1016/j.coi.2024.102458.
17. Baral P, Udit S, Chiu IM. Pain and immunity: implications for host defence. Nat Rev Immunol. 2019;19:433–47. https://doi.org/10.1038/s41577-019-0147-2.
18. Emanuel E, Arifuzzaman M, Artis D. Epithelial-neuronal-immune cell interactions: implications for immunity, inflammation, and tissue homeostasis at mucosal sites. J Allergy Clin Immunol. 2024;153:1169–80. https://doi.org/10.1016/j.jaci.2024.02.004.
19. Aarts P, Aitken JJ, van Straalen KR. Prevalence of central sensitization in patients with Hidradenitis Suppurativa. JAMA Dermatol. 2021;157:1209–12. https://doi.org/10.1001/jamadermatol.2021.2918.
20. Machado MO, Stergiopoulos V, Maes M, Kurdyak PA, Lin P-Y, Wang L-J, Shyu Y-C, Firth J, Koyanagi A, Solmi M, et al. Depression and anxiety in adults with Hidradenitis Suppurativa. JAMA Dermatol. 2019;155:939–45. https://doi.org/10.1001/jamadermatol.2019.0759.
21. Garg A, Neuren E, Cha D, Kirby JS, Ingram JR, Jemec GBE, Esmann S, Thorlacius L, Villumsen B, del Marmol V, et al. Evaluating patients' unmet needs in hidradenitis suppurativa: results from the Global Survey Of Impact and Healthcare Needs (VOICE) Project. J Am Acad Dermatol. 2020;82:366–76. https://doi.org/10.1016/j.jaad.2019.06.1301.
22. Vlassova N, Kuhn D, Okoye G. Hidradenitis Suppurativa disproportionately affects African Americans: a single-center retrospective analysis. Acta Derm Venereol. 2015;95:990–1. https://doi.org/10.2340/00015555-2176.
23. Surapaneni V, Milosavljevic MV, Orenstein LAV. Pain management in hidradenitis suppurativa. J Am Acad Dermatol. 2024;91:S52–63. https://doi.org/10.1016/j.jaad.2024.09.006.

24. Trupiano N, Young K, Echuri H, Maghfour J, Orenstein LAV, Hamzavi I. Exploring itch in hidradenitis suppurativa with lessons from atopic dermatitis and psoriasis. J Dermatol. 2025;52:239–46. https://doi.org/10.1111/1346-8138.17622.
25. Agarwal P, Lunge SB, Shetty NS, Karagaiah P, Daveluy S, Ortega-Loayza AG, Tzellos T, Szepietowski JC, Zouboulis CC, Grabbe S, et al. Itch in Hidradenitis Suppurativa/Acne Inversa: a systematic review. J Clin Med. 2022;11:3813. https://doi.org/10.3390/jcm11133813.
26. Kim BS. The translational revolution of itch. Neuron. 2022;110:2209–14. https://doi.org/10.1016/j.neuron.2022.03.031.
27. Bordon Y. JAK in the itch. Nat Rev Drug Discov. 2017;16:753. https://doi.org/10.1038/nrd.2017.204.
28. Chen GF, Cohen JM, Eisenstein A. Associations between hidradenitis suppurativa and asthma and allergic rhinitis: a case–control study in the All of Us research program. Int J Dermatol. 2024;63:e74–5. https://doi.org/10.1111/ijd.16994.
29. Miao X, Huang Y, Liu T-T, Guo R, Wang B, Wang X-L, Chen L-H, Zhou Y, Ji R-R, Liu T. TNF-α/TNFR1 signaling is required for the full expression of acute and chronic itch in mice via peripheral and central mechanisms. Neurosci Bull. 2018;34:42–53. https://doi.org/10.1007/s12264-017-0124-3.
30. Lee JY, Park CS, Seo KJ, Kim IY, Han S, Youn I, Yune TY. IL-6/JAK2/STAT3 axis mediates neuropathic pain by regulating astrocyte and microglia activation after spinal cord injury. Exp Neurol. 2023;370:114576. https://doi.org/10.1016/j.expneurol.2023.114576.
31. Atta AA, Ibrahim WW, Mohamed AF, Abdelkader NF. Microglia polarization in nociplastic pain: mechanisms and perspectives. Inflammopharmacology. 2023;31:1053–67. https://doi.org/10.1007/s10787-023-01216-x.
32. Obara I, Medrano MC, Signoret-Genest J, Jiménez-Díaz L, Géranton SM, Hunt SP. Inhibition of the mammalian target of rapamycin complex 1 signaling pathway reduces itch behaviour in mice. Pain. 2015;156:1519–29. https://doi.org/10.1097/j.pain.0000000000000197.
33. Karagianni F, Pavlidis A, Malakou LS, Piperi C, Papadavid E. Predominant role of mTOR signaling in skin diseases with therapeutic potential. Int J Mol Sci. 2022;23:1693. https://doi.org/10.3390/ijms23031693.
34. Govas P, Ketchum A, Kazi R, Gordon BR, Carroll BT. Pain intensity assessment scales for dermatologic surgery patients: a systematic review. Dermatologic Surg. 2022;48:232–8. https://doi.org/10.1097/dss.0000000000003353.
35. Haydek CG, Love E, Mollanazar NK, Rodriguez RV, Lee H, Yosipovitch G, Tharp MD, Hanifin JM, Chen K-H, Chen SC. Validation and banding of the ItchyQuant: a self-report itch severity scale. J Invest Dermatol. 2017;137:57–61. https://doi.org/10.1016/j.jid.2016.06.633.
36. Finlay AY, Khan GK. Dermatology Life Quality Index (DLQI)—a simple practical measure for routine clinical use. Clin Exp Dermatol. 1994;19:210–6. https://doi.org/10.1111/j.1365-2230.1994.tb01167.x.
37. Kirby JS, Thorlacius L, Villumsen B, Ingram JR, Garg A, Christensen KB, Butt M, Esmann S, Tan J, Jemec GBE. The Hidradenitis Suppurativa Quality of Life (HiSQOL) score: development and validation of a measure for clinical trials. Br J Dermatol. 2020;183:340–8. https://doi.org/10.1111/bjd.18692.
38. Alikhan A, Sayed C, Alavi A, Alhusayen R, Brassard A, Burkhart C, Crowell K, Eisen DB, Gottlieb AB, Hamzavi I, et al. North American clinical management guidelines for hidradenitis suppurativa: a publication from the United States and Canadian Hidradenitis Suppurativa Foundations Part II: topical, intralesional, and systemic medical management. J Am Acad Dermatol. 2019;81:91–101. https://doi.org/10.1016/j.jaad.2019.02.068.
39. Thorlacius L, Ingram JR, Villumsen B, Esmann S, Kirby JS, Gottlieb AB, Merola JF, Dellavalle R, Nielsen SM, Christensen R, et al. A core domain set for hidradenitis suppurativa trial outcomes: an international Delphi process. Br J Dermatol. 2018;179:642–50. https://doi.org/10.1111/bjd.16672.

40. Kimball AB, Okun MM, Williams DA, Gottlieb AB, Papp KA, Zouboulis CC, Armstrong AW, Kerdel F, Gold MH, Forman SB, et al. Two phase 3 trials of Adalimumab for Hidradenitis Suppurativa. N Engl J Med. 2016;375:422–34. https://doi.org/10.1056/nejmoa1504370.
41. Kimball AB, Jemec GBE, Alavi A, Reguiai Z, Gottlieb AB, Bechara FG, Paul C, Bourboulis EJG, Villani AP, Schwinn A, et al. Secukinumab in moderate-to-severe hidradenitis suppurativa (SUNSHINE and SUNRISE): week 16 and week 52 results of two identical, multicentre, randomised, placebo-controlled, double-blind phase 3 trials. Lancet. 2023;401:747–61. https://doi.org/10.1016/s0140-6736(23)00022-3.
42. Kimball AB, Jemec GBE, Sayed CJ, Kirby JS, Prens E, Ingram JR, Garg A, Gottlieb AB, Szepietowski JC, Bechara FG, et al. Efficacy and safety of bimekizumab in patients with moderate-to-severe hidradenitis suppurativa (BE HEARD I and BE HEARD II): two 48-week, randomised, double-blind, placebo-controlled, multicentre phase 3 trials. Lancet. 2024;403:2504–19. https://doi.org/10.1016/s0140-6736(24)00101-6.
43. Sarkissian SD, Hessam S, Kirby JS, Lowes MA, Mintoff D, Naik HB, Ring HC, Suyien NC, Frew JW. Identification of biomarkers and critical evaluation of biomarker validation in Hidradenitis Suppurativa. JAMA Dermatol. 2022;158:300–13. https://doi.org/10.1001/jamadermatol.2021.4926.
44. Nielsen RM, Andersen PL, Sigsgaard V, Riis PT, Jemec GB. Pain perception in patients with hidradenitis suppurativa. Br J Dermatol. 2020;182:166–74. https://doi.org/10.1111/bjd.17935.
45. Veehof MM, Oskam M-J, Schreurs KMG, Bohlmeijer ET. Acceptance-based interventions for the treatment of chronic pain: a systematic review and meta-analysis. J Int Assoc Study Pain. 2011; https://doi.org/10.1016/j.pain.2010.11.002.
46. Ehde DM, Dillworth TM, Turner JA. Cognitive-behavioral therapy for individuals with chronic pain: efficacy, innovations, and directions for research; 2014. https://doi.org/10.1037/a0035747.
47. Barron BA. J. D. Otis, managing chronic pain: a cognitive-behavioral therapy approach. J Occup Rehabil. 2009;19:113. https://doi.org/10.1007/s10926-008-9157-9.
48. Darnall BD. Psychological treatment for patients with chronic pain. American Psychological Association; 2018.
49. Beehler GP, Murphy JL, King PR, Dollar KM, Kearney LK, Haslam A, Wade M, Goldstein WR. Brief cognitive behavioral therapy for chronic pain. Clin J Pain. 2019;35:809–17. https://doi.org/10.1097/ajp.0000000000000747.
50. Petrosino S, Cristino L, Karsak M, Gaffal E, Ueda N, Tüting T, Bisogno T, Filippis DD, D'Amico A, Saturnino C, et al. Protective role of palmitoylethanolamide in contact allergic dermatitis. Allergy. 2010;65:698–711. https://doi.org/10.1111/j.1398-9995.2009.02254.x.
51. Szepietowski JC, Szepietowski T, Reich A. Efficacy and tolerance of the cream containing structured physiological lipids with endocannabinoids in the treatment of uremic pruritus: a preliminary study. Acta Dermatovenerol Croat. 2005;13:97–103.
52. Whiting PF, Wolff RF, Deshpande S, Nisio MD, Duffy S, Hernandez AV, Keurentjes JC, Lang S, Misso K, Ryder S, et al. Cannabinoids for medical use: a systematic review and meta-analysis. JAMA. 2015;313:2456–73. https://doi.org/10.1001/jama.2015.6358.
53. Ju ZY, Wang K, Cui HS, Yao Y, Liu SM, Zhou J, Chen TY, Xia J. Acupuncture for neuropathic pain in adults. Cochrane Database Syst Rev. 2017;2019:CD012057. https://doi.org/10.1002/14651858.cd012057.pub2.
54. Baicus C, Purcarea A, von Elm E, Delcea C, Furtunescu FL. Alpha-lipoic acid for diabetic peripheral neuropathy. Cochrane Database Syst Rev. 2024;2024:CD012967. https://doi.org/10.1002/14651858.cd012967.pub2.
55. Hsieh R-Y, Huang I-C, Chen C, Sung J-Y. Effects of oral alpha-Lipoic acid treatment on diabetic polyneuropathy: a meta-analysis and systematic review. Nutrients. 2023;15:3634. https://doi.org/10.3390/nu15163634.
56. Ziegler D, Ametov A, Barinov A, Dyck PJ, Gurieva I, Low PA, Munzel U, Yakhno N, Raz I, Novosadova M, et al. Oral treatment with α-Lipoic acid improves symptomatic diabetic polyneuropathy. Diabetes Care. 2006;29:2365–70. https://doi.org/10.2337/dc06-1216.

57. Fasipe B, Faria A, Laher I. Potential for novel therapeutic uses of alpha Lipoic acid. Curr Med Chem. 2022;30 https://doi.org/10.2174/0929867329666221006115329.
58. Han T, Bai J, Liu W, Hu Y. THERAPY OF ENDOCRINE DISEASE: a systematic review and meta-analysis of α-lipoic acid in the treatment of diabetic peripheral neuropathy. Eur J Endocrinol. 2012;167:465–71. https://doi.org/10.1530/eje-12-0555.
59. Lopresti AL, Smith SJ, Jackson-Michel S, Fairchild T. An investigation into the effects of a Curcumin extract (Curcugen®) on osteoarthritis pain of the knee: a randomised, double-blind, placebo-controlled study. Nutrients. 2021;14:41. https://doi.org/10.3390/nu14010041.
60. Bideshki MV, Jourabchi-Ghadim N, Radkhah N, Behzadi M, Asemani S, Jamilian P, Zarezadeh M. The efficacy of curcumin in relieving osteoarthritis: a meta-analysis of meta-analyses. Phytother Res. 2024;38:2875–91. https://doi.org/10.1002/ptr.8153.
61. Frew JW, Navrazhina K, Grand D, Sullivan-Whalen M, Gilleaudeau P, Garcet S, Ungar J, Krueger JG. The effect of subcutaneous brodalumab on clinical disease activity in hidradenitis suppurativa: an open-label cohort study. J Am Acad Dermatol. 2020;83:1341–8. https://doi.org/10.1016/j.jaad.2020.05.007.
62. Chu C-B, Yang C-C, Hsueh Y-Y, Chen P-C, Hong Y-K, Kuo Y-Y, Tsai S-J. Aberrant expression of interleukin-17A in mast cells contributes to the pathogenesis of hidradenitis suppurativa. Br J Dermatol. 2023;189:719–29. https://doi.org/10.1093/bjd/ljad273.
63. Alavi A, Hamzavi I, Brown K, Santos LL, Zhu Z, Liu H, Howell MD, Kirby JS. Janus kinase 1 inhibitor INCB054707 for patients with moderate-to-severe hidradenitis suppurativa: results from two phase II studies*. Br J Dermatol. 2022;186:803–13. https://doi.org/10.1111/bjd.20969.
64. Oprita G, Domocos D, Selescu T, Paduraru A, Tunaru S, Leffler A, Babes A, Babes R-M. Statins activate temperature-gated transient receptor potential ion channels. Eur J Pharmacol. 2025;1006:178206. https://doi.org/10.1016/j.ejphar.2025.178206.
65. Inagaki-Katashiba N, Ito T, Inaba M, Azuma Y, Tanaka A, Phan V, Kibata K, Satake A, Nomura S. Statins can suppress DC-mediated Th2 responses through the repression of OX40-ligand and CCL17 expression. Eur J Immunol. 2019;49:2051–62. https://doi.org/10.1002/eji.201847992.
66. Bucelli RC, Gonsiorek EA, Kim W-Y, Bruun D, Rabin RA, Higgins D, Lein PJ. Statins decrease expression of the proinflammatory neuropeptides calcitonin gene-related peptide and substance P in sensory neurons. J Pharmacol Exp Ther. 2008;324:1172–80. https://doi.org/10.1124/jpet.107.132795.
67. Arun B, Loffeld A. Long-standing hidradenitis suppurativa treated effectively with metformin. Clin Exp Dermatol. 2009;34:920–1. https://doi.org/10.1111/j.1365-2230.2008.03121.x.

Chapter 8
Treatment of HS with Topical Therapy

Lauren DeBusk, Angela Rosenberg, and Hadar Lev-Tov

Case Title A 29-year-old female presents with recurring lesions in her axilla and inframammary folds.

Case
It is Tuesday morning in the clinic, and your first patient is a 29-year-old female with a history of mild hidradenitis suppurativa (HS) affecting her axillae and inframammary folds. She has been experiencing intermittent painful nodules and is looking for topical treatment options to manage her symptoms. She asks about available topical therapies, their effectiveness, and potential side effects. How would you approach her treatment plan?

Board Review Question
Which of the following topical treatments is considered first-line for mild hidradenitis suppurativa?

A. Tretinoin cream 0.05%
B. Clindamycin 1% solution
C. Tacrolimus ointment
D. Silver sulfadiazine
E. Ruxolitinib cream

Hidradenitis suppurativa (HS) is a chronic, inflammatory skin disorder characterized by recurrent nodules, abscesses, and tunnel formation, primarily in

L. DeBusk (✉) · A. Rosenberg
Department of Dermatology, University of Texas Southwestern Medical Center, Dallas, TX, USA

H. Lev-Tov
Dr. Phillip Frost Department of Dermatology and Cutaneous Surgery, University of Miami, Miller School of Medicine, Miami, FL, USA

N. Brownstone (ed.), *Clinical Cases in Hidradenitis Suppurativa*, Clinical Cases in Dermatology, https://doi.org/10.1007/978-3-032-15200-8_8

intertriginous areas [1]. The pathophysiology involves follicular occlusion, immune dysregulation, and secondary bacterial dysbiosis, contributing to chronic inflammation and tissue damage [1, 2]. Systemic treatments are the cornerstone for moderate-to-severe HS and topical therapies provide a valuable option for mild cases and adjunctive management. Often, early stages of HS (Hurley Stage I) can be managed with topical therapy alone [1]. Topical treatment should also be considered in pregnant and breastfeeding women, as many of the systemic therapies available have known teratogenic effects or are used off-label during pregnancy and lactation [3]. Importantly, topical therapies should not be used as monotherapy in patients who present with many concurrent nodules and/or abscesses and are not useful to treat tunnels. Topical therapies for HS include topical antibiotics, antiseptics, keratolytics, retinoids, anti-inflammatory agents, and hormone receptor blockers [1]. This chapter explores the mechanisms, efficacy, and clinical application of topical agents in HS management.

Antibiotics (Clindamycin)

Clindamycin 1% as a lotion, solution, gel, or cream is the only topical antibiotic that has been studied in HS populations and is indicated for use in Hurley stage I or II disease [1, 4]. The proposed mechanism of action involves clindamycin binding to the bacterial 50S ribosomal subunit, disrupting protein synthesis in a manner similar to macrolides [4].

Large-scale clinical trials evaluating the efficacy of topical clindamycin in HS are lacking; however, limited clinical trial data supports its use in mild disease [4]. In 1983, a double-blinded, randomized, placebo-controlled trial evaluated the efficacy of topical clindamycin 0.1% in 27 patients with stage I or mild stage II HS. They found a reduction in the number of abscesses, nodules, and pustules at monthly evaluations during a 3-month course of treatment. Of note, the effect was most significant for superficial lesions, with the effect on deep lesions being very low [5]. In 1988, another small, double-blind, double dummy-controlled trial found no difference between the use of topical clindamycin versus oral tetracyclines in 46 patients with stage I or II disease [6].

The 2019 North American Clinical Guidelines for Hidradenitis Suppurativa recommend topical clindamycin 1% for reducing superficial lesions such as pustules but caution the risk of bacterial resistance when used alone [1]. Combination with a benzoyl peroxide wash may mitigate the risk of *Staphylococcus aureus* resistance [7].

Antiseptics

Antiseptic use in HS is supported only by weak anecdotal data and therefore is not included in recent guidelines. It is important to stress to the patient that HS is not related to personal hygiene. However, because bacterial dysbiosis exists in HS and is thought to exacerbate disease, use of antiseptics may be helpful. [8] Commonly used as adjunctive therapies, chlorhexidine wash, bleach baths, pyrithione zinc shampoo, and benzoyl peroxide (BPO) are valued for their anti-inflammatory effects and potential to minimize antibacterial resistance.

The selection of a specific antiseptic agent is typically based on clinical judgment and expert recommendations. A cross-sectional study evaluating adherence to antimicrobial washes among HS patients found that only 30% of the 54 individuals advised to use these washes incorporated them into their daily routine [9]. Key barriers identified in this study include affordability and patient's ability to find the washes in stores. These findings highlight the importance of counseling patients on antiseptic options and recommending therapies accessible to the individual patient.

Benzoyl peroxide wash works as an antimicrobial agent by releasing free oxygen radicals, which reduce the concentration of *Cutibacterium acnes* and other microorganisms on the skin [10]. Most commonly used in the treatment of acne, the role of benzoyl peroxide wash in HS to reduce bacterial load is supported by expert opinion [1]. Benzoyl peroxide in particular is recommended as an adjunctive treatment in patients using topical clindamycin to reduce risk of *Staphylococcus aureus* resistance [7]. Notably, benzoyl peroxide wash is available without prescription and is affordable.

Pyrithione zinc 1%, an anti-fungal agent commonly used in seborrheic dermatitis, has also been suggested as an inexpensive and safe topical cleanser for HS patients. Compared to chlorhexidine gluconate, pyrithione zinc has been shown to have greater bacterial suppression after 72 h when applied to the forearm [11]. In addition to antibacterial properties, proponents of pyrithione zinc washes highlight the added benefits of antiproliferative, anti-inflammatory and antiandrogenic properties of pyrithione zinc–based solutions [8, 12]. Pyrithione zinc shampoos are also three times less expensive than commonly used chlorhexidine washes and can be easily applied and rinsed off in hair bearing areas [8].

Importantly, all antiseptics mentioned above should be applied to wet skin, lathered on, allowed to dry on the skin for a few minutes and only then rinsed off, thoroughly.

Keratolytics

Resorcinol 15% cream functions primarily as a topical keratolytic agent and has emerged as a promising alternative to topical antibiotic therapy [13, 14]. Resorcinol has been shown to reduce pain and duration of abscesses in recurrent Hurley stage I or II disease when used twice daily during flares and once daily between flares [15]. A retrospective study evaluating the efficacy and safety of topical resorcinol 15% versus topical clindamycin 1% found that patients treated with resorcinol had a significant improvement in Hidradenitis Suppurativa Clinical Response, International Hidradenitis Suppurativa Severity Score System, and Pain Visual Analogue Scale from baseline compared with clindamycin at 12 weeks [16]. These findings support the use of resorcinol as a valid alternative to clindamycin.

The 2019 North American Clinical Guidelines for Hidradenitis Suppurativa recommend topical resorcinol 15% but caution that it may induce contact dermatitis [1]. Notably, resorcinol is not available as a prescription in the USA, requiring it to be compounded and therefore, often, unaffordable.

Topical retinoids, including tretinoin and adapalene, have also been used in HS topical therapy, although current North American and European guidelines do not discuss their use [1, 4, 17]. Limited data on the use of topical retinoids exists in the literature, with one case report of tretinoin in combination with other oral and topical therapies and three cases involving adapalene in combination with other agents [17]. Topical retinoids work by acting on retinoic acid receptors, which in turn promote proliferation and differentiation of epidermal cells, increasing follicular epithelial turnover, clearing mature comedones and suppressing microcomedo formation [17, 18].

Topical Corticosteroids

Topical steroids are not recommended for ongoing therapy in HS but may be useful for short term therapy during a flare [19, 20]. Flares are common in the disease course of HS and patients should be given a plan to address them. Topical corticosteroids work via anti-inflammatory, immunosuppressive, and anti-mitotic properties [21]. Anti-inflammatory mechanisms include vasoconstriction and the inhibition of phospholipase A2 release, along with inhibition of DNA and inflammatory transcription factors [21]. Immunosuppression is seen due to corticosteroid inhibition of the humoral system and suppression of immune cell maturation, differentiation, and proliferation [21]. Anti-mitotic effects are thought to be secondary to an increase in lipocortin in the epidermis and inhibition of cell proliferation and collagen synthesis in the dermis [21].

Topical therapies, low- to mid-potency topical corticosteroids, such as hydrocortisone 2.5%, desonide 0.05%, or triamcinolone 0.1% may be used short term to manage acute flares of HS [19]. These agents can reduce pain, erythema, and inflammation associated with individual nodules, particularly in Hurley Stage I disease. However, they are not recommended for long-term use due to the risk of skin atrophy (especially in skin folds that are the common location for HS lesions) and tachyphylaxis [21].

Novel Emerging Therapies

Ruxolitinib 1.5% cream, a topical Janus kinase (JAK) inhibitor selective to JAK1/2, has recently emerged as a potential treatment for mild-to-moderate HS [22]. JAK inhibition is thought to reduce inflammation in HS by inhibiting the JAK-STAT pathway, resulting in regulation of inflammatory cytokines including interleukin (IL) 2, IL-6, IL-10, IL-12, IL-23 and interferon-gamma [22, 23] In the phase 2 randomized, double-blind, and placebo-controlled trial (NCT05635838), 79.2% of participants with moderate HS using topical ruxolitinib 1.5% cream twice daily achieved HiSCR (Hidradenitis Suppurativa Clinical Response) versus 50% with placebo [24, 25]. The topical formulation was well tolerated, with minimal systemic absorption. Interim analysis of another ongoing phase 2 trial of ruxolitinib 1.5% cream showed that five of the six patients with Hurley stage I disease achieved HiSCR through 16 weeks of therapy [26, 27]. While not currently FDA approved for HS, ruxolitinib cream may represent a promising non-antibiotic option for patients who are not candidates for systemic therapy or who prefer to avoid long-term antibiotic use. Phase III trials are ongoing.

In a small, retrospective chart review, clascoterone 1% cream—a topical androgen receptor antagonist—was evaluated in 12 patients with mild HS. After a median of 12 weeks, 83% of patients reported clinical improvement, with reductions in nodule size, frequency of flares, and perilesional erythema. The treatment was well tolerated with no reported adverse effects, supporting its potential as a hormone-targeted topical option for residual nodular disease in mild HS [28]. Clascoterone is FDA approved for treatment of acne vulgaris which is often concomitant in people with HS and therefore, may simplify the treatment regimen.

Many alternative therapies are endorsed online by patient support organizations and on social media platforms but have not been subjected to scientific evaluations. These are mentioned here to equip the provider with awareness and some data about these treatments but should not be misconstrued as a recommendation for treatment. In a survey administered in online HS-related forums, commonly reported topical remedies included Vicks VapoRub, tea tree oil, witch hazel, bleach baths and warm compresses [29].Of these, participants most commonly rated Vicks VapoRub as good or excellent in treating nodules [29]. Vicks VapoRub, an over-the-counter topical ointment marketed as a cough suppressant, contains active ingredients such as camphor (4.8%), menthol (2.6%), and eucalyptus oil (1.2%), known for their analgesic and anti-inflammatory properties [30–35].

Practical Considerations and Patient Counseling

Successful management of HS with topical therapies requires patient-centered counseling on proper application techniques and strategies to promote adherence. Patients should be instructed to apply topical agents to clean and dry skin. For example, clindamycin solution should be applied twice daily with a cotton pad or clean fingertips to affected areas, while resorcinol may require specific instructions for use during flare versus maintenance phases. Incorporating treatment into daily hygiene routines—such as applying benzoyl peroxide wash in the shower—can improve compliance. Providers should also discuss realistic expectations regarding treatment timelines, as many agents may take several weeks to show full benefit.

Odor is a common concern for people with HS; however, antiperspirants have not been rigorously evaluated. It is our practice to suggest spray deodorants onto clothing for people who find these products to be irritating to the skin or worsening their disease.

Counseling should also address strategies to minimize irritation, particularly with agents known to cause dryness or contact dermatitis. Using a non-comedogenic moisturizer and spacing out applications during initial use can improve tolerability. In addition, cost and accessibility are major factors influencing adherence. Many HS patients face financial barriers or difficulty locating antiseptic washes or compounded formulations. Providers should offer affordable, over-the-counter options when possible—such as pyrithione zinc shampoo or generic benzoyl peroxide—and work with pharmacies or patient assistance programs to support access to prescription therapies. Addressing these practical considerations early can help empower patients to engage in consistent self-management and improve outcomes. Table 8.1 reviews the topical treatments used in treating HS.

Board Review Question Explanation

Which of the following topical treatments is considered first-line for mild hidradenitis suppurativa?

A. Tretinoin cream 0.05%.
B. Clindamycin 1% solution (Correct).

Table 8.1 Topical treatments used in the treatment of HS

Agent	Class	Formulations
Clindamycin 1%	Antibiotic	Lotion, solution, gel, and cream
Benzoyl peroxide 5–10%[a]	Antiseptic	Wash
Chlorhexidine 2–4%[a]	Antiseptic	Wash
Pyrithione zinc 1%[a]	Antiseptic	Shampoo
Resorcinol 15%[a]	Keratolytic	Cream
Tretinoin 0.01–0.1%	Retinoid	Cream, gel
Adapalene 0.1–0.3%	Retinoid	Cream, gel
Hydrocortisone 2.5%[a]	Corticosteroid	Cream
Desonide 0.05%[a]	Corticosteroid	Cream
Triamcinolone 0.1%	Corticosteroid	Cream
Ruxolitinib 1.5%[b]	Janus kinase (JAK) inhibitor	Cream
Clascoterone 1%[a]	Hormone receptor blocker	Cream

[a] Not FDA approved
[b] Not currently FDA approved, phase III trials ongoing

C. Tacrolimus ointment.
D. Silver sulfadiazine.
E. Ruxolitinib cream.

Answer Explanation
The correct answer is B. Clindamycin 1% solution. Topical clindamycin is considered a first-line treatment for mild HS, given its anti-inflammatory and antibacterial properties. Other options such as retinoids (A), tacrolimus (C), and silver sulfadiazine (D) are not typically first-line choices. Ruxolitinib (E) is still undergoing FDA approval, with phase III trials ongoing [1, 25, 27].

Key Takeaway Points
- HS is a chronic inflammatory disease with a relapsing course and the development of more effective topical therapies is an unmet need in HS therapy.
- Clindamycin is indicated for localized mild to moderate HS, typically applied twice daily for 3 months, with extended treatment if clinically necessary.
- Resorcinol, ruxolitinib, and clascoterone are emerging topical therapies and can be used as an alternative to topical antibiotic therapy.

References

1. Alikhan A, Sayed C, Alavi A, et al. North American clinical management guidelines for hidradenitis suppurativa: a publication from the United States and Canadian Hidradenitis Suppurativa Foundations: part II: topical, intralesional, and systemic medical management. J Am Acad Dermatol. 2019;81(1):91–101. https://doi.org/10.1016/j.jaad.2019.02.068.
2. Alavi A, Kirsner RS. Local wound care and topical management of hidradenitis Suppurativa. J Am Acad Dermatol. 2015;73(5 Suppl 1):S55–61. https://doi.org/10.1016/j.jaad.2015.07.048.
3. Özbek L, Güldan M, Alpsoy E, Vural S. Hidradenitis Suppurativa treatment during pregnancy and lactation: navigating challenges. Int J Dermatol Published online January 31, 2025. https://doi.org/10.1111/ijd.17672.
4. Zouboulis CC, Bechara FG, Benhadou F, et al. European S2k guidelines for hidradenitis suppurativa/acne inversa part 2: treatment. J Eur Acad Dermatol Venereol. Published online December 19. 2024; https://doi.org/10.1111/jdv.20472.
5. Clemmensen OJ. Topical treatment of hidradenitis suppurativa with clindamycin. Int J Dermatol. 1983;22(5):325–8. https://doi.org/10.1111/j.1365-4362.1983.tb02150.x.
6. Jemec GB, Wendelboe P. Topical clindamycin versus systemic tetracycline in the treatment of hidradenitis suppurativa. J Am Acad Dermatol. 1998;39(6):971–4. https://doi.org/10.1016/s0190-9622(98)70272-5.
7. Fischer AH, Haskin A, Okoye GA. Patterns of antimicrobial resistance in lesions of hidradenitis suppurativa. J Am Acad Dermatol. 2017;76(2):309–313.e2. https://doi.org/10.1016/j.jaad.2016.08.001.
8. Danesh MJ, Kimball AB. Pyrithione zinc as a general management strategy for hidradenitis suppurativa. J Am Acad Dermatol. 2015;73(5):e175. https://doi.org/10.1016/j.jaad.2015.07.026.
9. Leiphart P, Kitts S, Sciacca Kirby J. Adherence to over-the-counter antimicrobial washes in hidradenitis Suppurativa patients. Dermatol Basel Switz. 2019;235(5):440–1. https://doi.org/10.1159/000500827.

10. Reynolds RV, Yeung H, Cheng CE, et al. Guidelines of care for the management of acne vulgaris. J Am Acad Dermatol. 2024;90(5):1006.e1–1006.e30. https://doi.org/10.1016/j.jaad.2023.12.017.
11. Guthery E, Seal LA, Anderson EL. Zinc pyrithione in alcohol-based products for skin antisepsis: persistence of antimicrobial effects. Am J Infect Control. 2005;33(1):15–22. https://doi.org/10.1016/j.ajic.2004.07.012.
12. Gupta M, Mahajan VK, Mehta KS, Chauhan PS. Zinc therapy in dermatology: a review. Dermatol Res Pract. 2014;2014:709152. https://doi.org/10.1155/2014/709152.
13. Zouboulis CC, Desai N, Emtestam L, et al. European S1 guideline for the treatment of hidradenitis suppurativa/acne inversa. J Eur Acad Dermatol Venereol. 2015;29(4):619–44. https://doi.org/10.1111/jdv.12966.
14. Molinelli E, Brisigotti V, Simonetti O, et al. Efficacy and safety of topical resorcinol 15% as long-term treatment of mild-to-moderate hidradenitis Suppurativa: a valid alternative to clindamycin in the panorama of antibiotic resistance. Br J Dermatol. 2020;183(6):1117–9. https://doi.org/10.1111/bjd.19337.
15. Boer J, Jemec GBE. Resorcinol peels as a possible self-treatment of painful nodules in hidradenitis Suppurativa. Clin Exp Dermatol. 2010;35(1):36–40. https://doi.org/10.1111/j.1365-2230.2009.03377.x.
16. Molinelli E, Brisigotti V, Simonetti O, et al. Efficacy and safety of topical resorcinol 15% versus topical clindamycin 1% in the management of mild-to-moderate hidradenitis Suppurativa: a retrospective study. Dermatol Ther. 2022;35(6):e15439. https://doi.org/10.1111/dth.15439.
17. Molinelli E, Gioacchini H, Marani A, et al. Topical and systemic retinoids in the management of hidradenitis suppurativa: a comprehensive literature review. Dermatol Ther. 2024;14(5):1079–91. https://doi.org/10.1007/s13555-024-01169-1.
18. Thielitz A, Abdel-Naser MB, Fluhr JW, Zouboulis CC, Gollnick H. Topical retinoids in acne–an evidence-based overview. J Dtsch Dermatol Ges J Ger Soc Dermatol. 2008;6(12):1023–31. https://doi.org/10.1111/j.1610-0387.2008.06741.x.
19. Ingram JR, McPhee M. Management of hidradenitis Suppurativa: a U.K. survey of current practice. Br J Dermatol. 2015;173(4):1070–2. https://doi.org/10.1111/bjd.13866.
20. Davis SA, Lin HC, Balkrishnan R, Feldman SR. Hidradenitis Suppurativa Management in the United States: an analysis of the National Ambulatory Medical Care Survey and MarketScan Medicaid Databases. Skin Appendage Disord. 2015;1(2):65–73. https://doi.org/10.1159/000431037.
21. Gabros S, Nessel TA, Zito PM. Topical COrticosteroids. In: StatPearls [Internet]. StatPearls Publishing; 2025. Accessed 6 June 2025. https://www.ncbi.nlm.nih.gov/sites/books/NBK532940/.
22. Jaguan D, Nguyen KT, Goldfarb N. Selective small molecule inhibitors for hidradenitis Suppurativa: today and tomorrow. J Am Acad Dermatol. 2024;91(6S):S31–6. https://doi.org/10.1016/j.jaad.2024.09.014.
23. Spadafora M, Morsia S, Di Lernia VG, Kaleci S, Pellacani G, Longo C. Off-label use of topical Ruxolitinib in dermatology: a systematic literature review and current perspectives. Exp Dermatol. 2025;34(4):e70095. https://doi.org/10.1111/exd.70095.
24. Brunk D. Ruxolitinib cream shows promise for hidradenitis Suppurativa. Medscape Dermatology. AAD 2024. Accessed 2 June 2025. https://www.medscape.com/viewarticle/ruxolitinib-cream-shows-promise-hidradenitis-suppurativa-2024a100069e
25. Incyte Corporation. A phase 2, double-blind, randomized, vehicle-controlled, efficacy, and safety study of Ruxolitinib cream in participants with hidradenitis Suppurativa. clinicaltrials.gov; 2024. Accessed June 2, 2025. https://clinicaltrials.gov/study/NCT05635838
26. Schell SL, Sennett ML, Feehan RP, et al. Pilot study of topical ruxolitinib demonstrates efficacy and blunting of heterogeneous inflammatory processes in mild hidradenitis suppurativa. Br J Dermatol. 2025;192(5):845–56. https://doi.org/10.1093/bjd/ljae495.

27. Zaenglein A. Exploratory trial of Ruxolitinib 1.5% cream for the treatment of early stage hidradenitis Suppurativa. clinicaltrials.gov; 2024. Accessed 2 June 2025. https://clinicaltrialsgov/study/NCT04414514
28. Hargis A, Yaghi M, Maskan Bermudez N, Lev-Tov H. Clascoterone in the treatment of mild hidradenitis Suppurativa. J Am Acad Dermatol. 2024;90(1):142–4. https://doi.org/10.1016/j.jaad.2023.08.064.
29. Poondru S, Scott K, Riley JM. Patient perspectives of wound care management in hidradenitis Suppurativa. Arch Dermatol Res. 2023;315(6):1847–50. https://doi.org/10.1007/s00403-023-02576-8.
30. Vicks VapoRub Topical Ointment Drug Facts [package insert]. Accessed 6 June 2025. https://assets.ctfassets.net/nvoox4konz4a/2UQyJBdjHzFWUzLsLPELjn/efb8f4729c2477450e30c1defa14e144/VapoRub-Topical-Ointment-Drug-Facts.pdf.
31. Cheng H, An X. Cold stimuli, hot topic: An updated review on the biological activity of menthol in relation to inflammation. Front Immunol. 2022;13:1023746. https://doi.org/10.3389/fimmu.2022.1023746.
32. Silva J, Abebe W, Sousa SM, Duarte VG, Machado MIL, Matos FJA. Analgesic and anti-inflammatory effects of essential oils of eucalyptus. J Ethnopharmacol. 2003;89(2–3):277–83. https://doi.org/10.1016/j.jep.2003.09.007.
33. Xu H, Blair NT, Clapham DE. Camphor activates and strongly desensitizes the transient receptor potential vanilloid subtype 1 channel in a vanilloid-independent mechanism. J Neurosci. 2005;25(39):8924–37. https://doi.org/10.1523/JNEUROSCI.2574-05.2005.
34. Wu D, Li M, Gong J, Huang W, Zeng W, Jiang Y. Analysis of pharmacological effects and mechanisms of compound essential oils via GC-MS and network pharmacology. Biomed Chromatogr. 2024;38(12):e6033. https://doi.org/10.1002/bmc.6033.
35. Duda-Madej A, Viscardi S, Grabarczyk M, et al. Is camphor the future in supporting therapy for skin infections? Pharmaceuticals. 2024;17(6):715. https://doi.org/10.3390/ph17060715.

Chapter 9
Treatment of HS with Systemic Antibiotics

Claire S. Chung, Kenan Kherallah, Raveena Ghanshani, Vivian Y. Shi, Jennifer L. Hsiao, and Katrina H. Lee

Case Title A 32-year-old female with Hurley stage II HS.

Case

A 32-year-old female with Hurley stage II hidradenitis suppurativa on topical clindamycin, spironolactone, and adalimumab 80 mg every 2 weeks presents to clinic with a 3-day flare after traveling to the desert. Physical examination reveals two inflamed nodules. Her last flare 6 months prior was treated with doxycycline, which caused severe nausea. She was previously unable to tolerate intralesional corticosteroid injections due to pain with injections. What alternative antibiotics could be prescribed to help manage her current flare?

Board Review Question

A 32-year-old pregnant female with type I diabetes presents with an HS flare; her last flare was 7 months ago. You would like to start her on an oral antibiotic to help with her flare symptoms. She has a penicillin and sulfa allergy. Which of the following is the most appropriate next step in managing this patient's condition?

A. Start doxycycline for a 3-month course.
B. Prescribe amoxicillin-clavulanate to use for 2 weeks as needed for flare.
C. Prescribe trimethoprim-sulfamethoxazole to use for 2 weeks as needed for flare.

C. S. Chung · K. Kherallah · R. Ghanshani
Keck School of Medicine, University of Southern California, Los Angeles, CA, USA
e-mail: cschung@usc.edu; kheralla@usc.edu

V. Y. Shi
Department of Dermatology, University of Washington, Seattle, WA, USA

J. L. Hsiao (✉) · K. H. Lee
Department of Dermatology, Keck School of Medicine, University of Southern California, Los Angeles, CA, USA

N. Brownstone (ed.), *Clinical Cases in Hidradenitis Suppurativa*, Clinical Cases in Dermatology, https://doi.org/10.1007/978-3-032-15200-8_9

D. Prescribe oral clindamycin to use for 2 weeks as needed for flare.
E. Start oral clindamycin and rifampin together for a 3-month course.

Introduction

Systemic antibiotics are a key therapeutic class for hidradenitis suppurativa (HS) management [1]. Although HS is an inflammatory and non-infectious condition, systemic antibiotics may be useful to treat HS symptoms due to their anti-inflammatory effects [2]. Current recommendations suggest that systemic antibiotics should not be utilized as a long-term therapy for HS due to concerns for resistance. Instead, they should be reserved for short-term use to mitigate an HS flare or used as a bridge to a long-term therapeutic option. Systemic antibiotics may be administered as a single agent (monotherapy), in combination with other antibiotics (combination therapy), or in severe cases, intravenously. The following chapter discusses the current recommendations on systemic antibiotic use in the management of HS.

Best Practices: Practical Management of HS with Systemic Antibiotics

Systemic antibiotics often offer patients rapid improvement in pain and drainage, particularly during flares [1, 3]. In managing flares, a recommended strategy is to use 2 weeks of oral antibiotics, with consideration for a concomitant prednisone taper for debilitating widespread flares [4]. Antibiotics are also used as adjuvant therapy in severe or refractory cases as part of a multimodal approach to care. However, prolonged use of systemic antibiotics is associated with significant risks, including the development of antibiotic resistance. Therefore, the overall goal for treating HS is a long-term management plan that minimizes dependence on systemic antibiotics. In this context, antibiotics are best viewed as a "bridge" therapy over 2–3 months, ideally providing faster-onset short-term control of symptoms while patients transition to more definitive treatments, such as biologics or surgery (Table 9.1). In very severe cases, intravenous ertapenem may be considered as a rescue therapy with a similar goal of bridging patients to definitive long-term interventions [5, 6]. In patients with chronic draining tunnels, systemic antibiotics alone may be inadequate, especially in the setting of bacterial biofilm formation; these patients often require definitive surgical removal of the affected tissue [7]. In addition, despite their efficacy, antibiotics may cause significant gastrointestinal discomfort. Therefore, patient-oriented tips, such as advising co-administration with food, recommending pre- or probiotics, and introducing antibiotics in a stepwise manner over the first few days when a combination antibiotic regimen is prescribed (i.e. starting with clindamycin for 1 week, then layering in rifampin during week 2), can be helpful in promoting medication adherence.

Table 9.1 Practical considerations for systemic antibiotic use

Strategies for systemic antibiotic use	Time frame for use	Options for use	Special considerations
Monotherapy: Flare treatment or as a bridge to long-term therapeutic option for mild to moderate HS	2 weeks for flare 12 weeks as bridge therapy	Doxycycline (100 mg BID)	Avoid use in children <8 years old or pregnant women
		TMP-SMX (160/800 mg BID)	Avoid in pregnant women during the first trimester Increased risk of myelosuppression if taken with methotrexate
		Amoxicillin-Clavulanate (875/125 mg BID)	Reduced dosing for renal insufficiency
		Dapsone (50–150 mg daily)	Avoid in patients with G6PD deficiency
		Cephalexin (500 mg BID)	Use cautiously in patients with penicillin allergies
		Cefdinir (300 mg BID)	
		Clindamycin (300 mg BID)	Increased risk for CDI
		Rifampin (300 mg BID)	Avoid in pregnancy Adjust dosing in patients taking other medications metabolized by CYP450
Combination therapy: Bridge to long-term therapeutic option, moderate to severe HS	12 weeks	Clindamycin (300 mg BID) + Rifampin (300 mg BID)	Consider clindamycin monotherapy instead
		TMP-SMX (160/800 mg BID) + cephalexin (500 mg BID)	
	6–12 weeks	Rifampin (300 mg BID) + Moxifloxacin (400 mg daily) + metronidazole (500 mg TID)	Avoid combining with QT-prolonging medications
	6–12 weeks	Ciprofloxacin (500 mg BID) + Metronidazole (500 mg BID)	Avoid in older patients taking corticosteroids Preferred treatment duration <6 weeks

(continued)

Table 9.1 (continued)

Strategies for systemic antibiotic use	Time frame for use	Options for use	Special considerations
Rescue therapy: Bridge to surgery or other long-term therapeutic option for severe, recalcitrant HS	6–12 weeks	IV ertapenem (1 g daily)	Consider monitoring renal, hepatic, hematopoietic function May rarely (<1%) cause neurotoxicity; exercise caution in patients with renal insufficiency, pre-existing neurological disease, and hypoalbuminemia [33] Rapid recurrence of symptoms when discontinued
		IV ceftriaxone (1 g daily)	May be used as induction therapy prior to transition to PO antibiotics
		Linezolid (600 mg BID)	Monitor CBC weekly and for signs of clonus Avoid tyramine-rich foods due to risk of hypertensive crisis

Abbreviations: *HS* hidradenitis suppurativa, *mg* milligram, *g* gram, *BID* twice daily, *TID* three times daily, *TMP-SMX* trimethoprim-sulfamethoxazole, *G6PD* glucose-6-phosphate dehydrogenase, *CDI Clostridium difficile* infection, *CYP450* cytochrome P450, *IV* intravenous, *PO* oral, *CBC* complete blood count

Single Antibiotic Therapy

Tetracyclines

Tetracyclines, such as doxycycline and minocycline, have been shown to benefit patients with HS and are recommended by both the North American (NA) guidelines and European S2k clinical management guidelines as a first-line therapy for mild to moderate HS [1, 3]. A prospective study of 108 patients with HS who were initiated on tetracycline 500 mg ($n = 32$), doxycycline 100 mg ($n = 31$), or lymecycline 300 mg ($n = 45$) twice daily, found a statistically significant mean reduction in their Sartorius Score (8.13 points from baseline). There was no statistically significant difference in score or score reduction between the three groups. Furthermore, the mean Dermatology Life Quality Index (DLQI) and pain Numerical Rating Scale (NRS) scores decreased significantly [8]. Another prospective cohort study of 283 patients comparing the efficacy of tetracyclines and clindamycin/rifampicin combination therapy in HS found that tetracycline therapy (tetracycline 500 mg twice daily, doxycycline 100 mg once daily, or minocycline 100 mg once daily) resulted in a statistically significant decrease in the number of lesions (abscesses, inflammatory nodules, and draining tunnels), pain, pruritus, and International Hidradenitis Suppurativa Severity Scoring System (IHS4) score. There was no significant difference in efficacy between the tetracycline and clindamycin/rifampicin groups [9].

Amoxicillin-Clavulanate

A prospective observational study of 44 patients evaluated the combination of amoxicillin-clavulanate (875/125 mg twice daily) with a prednisone taper (starting at 40 mg daily and decreasing by 10 mg every 3 days). Both mean DLQI and HS pain scores of patients decreased significantly following treatment [4]. Broad-spectrum antibiotics like amoxicillin-clavulanate may have lower resistance rates compared to the more commonly prescribed tetracyclines. One study evaluated antibiotic resistance of pathogens isolated from the lesions of 69 patients with HS, and found the resistance rate against amoxicillin-clavulanate to be 11.9% compared to 64.4% against tetracyclines [10]. One case study describes the use of amoxicillin-clavulanate perioperatively for several weeks as a bridge to surgical excision and for 4 weeks post-operatively; the patient remained in remission more than 12 months later [11].

Trimethoprim-Sulfamethoxazole

One retrospective study evaluated 18 patients with HS who were treated with trimethoprim-sulfamethoxazole (TMP-SMX). Fifty percent of patients had an excellent response (defined as a HS Physician's Global Assessment [HS-PGA] score of 1 [clear] or 2 [minimal]) and 38.9% had a partial response (defined as any improvement to the HS-PGA score). Most patients were on one double strength (160/800 mg) tablet twice daily. Length of treatment ranged from 2 months to several years. Of note, 16/18 patients (89%) in the study were on concomitant non-antibiotic therapies, 7 of whom were on a biologic [12]. Lastly, TMP-SMX should also be avoided in patients on concomitant methotrexate therapy due to associations with severe myelosuppression and nephrotoxicity.

Cephalosporins

Cephalosporins, including cephalexin and cefdinir, may also be used in the treatment of HS as either monotherapy or in combination with other antibiotics. A survey of HS experts found that cephalosporins were frequently used for HS flares [13]. Cephalexin 500 mg twice daily or cefdinir 300 mg twice daily may be considered.

Dapsone

Dapsone is a sulfone drug that has both anti-inflammatory and antimicrobial properties [14]. The NA guidelines and European S2k guidelines for treatment of HS both cite dapsone as a third-line agent in patients with mild to moderate disease [1, 3, 15]. A retrospective case series of 56 patients with Hurley stage I or II HS found that 62.5% of patients achieved HS Clinical Response (HiSCR, or at least 50% reduction in abscess and inflammatory nodule count with no increase in number of abscesses or draining tunnels compared to baseline) after 12 weeks of treatment [16]. In another retrospective study of 25 patients with HS, 16/24 patients (64%) taking dapsone had clinician-reported improvement [17]. The prescribed dose of dapsone ranged from 50 to 150 mg daily in these studies [16, 17]. Dapsone should be avoided in patients with known glucose-6-phosphate dehydrogenase (G6PD) deficiency due to risk of hemolysis.

Combination Antibiotic Therapy

Combination antibiotic therapy may be considered in patients with moderate to severe disease or in cases where monotherapy is insufficient to achieve clinical improvement [1].

Clindamycin and Rifampin

Clindamycin and rifampin combination therapy is recommended by the NA guidelines for mild to moderate disease or as adjuvant therapy in severe disease (both at a dose of 300 mg twice daily for a duration of 8–12 weeks) [1]. This combination therapy is one of the most widely studied antibiotic regimens for HS; however, recent data suggests that monotherapy clindamycin may be sufficient. A retrospective study of 60 HS patients found that clindamycin monotherapy (150 mg 4 times daily) was noninferior to combination clindamycin/rifampin for HS with no significant difference in IHS4 scores after 8 weeks of treatment [18]. In addition, another study evaluating osteoarticular infections found that mean serum concentrations of clindamycin when combined with rifampin were 0.79 ± 0.3 μg/ml, compared to 4.7 ± 1.2 μg/ml when combined with levofloxacin, suggesting that rifampin affects the pharmacokinetics of clindamycin leading to serum levels below recommended therapeutic levels [19]. Thus, at this point in time, clindamycin monotherapy (300 mg twice a day) should be strongly considered in lieu of clindamycin and rifampin combination therapy. It should be noted that clindamycin use is associated with higher risk of developing *Clostridium difficile* infection [20]. If rifampin is utilized, thorough medication reconciliation is advised given rifampin is an inducer of cytochrome P450 (CYP450) and may affect the metabolism of concurrent medications such as oral contraceptives and warfarin [21].

Trimethoprim-Sulfamethoxazole and Cephalexin

A combination of trimethoprim-sulfamethoxazole (TMP-SMX) and cephalexin may also be used to treat HS. In one case series, 16 patients, primarily with Hurley stage II ($n = 7$) or III ($n = 8$) disease, were treated with a combination of TMP-SMX and cephalexin for 3 months. Following treatment, 75% of patients showed improvement based on physician assessments and 68.8% of patients had self-reported improvement. Most patients received a regimen of TMP-SMX 160/800 mg twice daily and cephalexin 500 mg twice daily, and 2/16 patients (12.5%) received half this dose [22]. Although commonly prescribed to treat dermatological conditions, TMP-SMX and cephalexin both have potential for renal toxicity and their doses should be adjusted in those with renal insufficiency [23]. Combination therapy with TMP-SMX and cephalexin can be considered in patients with HS who have failed other systemic antibiotic treatments, but further research is needed to study its efficacy compared to other therapies.

Ciprofloxacin and Metronidazole

The combination of ciprofloxacin and metronidazole can also be employed in the management of HS and has also been used in combination to treat other inflammatory conditions such as Crohn's disease [24]. A study examining the microbial profile of HS observed that several fluoroquinolones, including ciprofloxacin, were among the most effective antibiotics against bacteria isolated from HS lesions [25]. Although optimal HS dosing has not been studied, a regimen of ciprofloxacin 500 mg twice daily and metronidazole 500 mg twice daily may be considered.

Rifampin, Moxifloxacin, Metronidazole

A combination of rifampin, moxifloxacin, and metronidazole has been used in combination to treat HS, typically as a third-line therapy or a bridge to surgery, according to the NA guidelines [1]. A retrospective study of patients with Hurley stage I ($n = 6$), II ($n = 10$), and III ($n = 12$) HS who received treatment with a combination of rifampin 10 mg/kg once daily, moxifloxacin 400 mg daily, and metronidazole

500 mg three times daily saw complete remission in 16/28 patients (57%). Most of those who achieved complete remission had Hurley stage I (6/6) or II (8/10) disease; partial response was observed in the remaining 12 patients [26]. A prospective cohort study of 28 patients treated for 12 weeks with combination therapy consisting of rifampin (10 mg/kg once daily), moxifloxacin (400 mg once daily, or pristinamycin 1 g three times daily if contraindicated), and metronidazole (250–500 mg) found a significant decrease in the median Sartorius score from 14 to 0, with 75% ($n = 21$) achieving clinical remission (defined as Sartorius score of 0). After 1 year, the median number of HS flares dropped substantially from 21 to 1 per year [27].

Intravenous Antibiotics

Although more difficult to coordinate access, intravenous (IV) antibiotics may be appropriate in some cases of severe HS. IV ceftriaxone (1 g daily) has been used as part of induction therapy for severe recalcitrant HS, particularly as a bridge to long-term treatment options [28].

Ertapenem is a carbapenem antibiotic that has shown high efficacy in treating HS, but should primarily be used for severe, recalcitrant HS [1, 3]. Its use is limited by the practical challenges of IV administration and concern for antibiotic resistance. As a result, the NA guidelines recommend that ertapenem be reserved as a third-line therapy for a single 6-week course as rescue therapy or during surgical planning [1]. If necessary, this course may be extended up to 12–16 weeks. A 2024 retrospective study of 98 patients treated with IV ertapenem for a mean of 13 weeks found significant reduction to mean HS-PGA scores and pain scores, as well as several inflammatory markers (C-reactive protein, interleukin-6, and leukocytes) [29]. Literature on ertapenem's pharmacokinetics suggests that intramuscular (IM) ertapenem therapy has a relative bioavailability of 92% compared to the IV route [30]. In a study of 15 patients with moderate to severe HS where 9/15 received IV ertapenem, 5/15 received IM ertapenem, and 1/15 received a combination of both, researchers found that patients in the IM group experienced significant reductions in their IHS4 and pain visual analog scores (VAS), comparable to that of their IV counterparts [31]. One benefit of IM administration is the avoidance of a peripherally inserted central catheter (PICC); however, some patients may not be able to tolerate daily IM injections.

Anecdotally, linezolid has been reported to have benefit in HS and is typically reserved for severe, recalcitrant cases [1]. Published literature is currently limited to a single case report. IV linezolid in combination with meropenem demonstrated rapid remission in a patient with Hurley stage III HS [32]. Oral linezolid at a dose of 600 mg twice daily can also be considered for severe, recalcitrant cases of HS.

Conclusion

Managing HS involves careful utilization of a variety of treatment modalities, with consideration for sustainability and safety of therapies. Systemic antibiotics play a key role in controlling acute flares or serving as a bridge to longer-term therapies. However, the goal is to establish a stable treatment regimen that minimizes prolonged antibiotic use to reduce the risk of antibiotic resistance. Selecting the most appropriate therapy requires not only an understanding of the treatment options available, but also consideration of the individual patient's disease severity, comorbidities, and long-term management needs. Table 9.1 summarizes the practical considerations for systemic antibiotic use in HS.

Board Review Question Explanation
A 32-year-old pregnant female with type I diabetes presents with an HS flare, her last flare was 7 months ago. You would like to start her on an oral antibiotic to help with her flare symptoms. She has a penicillin and sulfa allergy. Which of the following is the most appropriate next step in managing this patient's condition?

A. Start doxycycline for a 3-month course.
B. Prescribe amoxicillin-clavulanate to use for 2 weeks as needed for flare.
C. Prescribe trimethoprim-sulfamethoxazole to use for 2 weeks as needed for flare.
D. Prescribe oral clindamycin to use for 2 weeks as needed for flare. (Correct)
E. Start oral clindamycin and rifampin together for a 3-month course.

Answer Explanation
The correct answer is D) Prescribe oral clindamycin to use for 2 weeks as needed for flare. Clindamycin is considered a first-line antibiotic therapy in treating HS and is safe to use in pregnant individuals. Tetracyclines should not be used during pregnancy due to the risk of dental staining to the fetus. Amoxicillin-clavulanate and trimethoprim-sulfamethoxazole should both be avoided in this case due to her penicillin and sulfa antibiotic allergies, respectively. Systemic prednisone is not recommended due to the patient's concomitant type I diabetes. Therefore, the most appropriate answer choice is to initiate oral clindamycin to treat this patient's HS flare.

Key Takeaway Points
- Systemic antibiotics play a crucial role in managing hidradenitis suppurativa as a treatment for flares, bridge to longer-term therapeutic options, and rescue therapy for severe, recalcitrant HS.
- Single antibiotic therapies that may be utilized for HS include tetracyclines, cephalosporins, trimethoprim-sulfamethoxazole, amoxicillin-clavulanate, and dapsone.

- Combination antibiotic therapies may be considered when patients have moderate to severe HS or have failed single antibiotic treatments.
- IV ertapenem and IV/oral linezolid are reserved as rescue therapy options for severe, recalcitrant HS.

References

1. Alikhan A, Sayed C, Alavi A, et al. North American clinical management guidelines for hidradenitis suppurativa: a publication from the United States and Canadian Hidradenitis Suppurativa Foundations. J Am Acad Dermatol. 2019;81:91–101. https://doi.org/10.1016/j.jaad.2019.02.068.
2. Molinelli E, De Simoni E, Candelora M, et al. Systemic antibiotic therapy in Hidradenitis Suppurativa: a review on treatment landscape and current issues. Antibiotics. 2023;12:978. https://doi.org/10.3390/antibiotics12060978.
3. European S2k guidelines for hidradenitis suppurativa/acne inversa part 2: Treatment – Zouboulis. J Eur Acad Dermatol Venereol. https://onlinelibrary-wiley-com.libproxy1.usc.edu/doi/10.1111/jdv.20472. Accessed 5 Jan 2025.
4. Gibson RS, Snyder CL, Porter ML, Kimball AB. Prednisone and amoxicillin/clavulanic acid for the treatment of hidradenitis suppurativa flares: a prospective observational study. Int J Womens Dermatol. 2024;10:e162. https://doi.org/10.1097/JW9.0000000000000162.
5. Join-Lambert O, Coignard-Biehler H, Jais J-P, et al. Efficacy of ertapenem in severe hidradenitis suppurativa: a pilot study in a cohort of 30 consecutive patients. J Antimicrob Chemother. 2016;71:513–20. https://doi.org/10.1093/jac/dkv361.
6. Chahine AA, Nahhas AF, Braunberger TL, et al. Ertapenem rescue therapy in hidradenitis suppurativa. JAAD Case Rep. 2018;4:482–3. https://doi.org/10.1016/j.jdcr.2017.12.010.
7. Kathju S, Lasko L-A, Stoodley P. Considering hidradenitis suppurativa as a bacterial biofilm disease. FEMS Immunol Med Microbiol. 2012;65:385–9. https://doi.org/10.1111/j.1574-695X.2012.00946.x.
8. Jørgensen A-HR, Yao Y, Thomsen SF, Ring HC. Treatment of hidradenitis suppurativa with tetracycline, doxycycline, or lymecycline: a prospective study. Int J Dermatol. 2021;60:785–91. https://doi.org/10.1111/ijd.15459.
9. van Straalen KR, Tzellos T, Guillem P, et al. The efficacy and tolerability of tetracyclines and clindamycin plus rifampicin for the treatment of hidradenitis suppurativa: results of a prospective European cohort study. J Am Acad Dermatol. 2021;85:369–78. https://doi.org/10.1016/j.jaad.2020.12.089.
10. Matusiak Ł, Bieniek A, Szepietowski JC. Bacteriology of hidradenitis Suppurativa—which antibiotics are the treatment of choice? Acta Derm Venereol. 2014;94:699–702. https://doi.org/10.2340/00015555-1841.
11. Nedomansky J, Weiss D, Willinger B, et al. Acne inversa complicated by Actinomyces neuii. Infection. 2016;44:247–9. https://doi.org/10.1007/s15010-015-0814-6.
12. Park M. Trimethoprim-Sulfamethoxazole as a mono-antibiotic therapy for Hidradenitis Suppurativa. 2024. https://journals-sagepub-com.libproxy2.usc.edu/doi/epub/10.1177/12034754241247520. Accessed 29 Nov 2024.
13. Masson R, Park S, Shi VY, et al. Expert practices in hidradenitis Suppurativa flare management: a cross-sectional survey study. Skin Appendage Disord. 2024;10:224–8. https://doi.org/10.1159/000536094.
14. Wozel G, Blasum C. Dapsone in dermatology and beyond. Arch Dermatol Res. 2014;306:103–24. https://doi.org/10.1007/s00403-013-1409-7.
15. Zouboulis CC, Desai N, Emtestam L, et al. European S1 guideline for the treatment of hidradenitis suppurativa/acne inversa. J Eur Acad Dermatol Venereol. 2015;29:619–44. https://doi.org/10.1111/jdv.12966.

16. López-Llunell C, Riera-Martí N, Gamissans M, Romaní J. Dapsone in hidradenitis suppurativa: a case series of 56 patients. Dermatol Ther. 2021;34:e15161. https://doi.org/10.1111/dth.15161.
17. Murray G, Hollywood A, Kirby B, Hughes R. Dapsone therapy for hidradenitis suppurativa. Br J Dermatol. 2020;183:767–8. https://doi.org/10.1111/bjd.19136.
18. Caposiena Caro RD, Cannizzaro MV, Botti E, et al. Clindamycin versus clindamycin plus rifampicin in hidradenitis suppurativa treatment: clinical and ultrasound observations. J Am Acad Dermatol. 2019;80:1314–21. https://doi.org/10.1016/j.jaad.2018.11.035.
19. Bernard A, Kermarrec G, Parize P, et al. Dramatic reduction of clindamycin serum concentration in staphylococcal osteoarticular infection patients treated with the oral clindamycin-rifampicin combination. J Infect. 2015;71:200–6. https://doi.org/10.1016/j.jinf.2015.03.013.
20. Miller AC, Arakkal AT, Sewell DK, et al. Comparison of different antibiotics and the risk for community-associated clostridioides difficile infection: a case–control study. Open Forum Infect Dis. 2023;10:ofad413. https://doi.org/10.1093/ofid/ofad413.
21. Niemi M, Backman JT, Fromm MF, et al. Pharmacokinetic interactions with rifampicin. Clin Pharmacokinet. 2003;42:819–50. https://doi.org/10.2165/00003088-200342090-00003.
22. Masson R, Seivright J, Shih T, et al. Trimethoprim/sulfamethoxazole and cephalexin combination therapy in hidradenitis suppurativa patients: a series of 16 cases. JAAD Case Rep. 2023;37:1–4. https://doi.org/10.1016/j.jdcr.2023.04.025.
23. Chung CS, Park SE, Hsiao JL, Lee KH. A review of hidradenitis Suppurativa in special populations: considerations in children, pregnant and breastfeeding women, and the elderly. Dermatol Ther. 2024;14:2407–25. https://doi.org/10.1007/s13555-024-01249-2.
24. Greenbloom SL, Steinhart AH, Greenberg GR. Combination ciprofloxacin and metronidazole for active Crohn's disease. Can J Gastroenterol. 1998;12:53–6. https://doi.org/10.1155/1998/349460.
25. Hessam S, Sand M, Georgas D, et al. Microbial profile and antimicrobial susceptibility of bacteria found in inflammatory hidradenitis Suppurativa lesions. Skin Pharmacol Physiol. 2016;29:161–7. https://doi.org/10.1159/000446812.
26. Join-Lambert O, Coignard H, Jais J-P, et al. Efficacy of rifampin-Moxifloxacin-metronidazole combination therapy in hidradenitis Suppurativa. Dermatology. 2010;222:49–58. https://doi.org/10.1159/000321716.
27. Delage M, Jais J-P, Lam T, et al. Rifampin-moxifloxacin-metronidazole combination therapy for severe Hurley stage 1 hidradenitis suppurativa: prospective short-term trial and 1-year follow-up in 28 consecutive patients. J Am Acad Dermatol. 2023;88:94–100. https://doi.org/10.1016/j.jaad.2020.01.007.
28. Nassif A. Complete remission of severe hidradenitis suppurativa obtained in 4 patients using wide-spectrum antimicrobial treatment. J Am Acad Dermatol. 2012;66:AB46. https://doi.org/10.1016/j.jaad.2011.11.202.
29. Nosrati A, Ch'en PY, Torpey ME, et al. Efficacy and durability of intravenous Ertapenem therapy for recalcitrant hidradenitis Suppurativa. JAMA Dermatol. 2024;160:312–8. https://doi.org/10.1001/jamadermatol.2023.6201.
30. Musson DG, Majumdar A, Birk K, et al. Pharmacokinetics of intramuscularly administered Ertapenem. Antimicrob Agents Chemother. 2003;47:1732–5. https://doi.org/10.1128/AAC.47.5.1732-1735.2003.
31. Segura Palacios JM, Soto Moreno A, Valladares Millán I, et al. Intramuscular ertapenem for the treatment of severe cases hidradenitis suppurativa. J Dermatol Treat. 2023;34:2179368. https://doi.org/10.1080/09546634.2023.2179368.
32. Scheinfeld N. Extensive hidradenitis suppurativa (HS) hurly stage III disease treated with intravenous (IV) linezolid and meropenem with rapid remission. Dermatol Online J. 2015;21 https://doi.org/10.5070/D3212025709.
33. Wang C, Zhou Y, Zhou Y, Ye C. Ertapenem-induced neurotoxicity: a literature review of clinical characteristics and treatment outcomes. Infect Drug Resist. 2023;16:3649–58. https://doi.org/10.2147/IDR.S406852.

Chapter 10
Treatment of Hidradenitis Suppurativa with Non-biologic, Non-antibiotic Systemic Therapies

Kenan Kherallah, Claire S. Chung, Raveena Ghanshani, Vivian Y. Shi, Jennifer L. Hsiao, and Katrina H. Lee

Case Title Systemic Therapy Selection in Hidradenitis Suppurativa Beyond Antibiotics

Case

A 34-year-old female with a history of obesity, type 2 diabetes, hypertension, and mild hidradenitis suppurativa presents with two inflammatory nodules in her axilla. She recently completed a 3-month course of oral doxycycline; however, she continues to have disease activity. What systemic therapies can be discussed with the patient? If her disease progresses, what non-biologic immunomodulators could be discussed with her? Finally, what are some non-antibiotic treatment options that can be used for HS flares or as a bridge to longer-term therapeutic options?

Board Review Question

A 42-year-old male with a history of obesity and hypertension presents with Hurley Stage II hidradenitis suppurativa involving his bilateral axillae and groin. He is overall well controlled on adalimumab 80 mg every 2 weeks and finasteride 5 mg daily but continues to experience very mild flares despite recently completing a 3-month course of doxycycline. Laboratory studies reveal elevated fasting insulin levels and HbA1c of 7.5%. Which of the following systemic therapies is the most appropriate next step in his management?

K. Kherallah · C. S. Chung · R. Ghanshani
Keck School of Medicine, University of Southern California, Los Angeles, CA, USA

V. Y. Shi
Department of Dermatology, University of Washington, Seattle, WA, USA

J. L. Hsiao (✉) · K. H. Lee
Department of Dermatology, Keck School of Medicine, University of Southern California, Los Angeles, CA, USA

N. Brownstone (ed.), *Clinical Cases in Hidradenitis Suppurativa*, Clinical Cases in Dermatology, https://doi.org/10.1007/978-3-032-15200-8_10

A. Acitretin
B. Drospirenone
C. Metformin
D. Prednisone
E. Spironolactone

Introduction

Management of hidradenitis suppurativa (HS) requires a multimodal approach tailored to disease severity, patient characteristics, and prior treatment responses. The heterogeneous nature of HS and its links to metabolic syndrome, polycystic ovarian syndrome (PCOS), and inflammatory bowel disease highlight the need for personalized therapies that address both HS disease activity and systemic comorbidities. Achieving sustained control often requires combining therapies to balance efficacy and safety. This chapter explores systemic, non-antibiotic, and non-biologic HS therapies, focusing on hormonal modulators, metabolic treatments, oral retinoids, and non-biologic immunomodulators.

Hormonal Modulators

HS is believed to be influenced by hormonal factors, which may play a significant role in its pathogenesis and progression. Though their exact role remains unclear, androgens may contribute to disease activity by promoting follicular occlusion through increased keratinocyte proliferation and follicular plugging. The primary defect in HS pathophysiology is thought to lie in the hair follicle, where occlusion leads to follicular rupture and an exaggerated immune response, ultimately driving inflammation and lesion formation [1]. Furthermore, frequent post-pubertal onset, occurrence of premenstrual flares in ovulating women, and the observation that HS disease activity changes during pregnancy, highlight the significant influence hormones may have on disease activity [2, 3]. Additionally, exogenous testosterone use has been reported to worsen HS [4]. Hormonal modulating therapies, including spironolactone, oral contraceptive pills (OCPs), and finasteride have been shown to have efficacy in HS.

Spironolactone, a potassium-sparing diuretic with anti-androgenic properties, is widely used in women with HS and supported by expert consensus [5]. Typical dosing ranges from 50 mg to 200 mg daily. It is thought to improve HS by blocking androgen receptors and reducing androgen production, thereby decreasing inflammatory nodule formation [6]. In a retrospective review of 53 patients, 84% of female patients with HS on spironolactone showed improvement after 3 months, with 81% maintaining improvement at 6 months [7]. However, patients with Hurley stage III disease may have lower response rates, thus adjunctive use with biologics or other immunomodulators in more advanced disease is often required [8]. Spironolactone may be especially beneficial in patients with HS and concomitant PCOS. Clinicians should consider monitoring for hyperkalemia, especially in those with renal dysfunction, on concomitant potassium-sparing medications, or over 65 years old, as one study has shown an increased incidence of hyperkalemia with spironolactone in this age group [9, 10]. Side effects such as menstrual irregularities can often be managed by combining spironolactone with an OCP.

Notably, OCPs can also serve as a treatment option for women with HS. Combined OCPs containing estrogen and a third- or fourth-generation progestin with lower androgenic activity, such as norgestimate or drospirenone, are particularly helpful. A retrospective cohort study of 89 women with HS found that OCPs significantly reduced disease severity, including total abscess and inflammatory nodule count. Factors associated with improved response to OCPs included the use of concomitant therapies, such as oral doxycycline, shorter disease duration, and the presence of HS flares with menstruation [11]. OCPs can also be particularly beneficial in patients who experience irregular periods, those with PCOS, and for those who desire contraception. Patients should be screened for contraindications such as migraines with aura (which is an absolute contraindication), active smoking status in women over 35 years old, unmanaged hypertension, history of thromboembolic events, and breast cancer prior to starting an OCP [12]. If a patient is unable to tolerate an estrogen-containing OCP, the drospirenone-only mini pill may be considered as an alternative [13]. Patients on concomitant OCPs and rifampin (an antibiotic commonly used with clindamycin for HS) should be advised that rifampin (a CYP3A4 inducer) may reduce the contraceptive effectiveness of OCPs [14].

Finasteride, a 5-alpha reductase inhibitor, reduces the conversion of testosterone to dihydrotestosterone (DHT) and is thought to potentially alter the end-organ sensitivity of the follicular pilosebaceous unit [15]. It is commonly used for benign prostatic hyperplasia and androgenetic alopecia in males, as well as hirsutism in females. A 5 to 10 mg daily dose has also been used off-label for HS, typically in males and post-menopausal women [16]. Evidence for finasteride in HS management is limited but promising, particularly in patients with refractory disease or contraindications to spironolactone. A retrospective study of 20 women with HS (mean age 34.3 ± 13.5 years), who had poor responsiveness to or contraindications for spironolactone and were treated with finasteride 5 mg/day, reported an overall patient satisfaction rate of 50%, with 80% experiencing no side effects. Minor side effects, including headache or menstrual irregularities, were observed in 20% of patients [17]. Furthermore, a case series of seven patients (five female, two male) showed significant symptom improvement within 2–8 weeks on finasteride 5 mg/day, including reduced pain, erythema, and drainage as well as healing of lesions. Some patients achieved prolonged remission lasting 8–18 months after 6–16 weeks of treatment, while others experienced recurrence that was managed successfully with reintroduction of the drug [15]. Clinicians should counsel patients on potential adverse effects, including sexual dysfunction—reported in approximately 2.1% to 3.8% of male patients—as well as reduced libido and mood changes. Notably, these sexual side effects are not believed to be dose-dependent [18]. Use of finasteride should be avoided in women of childbearing age due to teratogenicity, but if prescribed, reliable contraception is essential [19].

Metabolic

Patients with HS have increased risk of metabolic abnormalities, including central obesity, hyperlipidemia, hyperglycemia, and hypertension [20]. This constellation of comorbidities frequently fulfills the criteria for metabolic syndrome, which is more prevalent and develops at a younger age in patients with HS compared to the general population. Metabolic modulators have emerged as promising therapeutic options for HS management, particularly if patients also have other metabolic comorbidities [21].

Although indicated for type 2 diabetes, metformin has shown benefit for HS and can also be utilized in patients who do not have concomitant insulin resistance or diabetes [22]. Typical dosing ranges from 500 mg to 2000 mg daily. While the exact mechanism of metformin's effect on HS is unknown, it is hypothesized that the improvement in insulin sensitivity and reduction in hyperinsulinemia may lower androgen production and systemic inflammation [23]. Additionally, metformin inhibits the mTOR pathway, further contributing to its anti-inflammatory effects [24]. In a prospective cohort study of 25 patients with refractory HS, metformin was up-titrated from 500 mg once daily in the first week to 500 mg twice daily in the second week, and 500 mg three times daily from the third week onward, resulting in 72% of patients showing clinical improvement with a mean Dermatology Life Quality Index (DLQI) reduction of 7.6 [25]. Furthermore, in a retrospective analysis of 53 patients, the majority (72%) with Hurley Stage II HS, treated with an average of 1500 mg/day of metformin for an average of 11.3 months reported a 68% response rate, with 19% achieving complete lesion resolution [22]. A common side effect of metformin is gastrointestinal discomfort, which can be mitigated by gradual dose escalation. There is a rare risk of lactic acidosis in patients with renal impairment [22].

Preliminary data suggest that glucagon-like peptide-1 (GLP-1) receptor agonists, such as semaglutide (typically at a dose of 0.8–1.0 mg weekly), and liraglutide (typically at a dose of 3 mg daily), may reduce systemic inflammation associated with metabolic dysregulation in patients with HS [26, 27]. Their anti-inflammatory effects are attributed to the suppression of key inflammatory pathways involving TNF-α, IL-17, and NF-κB [28]. GLP-1 agonists may be particularly effective in patients who have comorbid obesity. In a study of 30 patients with HS and obesity treated with semaglutide at a mean weekly dose of 0.8 mg for an average of 8.2 months, 33% achieved a clinically significant improvement in DLQI, and 33% experienced greater than 10 kg weight loss; a limitation of the study was that patients were allowed to be on concomitant medications including biologics [29]. In another study of 45 obese patients with HS, semaglutide was initiated at a mean dose of 0.52 ± 0.47 mg/week and titrated to 1.11 ± 0.82 mg/week at 6 months and 1.36 ± 0.86 mg/week at 12 months. HS improvement, defined as a greater than 50% reduction in inflammatory lesions, no new lesions, and reduced need for rescue therapy, was observed in 60% of patients. Patients also experienced a mean weight loss of 10.1 ± 15.4 pounds at 12 months. While semaglutide was associated with improvement, statistical significance for the overall response rate was not explicitly reported [30]. While gastrointestinal symptoms are common during initiation of a GLP-1 agonist, these side effects are generally transient [31]. Patients initiated on GLP-1 agonists should be counseled on the potential for increased skin sagging and friction with significant weight loss, which may potentially exacerbate HS activity. Further large-scale, prospective studies evaluating the efficacy of GLP-1 agonists for HS are needed.

Oral Retinoids

Oral retinoids, including acitretin and isotretinoin, are systemic agents derived from vitamin A that have been utilized in the management of HS. While not entirely elucidated, oral retinoids act by normalizing keratinocyte differentiation, targeting follicular plugging, reducing sebaceous gland size, and modulating inflammation [32]. Generally, they are used as adjunctive therapies for HS, and are particularly useful in patients with comorbid moderate-to-severe acne.

Acitretin, a second-generation oral retinoid, has demonstrated efficacy in the treatment of HS. One study showed that 12 patients with severe HS, treated with doses ranging from 0.25 to 0.88 mg/kg/day, achieved remission and a significant decrease in pain. Nine of these patients experienced long-lasting improvement, particularly in pain reduction from nodules [33]. Additionally, one study of 17 patients reported that, at a mean dose of 0.56 mg/kg/day, 47% of patients achieved a clinical response to acitretin after 9 months, with a greater than 50% reduction in the HS Severity Index from baseline. Despite this, the medication's limitations were evident, as 47% discontinued the drug primarily due to ineffectiveness ($n = 5$) and adverse events, including retinoid-induced dermatitis ($n = 2$) and severe hair loss ($n = 1$) [34]. In addition, acitretin is contraindicated in women of child-bearing age.

Isotretinoin, a first-generation retinoid, is widely used for acne. Isotretinoin has also been explored as an off-label treatment for HS, particularly due to its anti-inflammatory and sebaceous gland-suppressing properties. One study showed that isotretinoin at a mean dose of 0.45 mg/kg/day was effective for mild to moderate HS, particularly in younger female patients with a personal history of acne and weight below 75 kg. Among complete responders, 67% weighed under 75 kg, and the average age was 31.1 years, compared to 38.5 years in non-responders. However, its efficacy appears limited in patients with Hurley stage III disease, who comprised 50% of the non-responders [35]. Notably, there are reports of isotretinoin leading to the worsening HS or triggering new-onset HS in some patients [36].

Side effects of oral retinoids include xerosis and cheilitis, hyperlipidemia, and hepatotoxicity. Teratogenicity from oral retinoids is a significant limitation, requiring strict contraception in women of childbearing potential during therapy and even many years after therapy with the use of acitretin [37]. Further research is needed to better define the role of oral retinoids in HS management and identify patient subgroups likely to benefit.

Non-biologic Immunomodulators

Non-biologic immunomodulators that play a role in HS management include Janus kinase (JAK) inhibitors, phosphodiesterase 4 (PDE4) inhibitors, and traditional immunosuppressants such as prednisone and cyclosporine.

JAK inhibitors target intracellular signaling pathways that mediate proinflammatory cytokine activity [38]. Upadacitinib, a JAK1 selective inhibitor, had a positive phase 2 trial for HS, achieving Hidradenitis Suppurativa Clinical Response 50 (HiSCR50) in 38.3% of patients and a 36.4% reduction in skin pain at 12 weeks, with sustained responses through 40 weeks. It was effective and well tolerated, including in patients with inadequate anti-tumor necrosis factor-alpha (TNF-α) responses [39]. In a retrospective study of 20 patients with HS on upadacitinib, 75% achieved HiSCR50 by week 4 on 15 mg daily, increasing to 100% by week 12 after escalation to 30 mg for non-responders. Patients with Hurley stage III disease showed higher HiSCR response rates, greater reductions in disease severity scores, and more significant improvements in quality of life and pain scores compared to those with less severe disease [40]. The most common side effects of upadacitinib across all clinical trials include upper respiratory tract-related infection, nasopharyngitis, and increase in blood creatine phosphokinase levels [41].

PDE4 inhibitors, such as apremilast and roflumilast, act by increasing intracellular cyclic adenosine monophosphate (cAMP), which suppresses the production of pro-inflammatory cytokines like TNF-α and IL-6 [42]. Apremilast, at a dosage of 30 mg twice daily, demonstrated efficacy in a phase 2 trial for mild-to-moderate HS, achieving HiSCR30 in 65% of patients by week 24. Significant improvements were observed in disease activity, pain, and quality of life [43]. In a prospective single-center study involving 16 patients with severe, refractory HS, oral roflumilast demonstrated efficacy at a dosage of 500 μg/day, improving disease severity (e.g., International Hidradenitis Suppurativa Severity Scoring System [IHS4]) and quality of life scores. Notably, weight loss was also observed, with patients experiencing a median reduction of 9 kg (range: 0–13.5 kg), highlighting potential additional benefits for those with obesity [44]. Common side effects of PDE4 inhibitors include diarrhea and nausea.

Bridge Therapies

Cyclosporine and prednisone are traditional immunosuppressants that are not appropriate long-term therapeutic options for HS. Cyclosporine has a role as a bridge therapy for severe disease to appropriate long-term treatments such as biologics and surgery, and prednisone is a useful therapy to mitigate acute flares.

Cyclosporine, a calcineurin inhibitor, suppresses T-cell activation and the production of pro-inflammatory cytokines, such as IL-2 and IFN-γ [45]. There are limited case reports and case series supporting the use of cyclosporine in HS, typically at a dose ranging from 2.0 to 5.0 mg/kg/day. In a case series of 18 patients with severe, refractory HS, cyclosporine led to improvement in 50% of cases, though most patients (39% of the total) experienced only slight improvement, defined as symptom relief but not a major response. While cyclosporine at lower dosages can be effective, higher dosages (5.0–6.0 mg/kg/day) may be needed for some individuals to achieve therapeutic responses, as discussed in the case series [46]. However, these higher doses increase the risk of nephrotoxicity, hypertension, and infections associated with the use of cyclosporine given that the US FDA maximum dose is 4 mg/kg/day. Regular monitoring of lipids, electrolytes, renal function, uric acid, and blood pressure is essential during cyclosporine therapy [47].

Systemic corticosteroids (including prednisone, prednisolone, methylprednisolone, betamethasone, dexamethasone) exert potent anti-inflammatory effects that can rapidly reduce inflammation and pain in HS flares, making them a valuable option for rescue therapy. A case series of three patients demonstrated that intermittent low-dose corticosteroid therapy, using betamethasone 5 mg twice weekly (each dose equivalent to ~31 mg prednisone), led to near-complete remission in severe HS, with significant reductions in inflammation and minimal side effects over 14–17 months of treatment. Adjuvant therapies included spironolactone (n = 1), zinc (n = 2), and acitretin (n = 1) [48]. While intermittent corticosteroid use can be beneficial, long-term use is often limited by side effects such as hyperglycemia, sleep disturbances, osteoporosis, weight gain, increased infection risk, and the potential for withdrawal flares, particularly with higher doses [48, 49]. Prednisone is therefore typically reserved for short-term use.

Conclusion

HS requires a multimodal treatment approach tailored to the patient's disease severity and individual comorbidities. Combination therapy, involving the use of hormonal modulators, metabolic agents, biologics, and non-biologic immunomodulators and immunosuppressants, is often necessary to address the multifaceted nature of HS. Table 10.1 summarizes and reviews non-biologic immunomodulator and immunosuppressant therapeutics for HS.

Board Review Question Explanation

A 42-year-old male with a history of obesity and hypertension presents with Hurley Stage II hidradenitis suppurativa involving his bilateral axillae and groin. He is overall well controlled on adalimumab 80 mg every 2 weeks and finasteride 5 mg daily, but continues to experience very mild flares despite recently completing a 3-month course of doxycycline. Laboratory studies reveal elevated fasting insulin levels and HbA1c of 7.5%. Which of the following systemic therapies is the most appropriate next step in his management?

A. Acitretin
B. Drospirenone

Table 10.1 Non-biologic immunomodulator and immunosuppressant therapeutics for hidradenitis suppurativa

Medication	FDA-approved indications[a]	HS dosing suggestions	Strategies for use	Special considerations
Upadacitinib	Ankylosing spondylitis AxSpA RA Psoriatic arthritis Atopic dermatitis Ulcerative colitis Crohn's disease Polyarticular juvenile idiopathic arthritis	15–45 mg/day	Moderate-to-severe HS Leverage use in patients with concomitant IBD or atopic dermatitis	Consider in biologic candidates with needle phobia Caution in patients with clot history, high cardiovascular burden, malignancy or infection risks CBC, LFTs, lipid panel monitoring after screening labs
Apremilast, roflumilast	Apremilast Psoriatic arthritis Plaque psoriasis Oral ulcers associated with Behcet disease Roflumilast COPD	Apremilast: 30 mg BID Roflumilast:500 μg/day	Mild-to-moderate HS Combination therapy with biologic in severe HS	Consider in patients with needle phobia Caution in patients with history of depression and/or suicidality
Prednisone	Various steroid responsive allergic, dermatologic, gastrointestinal, hematologic, ophthalmologic, neurologic, renal, pulmonary, rheumatologic diseases Endocrine conditions Palliation for neoplastic conditions Organ transplantation	Variable, consider two-week taper for HS flares starting dose of 20 to 60 mg per day; utilize for shortest duration possible	Acute HS flares Bridge therapy	Limit to short term use if possible Can consider combining with an oral antibiotic such as amoxicillin-clavulanic acid for HS flares Consider TMP-SMX if on prednisone ≥20 mg/day for ≥4 weeks. Consider PPI or H2-antagonist if history of ulcers, NSAID use, or other risk factors Consider calcium, vitamin D ± bisphosphonates if corticosteroid use ≥3 months and with other risk factors (increased age, prior fragility fracture, etc.)

(continued)

Table 10.1 (continued)

Medication	FDA-approved indications[a]	HS dosing suggestions	Strategies for use	Special considerations
Cyclosporine	RA Psoriasis Prophylaxis of kidney, liver, and heart rejection	2–5 mg/kg/day; shortest duration possible, recommended duration <1 year	Severe, recalcitrant HS Bridge therapy	Avoid in patients with renal insufficiency or uncontrolled hypertension Monitor renal function, CBC, lipid panel, serum magnesium, serum potassium, blood glucose, LFTs, uric acid

AxSpA Axial spondyloarthritis, *BID* twice daily dosage, *CBC* complete blood count, *COPD* chronic obstructive pulmonary disease, *H2-antagonist* histamine type 2 receptor antagonist, *IBD* inflammatory bowel disease, *LFTs* liver function tests, *mg/kg/day* milligrams per kilogram per day, *NSAID* nonsteroidal anti-inflammatory drug, *PPI* proton pump inhibitor, *RA* rheumatoid arthritis, *TMP-SMX* trimethoprim-sulfamethoxazole

[a]FDA approved indications as of Feb 20, 2025

C. Metformin (Correct)
D. Prednisone
E. Spironolactone

Answer Explanation

Metformin is particularly beneficial for patients with HS who have comorbid obesity, type 2 diabetes, pre-diabetes, or insulin resistance. However, it should be noted that metformin can still be utilized in patients without insulin resistance. Metformin improves insulin sensitivity, reduces hyperinsulinemia, and has anti-inflammatory effects, including inhibition of the mTOR pathway, which is implicated in HS pathogenesis. For this patient, metformin may help address both his metabolic dysfunction and his HS, making it the most suitable next adjunctive option in management.

Option A: Spironolactone is typically used in women, especially if there are signs of hyperandrogenic conditions.

Option B: Although prednisone can be used to treat acute flares of HS, it is not routinely used as a long-term option for patients with HS due to its extensive side effect profile. Further, this patient's hypertension and now diabetes (given HbA1c 7.5%) makes this option even less desirable.

Option D: Acitretin is a possibility to be considered, but based on the patient's HbA1c, metformin would be preferred over acitretin as a next-line therapy to add.

Option E: Drospirenone is typically used in female patients who are unable to tolerate combined OCPs.

Key Takeaway Points

- Medical HS management requires an individualized, multimodal approach that integrates therapies targeting inflammation, metabolic dysfunction, and/or hormonal influences.
- Anti-androgen therapies, such as spironolactone, oral contraceptives, and finasteride, have been shown to be helpful in HS.
- Agents like metformin and GLP-1 agonists address metabolic comorbidities while reducing systemic inflammation and HS disease activity. These therapies are particularly beneficial in patients with obesity, insulin resistance, or type 2 diabetes.
- Oral retinoids, including isotretinoin and acitretin, target follicular plugging, but have mixed efficacy data, and there are reports of oral retinoids inducing HS flares.
- Small molecule inhibitors such as upadacitinib and apremilast may be considered as long-term therapeutic options for HS.
- Cyclosporine may be considered as a bridge therapy for severe HS, and prednisone may be used as a flare treatment.

References

1. Prens E, Deckers I. Pathophysiology of hidradenitis suppurativa: an update. J Am Acad Dermatol. 2015;73(5, Supplement 1):S8–S11. https://doi.org/10.1016/j.jaad.2015.07.045.
2. Vossen ARJV, van Straalen KR, Prens EP, van der Zee HH. Menses and pregnancy affect symptoms in hidradenitis suppurativa: a cross-sectional study. J Am Acad Dermatol. 2017;76(1):155–6. https://doi.org/10.1016/j.jaad.2016.07.024.
3. Riis PT, Ring HC, Themstrup L, Jemec GB. The role of androgens and estrogens in Hidradenitis Suppurativa – a systematic review. Acta Dermatovenerol Croat. 2016;24(4):239–49.
4. Kamal K, Afzal N, Ziad A, Charrow A. Association between exogenous testosterone use and new diagnosis of hidradenitis suppurativa: a case series. JAAD Case Rep. 2024;44:27–9. https://doi.org/10.1016/j.jdcr.2023.11.012.
5. Alikhan A, Sayed C, Alavi A, et al. North American clinical management guidelines for hidradenitis suppurativa: a publication from the United States and Canadian Hidradenitis Suppurativa Foundations. J Am Acad Dermatol. 2019;81(1):91–101. https://doi.org/10.1016/j.jaad.2019.02.068.
6. Golbari NM, Porter ML, Kimball AB. Antiandrogen therapy with spironolactone for the treatment of hidradenitis suppurativa. J Am Acad Dermatol. 2019;80(1):114–9. https://doi.org/10.1016/j.jaad.2018.06.063.
7. Masson R, Park SE, Shih T, Hogeling M, Shi VY, Hsiao JL. Spironolactone in hidradenitis suppurativa: a single-center. Int J Womens Dermatol. 2024;10(1):e135. https://doi.org/10.1097/JW9.0000000000000135.
8. Gangidi SV, Greene RK, Olsen E, Jackson S, Nakamura M. Efficacy of spironolactone in treating hidradenitis suppurativa in women of childbearing age: a single-center retrospective analysis. Int J Womens Dermatol. 2024;10(3):e159. https://doi.org/10.1097/JW9.0000000000000159.
9. Wang Y, Lipner SR. Retrospective analysis of adverse events with spironolactone in females reported to the United States food and drug administration. Int J Womens Dermatol. 2020;6(4):272–6. https://doi.org/10.1016/j.ijwd.2020.05.002.

10. Collins M, Ali S, Wiss IMP. 33244 Increased risk of hyperkalemia in older women taking spironolactone for female pattern hair loss. J Am Acad Dermatol. 2022;87(3):AB70. https://doi.org/10.1016/j.jaad.2022.06.315.
11. Montero-Vilchez T, Valenzuela-Amigo A, Cuenca-Barrales C, Arias-Santiago S, Leyva-García A, Molina-Leyva A. The role of oral contraceptive pills in Hidradenitis Suppurativa: a cohort study. Life Basel Switz. 2021;11(7):697. https://doi.org/10.3390/life11070697.
12. Assiri GA, Bannan DF, Alshehri GH, Alshyhani M, Almatri W, Mahmoud MA. The contraindications to combined oral contraceptives among reproductive-aged women in an obstetrics and gynaecology clinic: a single-centre cross-sectional study. Int J Environ Res Public Health. 2022;19(3):1567. https://doi.org/10.3390/ijerph19031567.
13. Regidor PA, Schindler AE. Antiandrogenic and antimineralocorticoid health benefits of COC containing newer progestogens: dienogest and drospirenone. Oncotarget. 2017;8(47):83334–42. https://doi.org/10.18632/oncotarget.19833.
14. Zhanel GG, Siemens S, Slayter K, Mandell L. Antibiotic and oral contraceptive drug interactions: Is there a need for concern? Can J Infect Dis. 1999;10(6):429–33.
15. Joseph MA, Jayaseelan E, Ganapathi B, Stephen J. Hidradenitis suppurativa treated with finasteride. J Dermatol Treat. 2005;16(2):75–8. https://doi.org/10.1080/09546630510031403.
16. Khandalavala BN, Do MV. Finasteride in Hidradenitis Suppurativa. J Clin Aesthetic Dermatol. 2016;9(6):44–50.
17. Babbush KM, Andriano TM, Cohen SR. Antiandrogen therapy in hidradenitis suppurativa: finasteride for females. Clin Exp Dermatol. 2022;47(1):86–92. https://doi.org/10.1111/ced.14847.
18. Mysore V. Finasteride and sexual side effects. Indian Dermatol Online J. 2012;3(1):62–5. https://doi.org/10.4103/2229-5178.93496.
19. BinJadeed HF, Alajlan A. Pregnancy and neonatal outcome with maternal exposure to finasteride: case series. J Dermatol Dermatol Surg. 2021;25(2):84. https://doi.org/10.4103/jdds.jdds_33_21.
20. Shalom G, Freud T, Harman-Boehm I, Polishchuk I, Cohen AD. Hidradenitis suppurativa and metabolic syndrome: a comparative cross-sectional study of 3207 patients. Br J Dermatol. 2015;173(2):464–70. https://doi.org/10.1111/bjd.13777.
21. Witte K, Wolk K, Witte-Händel E, Krause T, Kokolakis G, Sabat R. Targeting metabolic syndrome in Hidradenitis Suppurativa by phytochemicals as a potential complementary therapeutic strategy. Nutrients. 2023;15(17):3797. https://doi.org/10.3390/nu15173797.
22. Jennings L, Hambly R, Hughes R, Moriarty B, Kirby B. Metformin use in hidradenitis suppurativa. J Dermatol Treat. 2020;31(3):261–3. https://doi.org/10.1080/09546634.2019.1592100.
23. Hambly R, Kearney N, Hughes R, Fletcher JM, Kirby B. Metformin treatment of Hidradenitis Suppurativa: effect on metabolic parameters, inflammation, cardiovascular risk biomarkers, and immune mediators. Int J Mol Sci. 2023;24(8):6969. https://doi.org/10.3390/ijms24086969.
24. Amin S, Lux A, O'Callaghan F. The journey of metformin from glycaemic control to mTOR inhibition and the suppression of tumour growth. Br J Clin Pharmacol. 2019;85(1):37–46. https://doi.org/10.1111/bcp.13780.
25. Verdolini R, Clayton N, Smith A, Alwash N, Mannello B. Metformin for the treatment of hidradenitis suppurativa: a little help along the way. J Eur Acad Dermatol Venereol. 2013;27(9):1101–8. https://doi.org/10.1111/j.1468-3083.2012.04668.x.
26. Semaglutide Improves Hidradenitis Suppurativa in Patients With Obesity. AJMC. September 24, 2024. Accessed 2 Dec 2024. https://www.ajmc.com/view/semaglutide-improves-hidradenitis-suppurativa-in-patients-with-obesity
27. Nicolau J, Nadal A, Sanchís P, Pujol A, Masmiquel L, Nadal C. Liraglutide for the treatment of obesity among patients with hidradenitis suppurativa. Med Clin (Barc). 2024;162(3):118–22. https://doi.org/10.1016/j.medcli.2023.11.007.
28. Krajewski PK, Złotowska A, Szepietowski JC. The therapeutic potential of GLP-1 receptor agonists in the management of Hidradenitis Suppurativa: a systematic review of anti-inflammatory and metabolic effects. J Clin Med. 2024;13(21):6292. https://doi.org/10.3390/jcm13216292.

29. Lyons D, Louly Nathan A, Pender E, et al. Semaglutide for weight loss in people with obesity as an adjunctive treatment for hidradenitis suppurativa: its impact on disease control and quality of life. Br J Dermatol. 2024;191(4):631–3. https://doi.org/10.1093/bjd/ljae216.
30. Posada Posada MI, Alora MB, Lima XTV. Impact of semaglutide use in obese and diabetic patients with hidradenitis suppurativa. J Eur Acad Dermatol Venereol. Published online October. 2024;19 https://doi.org/10.1111/jdv.20392.
31. Filippatos TD, Panagiotopoulou TV, Elisaf MS. Adverse effects of GLP-1 receptor agonists. Rev Diabet Stud. 2014;11(3):202–30. https://doi.org/10.1900/RDS.2014.11.202.
32. Scott-Emuakpor R, Vuthaluru K, Nagre A, Jawed I, Patel PA, Sidhu HK. Role of oral retinoids in treatment of acne vulgaris with a bioinformatics-based perspective of personalized medicine. Cureus. 2023;15(4):e38019. https://doi.org/10.7759/cureus.38019.
33. Boer J, Nazary M. Long-term results of acitretin therapy for hidradenitis suppurativa. Is acne inversa also a misnomer? Br J Dermatol. 2011;164(1):170–5. https://doi.org/10.1111/j.1365-2133.2010.10071.x.
34. Matusiak Ł, Bieniek A, Szepietowski JC. Acitretin treatment for hidradenitis suppurativa: a prospective series of 17 patients. Br J Dermatol. 2014;171(1):170–4. https://doi.org/10.1111/bjd.12884.
35. Huang CM, Kirchhof MG. A new perspective on isotretinoin treatment of Hidradenitis Suppurativa: a retrospective chart review of patient outcomes. Dermatol Basel Switz. 2017;233(2-3):120–5. https://doi.org/10.1159/000477207.
36. Gallagher CG, Kirthi SK, Cotter CC, Revuz JR, Tobin AMT. Could isotretinoin flare hidradenitis suppurativa? A case series. Clin Exp Dermatol. 2019;44(7):777–80. https://doi.org/10.1111/ced.13944.
37. Mills CM, Marks R. Adverse reactions to oral retinoids. An update. Drug Saf. 1993;9(4):280–90. https://doi.org/10.2165/00002018-199309040-00006.
38. Lin CM, Cooles FA, Isaacs JD. Basic Mechanisms of JAK Inhibition. Mediterr J Rheumatol. 2020;31(Suppl 1):100–4. https://doi.org/10.31138/mjr.31.1.100.
39. Kimball AB, Ackerman L, Schlosser BJ, et al. 43799 efficacy and safety of upadacitinib in moderate-to-severe Hidradenitis Suppurativa: a phase 2, randomized, placebo-controlled study. J Am Acad Dermatol. 2023;89(3):AB42. https://doi.org/10.1016/j.jaad.2023.07.172.
40. Kozera E, Flora A, Frew JW. Real-world safety and clinical response of Janus kinase inhibitor upadacitinib in the treatment of hidradenitis suppurativa: a retrospective cohort study. J Am Acad Dermatol. 2022;87(6):1440–2. https://doi.org/10.1016/j.jaad.2022.07.047.
41. Mohamed MF, Bhatnagar S, Parmentier JM, Nakasato P, Wung P. Upadacitinib: Mechanism of action, clinical, and translational science. Clin Transl Sci. 2023;17(1):e13688. https://doi.org/10.1111/cts.13688.
42. Fan T, Wang W, Wang Y, et al. PDE4 inhibitors: potential protective effects in inflammation and vascular diseases. Front Pharmacol. 2024;15:1407871. https://doi.org/10.3389/fphar.2024.1407871.
43. Kerdel FR, Azevedo FA, Kerdel Don C, Don FA, Fabbrocini G, Kerdel FA. Apremilast for the treatment of mild-to-moderate Hidradenitis Suppurativa in a prospective, open-label, phase 2 study. J Drugs Dermatol. 2019;18(2):170–6.
44. Nielsen VW, Holgersen NK, Ring HC, et al. 52267 Effectiveness and safety of oral roflumilast in patients with hidradenitis suppurativa: a prospective single-center study. J Am Acad Dermatol. 2024;91(3):AB192. https://doi.org/10.1016/j.jaad.2024.07.765.
45. Tsuda K, Yamanaka K, Kitagawa H, et al. Calcineurin inhibitors suppress cytokine production from memory T cells and differentiation of naïve T cells into cytokine-producing mature T cells. PLoS One. 2012;7(2):e31465. https://doi.org/10.1371/journal.pone.0031465.
46. Anderson MD, Zauli S, Bettoli V, Boer J, Jemec GBE. Cyclosporine treatment of severe Hidradenitis suppurativa – a case series. J Dermatol Treat. 2016;27(3):247–50. https://doi.org/10.3109/09546634.2015.1088128.

47. Tapia C, Nessel TA, Zito PM. Cyclosporine. In: StatPearls. StatPearls Publishing; 2025. Accessed 20 Feb 2025. http://www.ncbi.nlm.nih.gov/books/NBK482450/.
48. Erlendsson AM, Lönndahl L, Killasli H. Intermittent low-dose corticosteroid therapy for hidradenitis suppurativa: a case series. JAAD Case Rep. 2021;13:105–8. https://doi.org/10.1016/j.jdcr.2021.05.023.
49. Puckett Y, Gabbar A, Bokhari AA. Prednisone. In: StatPearls. StatPearls Publishing; 2024. Accessed 6 Dec 2024. http://www.ncbi.nlm.nih.gov/books/NBK534809/.

Chapter 11
Treatment of HS with TNF-Alpha Inhibitors

Radhika Gupta and Victoria Fang

Case Title A 25-year-old female presents for evaluation for biologic therapy given painful, recurrent abscesses in her groin and axillae.

Case

A 25-year-old female presents with a 5-year history of painful, recurrent boils in her underarms and groin. She has tried oral doxycycline, topical clindamycin lotion, and topical chlorhexidine wash in the past. She continues to get flares once per month, which significantly impacts her quality of life. She has never had an intralesional corticosteroid injection. On examination, when you palpate an active lesion, purulence drains from her skin more than 3 centimeters away. Is biologic therapy appropriate?

Board Review Question

A 27-year-old female with multiple sclerosis presents with several abscesses, scars, and draining tunnels in her axillae and her inguinal folds. She has been on several months of oral doxycycline and trialed a myriad of topicals with no relief. She is inquiring about adalimumab, after hearing from a close friend with HS about the significant improvement on the medication. What treatment regimen would you recommend to her?

A. Start guselkumab (anti-IL23) with close monitoring
B. Start infliximab (anti-TNF) with close monitoring
C. Start adalimumab (anti-TNF) with close monitoring

R. Gupta
Perelman School of Medicine, University of Pennsylvania, Philadelphia, PA, USA
e-mail: Radhika.Gupta@Pennmedicine.upenn.edu

V. Fang (✉)
Department of Dermatology, University of Pennsylvania, Philadelphia, PA, USA
e-mail: victoria.fang@pennmedicine.upenn.edu

N. Brownstone (ed.), *Clinical Cases in Hidradenitis Suppurativa*, Clinical Cases in Dermatology, https://doi.org/10.1007/978-3-032-15200-8_11

D. Start secukinumab (anti-IL17) with close monitoring
E. Avoid biologics and continue current management

Role of Anti-TNF Therapies in HS Treatment Paradigm

Introduction to TNF Inhibition

While the precise mechanism of immune dysregulation in patients with hidradenitis suppurativa (HS) is not well established, there has been significant research in the field over the past decade to better understand the composition of inflammatory infiltrates in HS skin. Skin and serum from HS patients demonstrate upregulation of cytokines such as TNF, IL-17, and IFN- γ compared to healthy volunteers. Levels of TNF are positively correlated with disease severity and anti-TNF treatment can reduce proinflammatory cytokines [1]. Large randomized controlled clinical trials demonstrating efficacy of the anti-TNF biologic adalimumab resulted in it becoming the first FDA approved therapy for moderate to severe hidradenitis suppurativa in 2015. TNF inhibitors have become mainstays in the treatment paradigm for patients with HS.

Role in Treatment Algorithm

Although some patients prefer an initial trial of non-biologic therapy (such as oral antibiotics, hormonal agents, and topicals), TNF inhibitor treatment is indicated in any patient with moderate to severe disease, and this should be offered in combination with other medical and surgical management.

Contraindications

TNF inhibitors are contraindicated in patients with tuberculosis, sepsis, opportunistic infections, multiple sclerosis, and congestive heart failure. Patients should be screened for hepatitis B, and if positive, need to be on anti-viral therapy throughout their course of TNF inhibitor therapy, as well as 6 months after cessation. Although published data to date has been reassuring regarding the malignancy risk associated with TNF inhibitors, they should generally be avoided or used with caution within 5 years of active malignancy (i.e., non-Hodgkin lymphomas, Hodgkin lymphomas, leukemia, melanoma, or malignant neoplasms).

Treatment Guidelines for Anti-TNF Therapies

Adalimumab

For most patients with moderate to severe HS who are being evaluated for biologic medications after failing non-biologic treatments, adalimumab is the first-line therapy. The data from the PIONEER I and II clinical trials consisting of >600 patients showed a HiSCR50 of 51% at week 12 among patients on weekly 40 mg adalimumab versus 27% among patients receiving placebo [2, 3]. In an extension study, the response to weekly adalimumab was sustained in >50% of patients through week 168; however, it is important to recognize that the disease course may wax and wane. In patients who experience at least some improvement on adalimumab but continue to have disease activity, increasing the dose to 80 mg weekly can be helpful [4, 5]. On the other hand, among patients who see no improvement by week 12, response is unlikely and switching to a different biologic is reasonable.

Adalimumab biosimilars have recently come to market. There is sparse data comparing biosimilars to adalimumab, and changing patients from a biosimilar to adalimumab is done on a case-by-case basis depending on efficacy and adverse effects.

Infliximab

If patients have an inadequate response to adalimumab by week 12 or lose their response, infliximab is used by HS experts as an effective next line of therapy (although it has not been studied in large, randomized controlled trials) [6]. One advantage of infliximab is the weight-based dosing with the ability to increase the dosing and frequency to as high as 10 mg/kg every 4 weeks. One study showed that 71% of patients treated with 7.5 mg every 4 weeks achieve a good clinical response by week 12. Of those with an inadequate response at that dose, 50% were able to achieve a good clinical response with escalation to 10 mg/kg every 4 weeks [7]. Overall, patients generally require at least moderately high doses of infliximab, beginning at 7.5 mg/kg every 6 weeks and escalating, as needed, to a maximum of 10 mg/kg every 4 weeks.

Development of Anti-drug Antibodies

Anti-adalimumab or anti-infliximab antibodies may develop and can lead to a decrease in efficacy. In patients who respond initially to the drug and later lose efficacy, clinicians should obtain a trough drug level and test for the presence of anti-drug antibodies. Presently, the goal TNF inhibitor trough level is 8-20 μg/mL. For patients losing efficacy due to anti-drug antibodies, concomitant methotrexate treatment (10–15 mg weekly) along with daily folic acid can rescue their response.

Certolizumab

Unlike other anti-TNF agents, certolizumab lacks the IgG Fc portion, preventing active transport through the placenta [8–11]. Although certolizumab has much less evidence for its efficacy in HS, its hypothesized safety in pregnancy makes it an attractive medication to consider for pregnant women. Generally, patients experiencing efficacy with adalimumab or infliximab can remain on these medications once pregnant. Special considerations are discussed below for this patient population.

Special Populations

Populations to be cautious of when considering TNF inhibitors include pregnant patients and pediatric patients.

- *Pregnant or breastfeeding patients:* Because it does not cross the placenta, certolizumab is generally the safest TNF inhibitor to use in pregnancy, but there is limited evidence for its efficacy. Both adalimumab and infliximab are generally safe to use during pregnancy, although a risks and benefits discussion is advised, especially during the third trimester given the risk of immunosuppression in the newborn. [15] Postpartum, newborns of mothers on TNF inhibitors should avoid live vaccines for 6–12 months [12]. TNF inhibitors are safe for use by breastfeeding patients since these agents have large molecular weights that prevent them from entering breast milk [13].
- *Pediatric patients:* The use of TNF inhibitors among pediatric patients with HS has not been well studied; however, adalimumab is the most widely used biologic in the pediatric population with over 16 years of safety data in a myriad of other indications. In 2016, adalimumab was approved for use in patients with HS aged 12 and older.

If a patient fails the anti-TNF agents, consider switching to another class of biologics such as IL-17 inhibitors. Secukinumab and bimekizumab were FDA approved in 2023, and 2024, respectively. For those with contraindications to IL17 inhibitors, IL-12/23 inhibitors, IL-1 inhibitors, and small molecule inhibitors (apremilast, JAK inhibitors), can be considered.

Educating Patients about Anti-TNF Therapies

Adverse Effects

Prior to initiating TNF inhibitors, patients should be counselled on the adverse effects associated with the therapies. These include:

- *Injection site reactions* often occur within the first month of treatment and last 3–5 days after each injection. These can be treated with topical steroids, antihistamines, NSAIDs, acetaminophen, and ice. Some patients have benefited from a citrate-free formulation of adalimumab.
- *Infusion reactions* have been published in some patients treated with infliximab. These can be treated with transfusion interruption, slower infusion rates, antihistamines, and acetaminophen. To prevent reactions in the future, antihistamines, acetaminophen, and corticosteroids may be administered prior to the infusion.
- *Immunologic reactions*, including antibody development, TNF inhibitor-induced psoriasis or drug-induced lupus, have been documented. In these cases, treatment for those conditions may be required, in addition, to switching to a different agent.
- *Opportunistic infections*, including tuberculosis and invasive fungal infections, may occur at a higher rate among patients on TNF inhibitors; though, they are rare. They are more often seen in patients on concurrent immunosuppressive therapies.
- Other rare but reported side effects include new-onset or exacerbation of central or peripheral nervous system demyelinating disease such as multiple sclerosis, new-onset or worsening heart failure, hepatitis B reactivation, hepatoxicity, lymphoma or other malignancies.

Laboratory Monitoring

Given the increased risk of opportunistic infections, patients should be screened for hepatitis B and tuberculosis prior to initiating a TNF inhibitor. Clinicians can also consider obtaining an HIV test in high risk populations as well as a pregnancy screen in patients of childbearing potential. Follow up laboratory monitoring is individualized, but an annual repeat TB screen is commonly employed. Otherwise, patients should avoid live vaccines at least 4–6 weeks prior to starting therapy and remain up to date with age-appropriate cancer screenings [14].

Duration of Treatment

Neither adalimumab nor infliximab provide complete or long-lasting disease remission and are usually continued for as long as they are effective for patients. Table 11.1 reviews the dosing guidelines for anti-TNF biologics.

Board Review Question Explanation
A 27-year-old female with multiple sclerosis presents with several abscesses, scars, and draining tunnels in her axillae and her inguinal folds. She has been on several months of oral doxycycline and has tried numerous topicals with no relief. She is inquiring about adalimumab, after hearing from a close friend with HS about the significant improvement on the medication. What treatment regimen would you recommend to her?

A. Start guselkumab (anti-IL23) with close monitoring
B. Start infliximab (anti-TNF) with close monitoring
C. Start adalimumab (anti-TNF) alone with close monitoring
D. Start secukinumab (anti-IL17) with close monitoring (Correct)
E. Avoid biologics and continue current management

Answer Explanation
Adalimumab and other anti-TNF therapies (choices B, C) are contraindicated in patients with multiple sclerosis (MS). For patients with MS and HS who meet the criteria for biologic therapy, it is preferred to offer medications from other drug classes such as the recently approved IL-17 inhibitors secukinumab or bimekizumab. Although anti-IL23 biologics (choice A) can be trialed in refractory HS patients, recent randomized controlled studies did not achieve statistical

Table 11.1 Dosing guidelines for anti-TNF biologics

Anti-TNF agent	Dosing recommendations
Adalimumab (FDA approved)	Loading dose of 160 mg subcutaneously (SC) on day 1, then 80 mg SC on day 15, then 40 mg SC weekly starting on day 29 for maintenance. Alternative dosing regimen: Loading dose of 160 mg SC on day 1, then 80 mg SC on day 15, then 80 mg SC every 2 weeks starting on day 29 for maintenance. Maintenance dosing can be escalated to 80 mg SC weekly for either regimen
Infliximab (not FDA approved)	Loading dose of 7.5 mg/kg at weeks 0, 2, and 6 followed by 7.5 mg/kg every 6 weeks for maintenance. Dose escalation, especially for patients who flare just before infusions: Increase dose and/or frequency to as high as 10 mg/kg every 4 weeks
Certolizumab (not FDA approved)	Loading dose of 400 mg at weeks 0, 2, and 4; maintenance dose of 200 mg every 2 weeks OR 400 mg every 4 weeks (depending on patient weight)
Golimumab (not FDA approved)	Loading dose of the higher of 200 mg or 2 mg/kg IV week 0 and week 2, with maintenance dose of the higher of 200 mg or 2 mg/kg every 4 weeks thereafter

significance compared with placebo, and no anti-IL23 medications are approved for HS. Among the answer choices presented, secukinumab is the only IL-17 inhibitor.

Key Take Away Points

- For patients with moderate to severe HS, offer adalimumab. Response should be monitored at 12 weeks; after which, partial responders may benefit from dose escalation and non-responders or those who lose their response may be transitioned to infliximab.
- Prior to starting anti-TNF therapies, patients should be screened for Hepatitis B and TB. Physicians should also ask about contraindications to anti-TNF therapies and consider anti-IL17 biologics for patients with contraindications.
- Patients should be counseled on the side effects of using anti-TNF therapies including injection site reactions, infusion reactions, development of antibodies, and increased risk of infections.

References

1. van der Zee HH, de Ruiter L, van den Broecke DG, Dik WA, Laman JD, Prens EP. Elevated levels of tumour necrosis factor (TNF)-alpha, interleukin (IL)-1beta and IL-10 in hidradenitis suppurativa skin: a rationale for targeting TNF-alpha and IL-1beta. Br J Dermatol. 2011;164(6):1292–8. https://doi.org/10.1111/j.1365-2133.2011.10254.x.
2. Zouboulis CC, Okun MM, Prens EP, et al. Long-term adalimumab efficacy in patients with moderate-to-severe hidradenitis suppurativa/acne inversa: 3-year results of a phase 3 open-label extension study. J Am Acad Dermatol. 2019;80(1):60–69 e2. https://doi.org/10.1016/j.jaad.2018.05.040.
3. Jemec GBE, Okun MM, Forman SB, et al. Adalimumab medium-term dosing strategy in moderate-to-severe hidradenitis suppurativa: integrated results from the phase III randomized placebo-controlled PIONEER trials. Br J Dermatol. 2019;181(5):967–75. https://doi.org/10.1111/bjd.17919.
4. Zouboulis CC, Hansen H, Caposiena Caro RD, et al. Adalimumab dose intensification in recalcitrant Hidradenitis Suppurativa/Acne Inversa. Dermatology. 2020;236(1):25–30. https://doi.org/10.1159/000503606.
5. Williams J, Guzik C, Wadhera A, Naik H. Increased doses of adalimumab are associated with clinical improvement of Hidradenitis Suppurativa. J Drugs Dermatol. 2023;22(6):615–8. https://doi.org/10.36849/JDD.6868.
6. Shih T, Lee K, Grogan T, De DR, Shi VY, Hsiao JL. Infliximab in hidradenitis suppurativa: a systematic review and meta-analysis. Dermatol Ther. 2022;35(9):e15691. https://doi.org/10.1111/dth.15691.
7. Ghias MH, Johnston AD, Kutner AJ, Micheletti RG, Hosgood HD, Cohen SR. High-dose, high-frequency infliximab: a novel treatment paradigm for hidradenitis suppurativa. J Am Acad Dermatol. 2020;82(5):1094–101. https://doi.org/10.1016/j.jaad.2019.09.071.
8. Holm JG, Jorgensen AR, Yao Y, Thomsen SF. Certolizumab pegol for hidradenitis suppurativa: case report and literature review. Dermatol Ther. 2020;33(6):e14494. https://doi.org/10.1111/dth.14494.
9. Shadid A, Alobaida S, Binamer Y. Certolizumab to treat hidradenitis suppurativa. Dermatol Rep. 2023;15(2):9566. https://doi.org/10.4081/dr.2022.9566.
10. Esme P, Akoglu G, Caliskan E. Rapid response to Certolizumab Pegol in hidradenitis Suppurativa: a case report. Skin Appendage Disord. 2021;7(1):58–61. https://doi.org/10.1159/000511284.

11. Tampouratzi E, Kanni T, Katsantonis J, Douvali T. Case report: treating a co-existence of hidradenitis suppurativa and psoriasis with different therapeutic approaches. F1000Res. 2019;8:2002. https://doi.org/10.12688/f1000research.21216.2.
12. Gisbert JP, Chaparro M. Vaccines in children exposed to biological agents in utero and/or during breastfeeding: are they effective and safe? J Crohns Colitis. 2023;17(6):995–1009. https://doi.org/10.1093/ecco-jcc/jjad005.
13. Chellappan B, Nguyen DDQ, Hoyer P, Ross L. Dermatologic management of Hidradenitis Suppurativa and Impact on pregnancy and breastfeeding. Cutis. 2022;109(3):160–2. https://doi.org/10.12788/cutis.0480.
14. Chat VS, Ellebrecht CT, Kingston P, et al. Vaccination recommendations for adults receiving biologics and oral therapies for psoriasis and psoriatic arthritis: Delphi consensus from the medical board of the National Psoriasis Foundation. J Am Acad Dermatol. 2024;90(6):1170–81. https://doi.org/10.1016/j.jaad.2023.12.070.
15. Collier EK, Seivright JR, Shi VY, Hsiao JL. Pregnancy and breastfeeding in hidradenitis suppurativa: a review of medication safety. Dermatol Ther. 2021;34(1):e14674.

Chapter 12
Treatment of HS with Secukinumab

Julienne Zhou and Graham H. Litchman

Case Title A 35 year-old female presents with chronic, painful, recurring "boils" under her arms and in her groin.

Case

You are seeing a 35-year-old female who complains of chronic, painful, recurrent "boils" under her arms and in her groin for the past several months. The lesions often drain pus and she has noticed scarring in these areas. On examination, you observe tender, erythematous nodules and abscesses, some of which have draining tunnels, in both the axillae and inguinal folds. The lesions have not improved despite multiple courses of oral antibiotics. The patient notes a history of smoking and obesity. She has been previously diagnosed with moderate-to-severe hidradenitis suppurativa (HS) and is interested in learning more about treatment options, particularly the use of biologics like secukinumab. How do you respond?

Board Review Question

Which of the following therapies targets IL-17A and has shown efficacy in reducing draining tunnels in recent clinical trials such as SUNRISE and SUNSHINE?

A. Adalimumab
B. Secukinumab
C. Ustekinumab
D. Methotrexate
E. Apremilast

J. Zhou
Touro University Nevada College of Osteopathic Medicine, Henderson, NV, USA

G. H. Litchman (✉)
Vivida Dermatology, Las Vegas, NV, USA

N. Brownstone (ed.), *Clinical Cases in Hidradenitis Suppurativa*, Clinical Cases in Dermatology, https://doi.org/10.1007/978-3-032-15200-8_12

Introduction

Hidradenitis suppurativa (HS) is a chronic, recurrent inflammatory skin disease that primarily affects apocrine gland-bearing areas, such as the axillae, groin, and inframammary regions. Characterized by painful nodules, abscesses, and sinus tracts, HS significantly impacts patients' quality of life, often leading to physical discomfort, malodor, and psychological distress [1]. The prevalence of HS is estimated to range from 1% to 4%, with a female predominance and a notable association with obesity, smoking, and metabolic syndrome [2].

The disease progresses through three stages as defined by the Hurley classification: Stage I involves isolated nodules and abscesses without sinus tracts; stage II presents with recurrent lesions and sinus tracts, often in multiple areas; and stage III includes diffuse involvement with interconnected sinus tracts and extensive scarring (Fig. 12.1) [3]. Despite advances in the understanding of HS, its pathogenesis remains incompletely understood, though it is widely recognized as a multifactorial disorder involving genetic predisposition, immune dysregulation, and environmental triggers [4].

The limited efficacy of existing treatments in managing severe HS has driven interest in targeted biologic therapies, including secukinumab. Secukinumab, a fully human monoclonal antibody targeting interleukin-17A (IL-17A), has emerged as a potential breakthrough in HS treatment due to its anti-inflammatory mechanism and its demonstrated efficacy in related diseases like psoriasis and ankylosing spondylitis. This chapter explores secukinumab's benefits, limitations, and its role in HS management.

Pathophysiology of HS and the Role of IL-17A

HS is driven by dysregulation of the innate and adaptive immune systems, particularly in the IL-23/IL-17 inflammatory axis. IL-17A, a cytokine central to neutrophil recruitment and activation, contributes to the chronic inflammation observed in HS

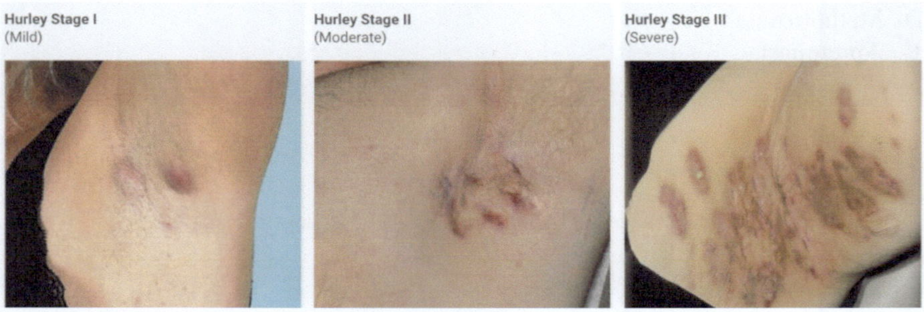

Fig. 12.1 Hurley staging system for HS

lesions, promoting abscess formation and tissue damage. Elevated IL-17A levels have been detected in HS lesional skin, correlating with disease severity [5]. This understanding has catalyzed the exploration of IL-17A inhibitors like secukinumab as a therapeutic option.

The Role of Draining Tunnels in HS

Draining tunnels, or sinus tracts, are among the most debilitating features of advanced HS. These lesions form as chronic inflammation leads to the breakdown of skin and subcutaneous tissue, creating interconnected channels that allow for persistent drainage of inflammatory material. Sinus tracts are associated with severe pain, recurrent infections, and malodor, which contribute to the psychosocial burden of HS [6]. Traditional treatments, including systemic antibiotics and TNF inhibitors, often fail to adequately address draining tunnels, necessitating the exploration of alternative therapies [7].

Secukinumab: A Breakthrough in HS Management

Secukinumab is a fully human monoclonal antibody targeting IL-17A and is FDA approved to treat HS. By inhibiting IL-17A, secukinumab reduces neutrophil recruitment and interrupts the inflammatory cascade that drives the formation of nodules, abscesses, and draining tunnels [8]. This specific mechanism offers an advantage over broad-spectrum immunosuppressants by minimizing side effects while effectively addressing key drivers of HS pathology [9]. The drug has already been FDA approved for the treatment of psoriasis, psoriatic arthritis, and ankylosing spondylitis, where it has demonstrated robust efficacy and a favorable safety profile [10].

In HS, secukinumab's efficacy has been evaluated in two pivotal Phase III trials: SUNSHINE and SUNRISE. These identical, randomized, double-blind, multicenter studies assessed the drug's performance in patients with moderate to severe HS over short-term (16-week) and long-term (1-year) periods. Both trials compared two dosing regimens: 300 mg every 2 weeks (Q2W) and every 4 weeks (Q4W), following an initial five-dose (Q1W) loading phase. The primary endpoint, HiSCR50 (50% reduction in abscess and nodule count without an increase in draining tunnels), was achieved in significantly more patients receiving secukinumab Q2W compared to placebo at week 16 [11].

In addition to meeting its primary endpoint, secukinumab reduced the formation and progression of draining tunnels, a symptom poorly managed by traditional therapies. Patients receiving secukinumab Q2W were less likely to experience an increase in the number of draining tunnels compared to those on placebo by week 16 [12]. This effect was sustained through week 52, with patients in both dosing groups showing stabilization or reduction in draining tunnels. These findings highlight secukinumab's potential to provide long-term control of one of HS's most challenging symptoms [13].

Sinus tract reduction is particularly important in HS management because these lesions are often refractory to conventional treatments and require invasive procedures, such as surgical excision or laser therapy, to achieve resolution. Secukinumab offers a non-surgical alternative for addressing sinus tracts, reducing the need for invasive interventions and improving patient outcomes [14]. Sustained control of disease activity over 1 year highlights secukinumab's potential as a long-term treatment option for refractory HS [15].

Comparison with Existing Therapies

Adalimumab, a TNF-α inhibitor, is currently the only FDA-approved biologic for HS which blocks TNF-α. While effective for some, approximately half of HS patients fail to achieve adequate response, underscoring the need for alternatives. Secukinumab offers a different mechanism, targeting IL-17A rather than TNF-α, potentially benefiting patients unresponsive to TNF inhibitors. Preliminary data suggest that secukinumab may provide greater efficacy in reducing draining tunnels and improving quality of life metrics [16].

Safety and Tolerability

Secukinumab has demonstrated a favorable safety profile in HS, consistent with its use in other indications such as psoriasis and ankylosing spondylitis. Adverse events reported in the SUNSHINE and SUNRISE trials were generally mild, including upper respiratory tract infections and injection site reactions [15]. Serious adverse events were rare and no new safety concerns were identified.

Compared to TNF inhibitors, secukinumab is associated with a lower risk of tuberculosis reactivation and other systemic infections, making it a safer option for patients with comorbidities or contraindications to TNF inhibition [4]. However, long-term safety data specific to HS are still emerging, necessitating ongoing monitoring and research.

Dosing Regimens

The approved dosing regimen for secukinumab in HS involves a loading phase of 300 mg administered weekly for 5 weeks (at weeks 0, 1, 2, 3, and 4), followed by maintenance doses every 4 weeks. For patients with inadequate response, increasing the frequency to every 2 weeks may enhance efficacy [17]. This flexible dosing strategy allows for tailored treatment, addressing varying levels of disease severity.

Combining secukinumab with adjunctive treatments, such as antibiotics or surgical interventions for severe sinus tracts, may enhance overall outcomes. Early integration into multidisciplinary management plans could maximize its benefits, particularly in stage II and III HS [18].

Benefits of Secukinumab

1. *Targeted Mechanism*: By selectively inhibiting IL-17A, secukinumab directly addresses the inflammatory pathways central to HS pathogenesis.
2. *Efficacy in Refractory Cases*: Secukinumab provides an option for patients unresponsive to TNF inhibitors, have relative contraindications to TNF inhibitors, or are unresponsive to other traditional systemic therapies.
3. *Impact on Draining Tunnels*: Reduction and stabilization of draining tunnels represent a significant advancement, addressing one of HS's most debilitating symptoms.
4. *Favorable Safety Profile*: With relatively mild side effects, secukinumab is well-tolerated, making it suitable for long-term use.

Limitations and Challenges

1. *Cost and Accessibility*: Like other biologics, secukinumab is expensive, potentially limiting access for uninsured or underinsured patients.
2. *Delayed Onset of Action*: While effective, secukinumab may take several weeks to achieve noticeable improvement, which can be challenging for patients seeking immediate relief.
3. *Incomplete Response in Some Patients*: A subset of patients may not achieve satisfactory outcomes, necessitating alternative or combination therapies.
4. *Need for Long-Term Data*: While short-term results are promising, data on the long-term efficacy and safety of secukinumab in HS remain limited.

Emerging Therapies and Future Directions

Secukinumab represents a significant advancement in HS treatment, and ongoing research is focused on expanding the therapeutic potential of secukinumab in HS, including:

- *Biomarker Identification*: Identifying predictors of response to secukinumab could help personalize treatment, improving efficacy and cost-effectiveness.
- *Combination Approaches*: Integrating secukinumab with emerging therapies, such as JAK inhibitors or microbiome-targeted interventions, may offer synergistic benefits.
- *Patient-Centered Outcomes*: Studies emphasizing quality of life, mental health, and patient-reported outcomes will further clarify secukinumab's role in comprehensive HS care.

Additionally, inhibitors of the JAK-STAT pathway, such as tofacitinib, are being investigated as additional therapeutic options for their ability to module immune responses in HS [19]. Similarly, therapies targeting the IL-23 pathway, including guselkumab, have shown early promise in reducing inflammation and lesion count [20].

Beyond biologics, research on the microbiome's role in HS is being recognized. Dysbiosis in lesional skin may exacerbate inflammation and contribute to disease progression. Future therapies could involve probiotics, prebiotics, or microbiota transplantation to restore microbial balance and improve clinical outcomes [21].

Addressing the Psychosocial Burden

The impact of HS extends beyond physical symptoms, as patients often experience depression and anxiety due to the visible and painful nature of the disease. Draining tunnels, in particular, contribute to feelings of embarrassment and social isolation. Comprehensive management strategies that combine biologic therapies with mental health support and patient education are essential for improving long-term outcomes [22]. Secukinumab's demonstrated ability to reduce draining tunnels and other symptoms has the potential to significantly enhance patients' quality of life.

Conclusion

Secukinumab is a promising advancement in the treatment of hidradenitis suppurativa as it was the first biologic approved for HS that specifically targets the IL-17 cytokine. By addressing the IL-17A-driven inflammatory cascade, secukinumab provides benefits for patients with moderate to severe HS, particularly those unresponsive to TNF inhibitors. Its efficacy in reducing draining tunnels is particularly noteworthy, addressing a critical unmet need in HS management, providing a non-surgical option for addressing one of the most challenging aspects of the disease. As research continues, the integration of novel biologic therapies with holistic patient care approaches will be critical for the advancement of treatment.

Board Review Question Explanation

Which of the following therapies targets IL-17A and has shown efficacy in reducing draining tunnels in recent clinical trials such as SUNRISE and SUNSHINE?

A. Adalimumab
B. Secukinumab (Correct)
C. Ustekinumab
D. Methotrexate
E. Apremilast

Answer Explanation

Secukinumab, a monoclonal antibody that selectively inhibits interleukin-17A (IL-17A), has demonstrated efficacy in treating moderate-to-severe hidradenitis suppurativa (HS). The SUNRISE and SUNSHINE clinical trials investigated secukinumab's role in reducing draining tunnels, a hallmark of severe HS, and showed promising results in reducing disease severity. IL-17A plays a significant role in the inflammatory cascade associated with HS, making secukinumab an effective targeted therapy.

- *Adalimumab:* A TNF-alpha inhibitor, adalimumab is FDA-approved for HS and often a first-line biologic for this condition. However, it does not target IL-17A.
- *Secukinumab:* Correct answer. Targets IL-17A and has shown efficacy in SUNRISE and SUNSHINE trials for HS.
- *Ustekinumab:* An IL-12/IL-23 inhibitor used for psoriasis and Crohn's disease but not shown to be effective for HS.
- *Methotrexate:* An immunosuppressant used for autoimmune diseases like rheumatoid arthritis, but it is not effective in treating HS or targeting IL-17A.
- *Apremilast:* A phosphodiesterase-4 (PDE4) inhibitor used for psoriasis and psoriatic arthritis, but it is not indicated for HS or IL-17A-related pathways.

Key Takeaway Points

- HS is a chronic, inflammatory skin disorder primarily affecting apocrine gland-bearing areas.
- HS typically presents with recurrent, painful nodules and abscesses in areas like the axillae and groin, with a tendency for scarring and sinus tract formation.
- Risk factors for HS include obesity, smoking, and a family history.
- The histopathological pattern of HS involves follicular occlusion, inflammation, and sinus tract formation.
- Secukinumab, an IL-17A inhibitor, offers a novel therapeutic option for moderate-to-severe HS patients with inadequate response to conventional therapies, particularly in cases with draining tunnels to help reduce inflammation and lesion formation.

References

1. Jemec GB. Clinical practice. Hidradenitis suppurativa. N Engl J Med. 2012;366(2):158–64. https://doi.org/10.1056/NEJMcp1014163.
2. Nguyen TV, Damiani G, Orenstein LA, Hamzavi IH, Jemec GB. Hidradenitis suppurativa: an update on pathogenesis, diagnosis, and treatment. J Am Acad Dermatol. 2021;84(5):1047–58. https://doi.org/10.1016/j.jaad.2020.07.081.
3. Hidradenitis Suppurativa Disease Staging. HS Disease Source. Accessed 14 Sept 2024. https://www.hsdiseasesource.com/hs-disease-staging.
4. Frew JW, Navrazhina K, Ingram JK, et al. Hidradenitis suppurativa: current understanding and research priorities. J Invest Dermatol. 2021;141(5):1121–30. https://doi.org/10.1016/j.jid.2020.10.029.
5. Hoffman LK, Ghias MH, Lowes MA. Pathophysiology of hidradenitis suppurativa. Semin Cutan Med Surg. 2017;36(2):47–54. https://doi.org/10.12788/j.sder.2017.006.
6. Vekic DA, Frew JW, Woods J, et al. Evaluating the burden of disease in hidradenitis suppurativa. Br J Dermatol. 2019;180(2):484–6. https://doi.org/10.1111/bjd.16690.
7. Saunte DM, Jemec GB. Hidradenitis suppurativa: advances in diagnosis and treatment. JAMA. 2017;318(20):2019–30. https://doi.org/10.1001/jama.2017.13714.
8. Menter A, Gelfand JM, Connor C, et al. Secukinumab in plaque psoriasis: long-term safety and efficacy in a randomized, double-blind, placebo-controlled trial. J Am Acad Dermatol. 2016;75(3):377–86. https://doi.org/10.1016/j.jaad.2016.06.001.
9. Kromann CB, Deckers IE, Esmann S, et al. Quality of life and disease impact in hidradenitis suppurativa. Dermatol. 2019;236(1):3–8. https://doi.org/10.1159/000495150.
10. Thaci D, Blauvelt A, Reich K, et al. Secukinumab is effective in hidradenitis suppurativa: results from SUNSHINE AND SUNRISE phase III studies. Br J Dermatol. 2023;188(5):724–35. https://doi.org/10.1111/bjd.21415.
11. FDA. Highlights of prescribing information for secukinumab (Cosentyx). FDAgov. Published 2022. Accessed Nov 2024. https://www.hsdiseasesource.com/hs-disease-staging.
12. Villani AP, Fabbrocini G, Cappelli A, et al. IL-17A inhibitors for hidradenitis suppurativa: emerging data and clinical considerations. Dermatol Ther. 2023;36(3):e16019. https://doi.org/10.1111/dth.16019.
13. Navrazhina K, Frew JW. Systemic therapies for hidradenitis suppurativa: current trends and future directions. Dermatol Ther. 2022;35(3):e15309. https://doi.org/10.1111/dth.15309.
14. Lavogiez C, Delaporte E, Darras-Vercambre S, et al. Hidradenitis suppurativa: pathogenesis and future perspectives. J Eur Acad Dermatol Venereol. 2016;30(6):987–95. https://doi.org/10.1111/jdv.13467.
15. Zouboulis CC, Kimball AB, Okun MM, et al. Secukinumab in hidradenitis Suppurativa: primary results from two phase 3, randomized, double-blind, placebo-controlled trials (SUNSHINE and SUNRISE). Lancet. 2023;401(10385):201–12. https://doi.org/10.1016/S0140-6736(22)02481-5.
16. Ingram JR, Woo PN, Chua SL, et al. Interventions for hidradenitis suppurativa: a cochrane systematic review incorporating GRADE assessment of evidence quality. Br J Dermatol. 2016;174(5):970–8. https://doi.org/10.1111/bjd.14425.
17. Ghias MH, Johnston AD, Kutner AJ, Murina A. Hidradenitis suppurativa and mental health: a scoping review and discussion. Dermatology. 2021;237(5):865–75. https://doi.org/10.1159/000512717.
18. Gottlieb AB, Armstrong AW, Le Bras MH, et al. A prospective, randomized study of secukinumab efficacy and safety in patients with moderate to severe psoriasis and psoriatic arthritis: impact on comorbid hidradenitis suppurativa. Arthritis Res Ther. 2017;19(1):132. https://doi.org/10.1186/s13075-017-1319-5.
19. Cleveland Clinic. Hidradenitis suppurativa: causes, symptoms, and treatments. Published 2024. Accessed Nov 2024. https://my.clevelandclinic.org/health/diseases/21693-hidradenitis-suppurativa.

20. Ring HC, Riis PT, Miller IM, et al. The microbiome of tunnels in hidradenitis suppurativa. Br J Dermatol. 2017;177(4):e203–5. https://doi.org/10.1111/bjd.15490.
21. Kelly G, Hughes R, McGarry T, et al. Dysregulated cytokine expression in hidradenitis suppurativa skin and the response to anti-TNF-α therapy. J Invest Dermatol. 2020;140(4):709–12. https://doi.org/10.1016/j.jid.2019.09.019.
22. van der Zee HH, de Ruiter L, Boer J, et al. Alterations in regulatory T-cell populations in hidradenitis suppurativa. Br J Dermatol. 2018;178(4):994–1002. https://doi.org/10.1111/bjd.16194.

Chapter 13
Treatment of HS with Bimekizumab

Lauren S. Jones and Cynthia L. Bartus

Case Title A 41-year-old female with a history of breast cancer presents with extensive history of recurrent abscesses and extensive scarring in the groin and axilla.

Case

A patient presents to your clinic with reports of recurrent abscesses and extensive scarring in her groin. She has had this condition for the past 20 years and was previously diagnosed with hidradenitis suppurativa (HS). Other significant past medical history includes stage I breast cancer diagnosed 2 years prior. She is in remission after a lumpectomy and local radiation. She has been to the emergency room numerous times seeking treatment for the abscesses. She has tried multiple treatments including oral steroids, topical and oral antibiotics, weight loss, and deroofing procedures. She previously tried adalimumab therapy in the past year but had minimal improvement of her abscesses on 6 months of therapy. The abscesses are painful, constantly draining, and impact her quality of life. On physical exam, you note 2 abscesses and 3 nodules in the groin. Sinus tract formation and purulent drainage is present. There is extensive scarring in the groin and bilateral axilla. Based on this presentation and history, a diagnosis of moderate-to-severe grade hidradenitis suppurativa is confirmed. The patient would like to know if there are any systemic medication options available to her given her prior history of breast cancer. How do you respond?

L. S. Jones (✉)
Lehigh Valley Health Network, Dermatology Residency Program, Allentown, PA, USA
e-mail: ljones@adaltd.com

C. L. Bartus
Lehigh Valley Health Network, Dermatology Residency Program,
Advanced Dermatology Associates, LTD., Allentown, PA, USA
e-mail: cbartus@adaltd.com

N. Brownstone (ed.), *Clinical Cases in Hidradenitis Suppurativa*, Clinical Cases in Dermatology, https://doi.org/10.1007/978-3-032-15200-8_13

Board Review Question
What is the mechanism of action of bimekizumab?

A. TNF-a inhibition
B. Only IL-17A inhibition
C. IL-12/23 inhibition
D. IL-17A/F inhibition
E. IL-31 inhibition

Practical Pearls for Treatment of HS with Bimekizumab

Patients with hidradenitis suppurativa (HS) often have prolonged, complicated clinical courses requiring trial and error of numerous therapies before achieving meaningful clinical improvement [1]. Effective treatment requires multiple specialists and multiple treatment modalities including topical, systemic, surgical, and laser therapies [2]. Traditional systemic treatment of HS has been limited to oral antibiotics and systemic steroids [2, 3]. Due to the lack of effective and sustainable systemic therapies, there has been significant research and clinical effort focused on the development of new therapies, including biologics, to target mediators of HS [3]. Biologics are defined as complex molecules derived from living organisms and include monoclonal antibodies, vaccines, gene therapy, and recombinant therapeutic proteins [4].

To date, there are three biologics approved for HS: adalimumab, secukinumab, and bimekizumab (Table 13.1). Adalimumab is a fully human, immunoglobulin G1 (IgG1) monoclonal antibody specific for tumor necrosis factor-alpha (TNF-a) and was first FDA approved for HS in 2015 [5]. Secukinumab is a human IgG1 monoclonal antibody that selectively binds to interleukin 17A (IL-17A) cytokine and inhibits interaction with IL-17 receptor complex. It was FDA-approved for HS in 2023 [5]. Bimekizumab, also known as bimekizumab (Bimzelx), is a recombinant, humanized IgG1/κ monoclonal antibody with identical-coupled antigen binding regions that selectively bind to interleukin 17A (IL-17A), IL17F, and IL-17-AF cytokines and subsequently inhibits the interaction with the IL-17 receptor complex [6]. Bimekizumab was FDA approved for hidradenitis suppurativa (HS) on in November 2024 [7]. It has four other indications including plaque psoriasis, psoriatic arthritis, non-radiographic axial spondylarthritis (nraxSpA), and ankylosing spondylitis [6]. Through multiple phase 2 and phase 3 trials, bimekizumab has been shown to be an effective and safe treatment option for patients with moderate-to-severe HS [8, 9]. The most reported treatment-emergent adverse event (TEAEs) is infection, most notably oral candidiasis [8–19].

Bimekizumab has been shown to be safe and effective in patients with psoriasis and psoriatic arthritis that previously failed other biologics including TNF-a inhibitors and other IL-17 inhibitors [13–19]. Additionally, the association of TNF-a inhibitors with the development of malignancy is unclear and available data is

Table 13.1 FDA-approved biologics for Hidradenitis Suppurativa (HS)

Name	Indication and usage for HS	MOA	Dosing	HiSCR50[b]	Adverse reactions	Warnings and precautions	Absolute contraindications
Adalimumab	Moderate-to-severe disease[a]; patients 12 years or older	Fully human, IgG1 monoclonal antibody specific for TNF-α	Adults: Loading dose: 160 mg Week 2: 80 mg Week 4 and subsequent/ maintenance doses: 40 mg every week or 80 mg every other week Adolescents 12 years of age and older: Adolescent Weight recommended dosage 30 kg (66 lbs) to less than 60 kg (132 lbs) Loading: 80 mg Day 8 and subsequent doses: 40 mg every other week 60 kg (132 lbs) and greater Loading dose: 160 mg (given in 1 day or split over two consecutive days) Week 2: 80 mg Week 4 and subsequent doses: 40 mg every week or 80 mg every other week	PIONEER I: Adalimumab 40 mg weekly—42% Placebo—26% (12 weeks) PIONEER II: Adalimumab 40 mg weekly—59% Placebo—28% (12 weeks)	Infection Headache Nasopharyngitis Cancer Psoriasis Worsening of existing disease/HS flare Anti-drug antibody development	Serious infections Invasive fungal infections Malignancies Anaphylaxis or serious hypersensitivity reactions Hepatitis B virus reactivation Demyelinating disease Cytopenias Heart failure Lupus-like syndrome	None

(continued)

Table 13.1 (continued)

Name	Indication and usage for HS	MOA	Dosing	HiSCR50[b]	Adverse reactions	Warnings and precautions	Absolute contraindications
Secukinumab	Adults with moderate-to-severe disease[a]	Human IgG1 monoclonal antibody that selectively binds to IL-17A cytokine, inhibits interaction with IL-17 receptor complex	300 mg administered by subcutaneous injection at weeks 0, 1, 2, 3, and 4 and every 4 weeks thereafter If a patient does not adequately respond, consider increasing the dosage to 300 mg every 2 weeks	SUNSHINE: Secukinumab 300 mg q4 weeks—41.3% Secukinumab 300 mg q2 week—44.5% Placebo—29.4% (week 16) SUNRISE: Secukinumab 300 mg q4 weeks—42.5% Secukinumab 300 mg q2 week—38.3% Placebo—26.1% (week 16)	Nasopharyngitis Diarrhea Upper respiratory tract infection	Infections Serious hypersensitivity reactions Tuberculosis Inflammatory bowel disease Eczematous eruptions Avoid use of live vaccines during treatment	Hypersensitivity reaction to secukinumab and/or inactive ingredients
Bimekizumab	Adults with moderate-to-severe disease[a]	Humanized IgG1/ κ monoclonal antibody with two identical antigen binding regions that selectively bind to IL-17A, IL17F, and IL-17-AF cytokines, inhibits interaction with IL-17 receptor complex	Administer 320 mg by subcutaneous injection at week 0, 2, 4, 6, 8, 10, 12, 14, and 16, then every 4 weeks thereafter	BE HEARD I: Bimekizumab-bkzx 320 mg q2 weeks until week 48 48% Placebo 29% (week 16) BE HEARD II: Bimekizumab-bkzx 320 mg q2 weeks until week 48–52% Placebo—32% (week 16)	Upper respiratory tract infections Oral candidiasis Headache Injection site reactions Tinea infections Gastroenteritis Herpes simplex infections Acne Folliculitis Other candida infections Fatigue	Suicidal ideation and behavior Infections Tuberculosis Liver biochemical abnormalities—elevated transaminases Inflammatory bowel disease Avoid use of live vaccines during treatment	None

Abbreviations: *HiSCR* Hidradenitis Suppurativa Clinical Response, *TNF-a* tumor necrosis factor-alpha, *IL17A* interleukin-17A, *IL 17A/F* interleukin-17A/F

[a]Moderate-to-severe disease as determined by the inflammatory component of disease, requiring a minimum combined number of abscesses (A) and inflammatory nodules (N), known as the abscess and nodule count, of 3 to 5, or at least 6 months of Hurley Stage II or Stage III disease

[b]HiSCR is defined as at least a 50% reduction in total abscess and inflammatory nodule count with no increase in abscess count and no increase in draining fistula count relative to baseline

inconsistent, with some research citing increased risk of lymphoma and non-melanoma skin cancer, whereas others suggest comparable rates to the general population [20, 21]. Therefore, until this relationship is better understood, bimekizumab may serve as an alternative treatment option for patients who have a history of malignancy such as lymphoma and/or who developed malignancy while undergoing TNF-a treatment [20, 21].

Safety and Efficacy of Bimekizumab

The safety and efficacy of bimekizumab was primarily evaluated through two phase 3 clinical trials, BE HEARD I and II [8]. These trials were randomized, double-blinded, placebo-controlled, multicenter, phase 3 trials conducted over 48 weeks. The design of the trials was almost identical. They both included patients who were 18 years or older with moderate-to-severe HS as defined as at least five inflammatory skin lesions (abscesses and/or inflammatory nodules) in at least two separate anatomical locations and diagnosed greater than 6 months prior to the baseline visit. Patients were allowed to continue oral antibiotic treatment during the trial if they were on a stable dose. Patients were randomized between four clinical pathways: (1) bimekizumab 320 mg every 2 weeks to week 48; (2) bimekizumab 320 mg every 2 weeks to week 16, followed by every 4 weeks to week 48; (3) bimekizumab 320 mg every 4 weeks to week 48; and (4) placebo to week 16 followed by bimekizumab 320 mg every 2 weeks to week 48.

The primary outcome of the trials was hidradenitis suppurativa clinical response 50 (HiSCR50), which is defined as a reduction in lesion count of at least 50% from baseline at week 16. Secondary outcomes included hidradenitis suppurativa clinical response 75 (HiSCR75, defined as a reduction in lesion count of at least 75% from baseline at week 16) flare count at week 16 (BE HEARD II only, >/=25% increase in abscess and inflammatory nodule count with an increase of at least two abscess and inflammatory nodules relative to baseline), absolute change in Dermatology Life Quality Index (DLQI), and skin lesion count at week 16. Skin pain was a secondary outcome assessed using the validated survey tool, Hidradenitis Suppurativa Symptom Daily Diary (HSSDD).

In both trials, the primary efficacy endpoint of HiSCR50 was met by all bimekizumab treatment groups. In BE HEARD I, HiSCR50 was significantly higher in the 2-week dosing group as compared to placebo. HiSCR50 for 4-week dosing was superior to placebo, but did not reach statistical significance. In BE HEARD II, HiSCR50 was also significantly higher in both 2-week and 4-week dosing groups as compared to placebo. These responses were durable up to week 48. Patients switching from placebo to bimekizumab dosing every 2 weeks had notable improvements in HiSCR50 and HiSCR75 shortly after switching.

Regarding secondary outcomes, in BE HEARD I, HiSCR 75 was met by all bimekizumab treatment groups, and it was significantly higher in the 2-week group compared to placebo. In BE HEARD II, HiSCR75 for the 2-week and 4-week groups was significantly higher compared to placebo. In BE HEARD II, flare count was decreased in both bimekizumab treatment groups but did not reach statistical significance. In both trials, other secondary outcomes including DLQI total score change, and HSSD outcomes improved across all bimekizumab treatment groups as compared to placebo.

Safety was assessed biweekly and continued until week 20. Treatment-emergent adverse events (TEAEs) were measured for all study groups from baseline to week 16 and for bimekizumab-treatment groups from week 0 to week 48. Specific safety events of interest to the researchers included infection, neutropenia, hypersensitivity reactions, suicidal ideation and behavior, major adverse cardiac events, hepatic inflammation, malignancies, and inflammatory bowel disease (IBD). Overall, bimekizumab was well tolerated and phase 3 safety data was consistent with phase 2 trials. In both phase 3 trials, the most common TEAE at weeks 16 and 48 was hidradenitis, defined as flaring or worsening of hidradenitis. Other common TEAEs included coronavirus infection, oral candidiasis (mild-to-moderate), diarrhea, and headache. While serious TEAEs were limited in both trials, they were higher in the bimekizumab treatment groups (8% BE HEARD I, 5% BE HEARD II at week 48) as compared to placebo (0 in both trials at week 16). Rates of discontinuation due to TEAEs were higher in bimekizumab treatment groups and were similar between trials, 8% BE HEARD I, 5% BE HEARD II at week 48.

Severe TEAEs were < 10% for both trials at week 48. Across both trials, only 1 death was reported. It was secondary to congestive heart failure in a patient with a history of cardiac disease and the patient was enrolled in the bimekizumab every 2 weeks treatment group of BE HEARD I (considered to be unrelated to bimekizumab by researchers). Hypersensitivity reactions were reported in 21% of BE HEARD I and 17% of BE HEARD II. Dermatitis and eczema were the most common hypersensitivity reactions, no anaphylaxis events after treatment with bimekizumab were reported. At week 48, suicidal ideation/behavior was seen in 1% BE HEARD I and < 1% BE HEARD II. Adjudicated major adverse cardiac events were low and reported in <1% of BE HEARD I at week 48 (0 BE HEARD II). Hepatic enzyme changes, malignancies, and irritable bowel disease (IBD) were reported in <1% of patients. No flares of IBD while on bimekizumab treatment were reported in patients with existing disease at time of enrollment.

Overall, these phase 3 trials show bimekizumab proved to be efficacious in significantly improving HiSCR50 and secondary outcomes with a favorable TEAE profile. These findings support bimekizumab as a safe treatment option for patients with moderate-to-severe HS.

Adverse Event Profile of Bimekizumab

The most reported adverse event associated with bimekizumab treatment is infection, most notably viral and fungal infections [6, 8–19]. The adverse event profile of bimekizumab is similar in all clinical indications [6]. Across the multiple phase 3 trials conducted investigating bimekizumab as a treatment for plaque psoriasis, psoriatic arthritis, and axSpA, the TEAE profile was favorable overall [6, 10–13, 16]. The most common TEAEs reported include nasopharyngitis, oral candidiasis, and upper respiratory infections [6, 10–13, 16].

Additional adverse events (IBD, liver abnormalities, suicidal ideation) were reported in small numbers with comparable rates to controls across the multiple clinical trials investigating use of bimekizumab for autoinflammatory conditions [6, 8–13]. Follow-up studies in psoriasis and psoriatic arthritis have shown no increased risk of TEAEs with a longer exposure period of 2 years to bimekizumab treatment [12, 13]. Additionally, in pooled data analysis from 5-phase 3/3b trials investigating the treatment of plaque psoriasis with bimekizumab, the exposure adjusted incidence rates of hepatic TEAEs did not increase over the 2-year study period and rates were comparable to placebo, adalimumab, secukinumab, and ustekinumab [12].

Prior to the BE HEARD trials, a double-blind, randomized, placebo-controlled, phase 2 clinical trial was conducted to investigate the efficacy and safety of bimekizumab in patients with moderate-to-severe HS [9]. The trial compared bimekizumab to adalimumab and placebo. The incidence of TEAEs was similar between treatment groups. The most common TEAEs were infections including oral and vulvovaginal candidiasis; all cases were localized and responded to treatment. Additional common TEAEs included headache, gastroenteritis, headache, and hidradenitis flaring during treatment. The rate of serious TEAEs was low and none led to discontinuation. There were no cases of IBD or suicidal ideation/behavior reported.

Efficacy of Bimekizumab When Patients Fail Other Biologics

There is limited data regarding efficacy of bimekizumab in patients with HS who have failed to improve on other biologics. In the BE HEARD I and BE HEARD II trials, previous biologic therapy was reported in more than 10% of patients in each treatment group [9]. However, failure of prior biologic therapy was not specified and outcomes for these patients as compared to biologic-naive patients were not reported.

Despite the lack of data in HS patients, there is available data from studies investigating the use of bimekizumab after prior biologic failure in patients with psoriasis and psoriatic arthritis [13–15]. The phase 3, double-blind, placebo-controlled trials, BE COMPLETE and BE VITAL, showed that in patients who had a history of psoriatic arthritis and/or psoriasis, and prior inadequate response or intolerance to TNF-a inhibitors, bimekizumab proved to be significantly more effective in improving skin and joint disease as compared to placebo and was well-tolerated [14, 17]. Additionally, further research has shown that the efficacy of bimekizumab is sustained for up to 2 years in previously biologic-naive patients and TNF-a-resistant patients [13].

A 16-week multi-center retrospective review investigated the use of bimekizumab for the treatment of plaque psoriasis in patients with prior exposure to interleukin-17 inhibitors (IL-17i) [15]. The baseline of Investigator Global Assessment

(IGA) for the majority of patients was 3 and the most common previous IL-17i used was secukinumab, followed by ixekizumab, and brodalumab. The study showed that a majority of prior IL-17i non-responders achieved IGA 0/1 or Psoriasis Area and Severity Index (PASI) 90 after 16 weeks of treatment with bimekizumab [15]. The real-world study was limited by a small sample size but showed favorable outcomes after treatment with bimekizumab in patients with a history of plaque psoriasis and prior biologic treatment failure.

Another study investigated bimekizumab efficacy and safety in patients with moderate-to-severe plaque psoriasis who switched from adalimumab, ustekinumab, and secukinumab by analyzing data from phase 3/3b trials (BE SURE, BE VIVID, BE BRIGHT, BE RADIANT) [19]. They found that once switched to bimekizumab, patients rapidly improved within 4 weeks and had sustained clinical responses over the study period. After 4 weeks of bimekizumab treatment, prior PASI90 non-responders achieved PASI90 after switching from adalimumab (67%), ustekinumab (79%), and secukinumab (53%). PASI90 response continued to increase after 48 weeks of bimekizumab treatment. Safety profiles were similar between all classes of biologics and most TEAEs were mild or moderate.

Despite the lack of data regarding efficacy of bimekizumab in patients with HS who had treatment failure on other biologics, research in patients with psoriasis and psoriatic arthritis suggests that bimekizumab is a safe and efficacious option for patients who do not respond to other biologics.

Board Review Question Explanation
What is the mechanism of action of bimekizumab?

A. TNF-a inhibition
B. IL-17A only inhibition
C. IL-12/23 inhibition
D. IL-17A/F inhibition (Correct)
E. IL-31 inhibition

Answer Explanation
Bimekizumab is a monoclonal IgG1 antibody that selectively inhibits IL-17A, IL-17F and IL-17 AF cytokines. Secukinumab is a monoclonal antibody that selectively inhibits IL-17A alone.

Key Takeaway Points
- Bimekizumab is a monoclonal IgG1 antibody that selectively inhibits IL-17A and IL-17F.
- In addition to psoriatic arthritis, plaque psoriasis, ankylosing spondylitis, and non-radiographic axial spondylarthritis, bimekizumab is now approved for moderate-to-severe HS.
- Bimekizumab is significantly more effective than placebo and has similar safety and efficacy when compared to established HS treatments including secukinumab and adalimumab.

- The most common adverse effects of bimekizumab include worsening of HS, viral infections, oral candidiasis (mild-to-moderate), diarrhea, and headache.
- Data from studies of patients with plaque psoriasis and psoriatic arthritis suggest that bimekizumab may be an efficacious and safe treatment option for patients who fail treatment on other biologics including TNF-a inhibitors and other IL-17 inhibitors.

References

1. Daveluy S, Okoye GA. Quality of life and the patient journey in hidradenitis suppurativa. J Am Acad Dermatol. 2024;91(6S):S8–S11. https://doi.org/10.1016/j.jaad.2024.09.008.
2. Dagenet CB, Lee KH, Fragoso NM, Shi VY. Approach to the patient with hidradenitis suppurativa: evaluating severity to guide therapy. J Am Acad Dermatol. 2024;91(6S):S22–6. https://doi.org/10.1016/j.jaad.2024.09.007.
3. Sayed CJ, Hsiao JL. Navigating the current revolution in hidradenitis suppurativa care and research. J Am Acad Dermatol. 2024;91(6S):S1–2. https://doi.org/10.1016/j.jaad.2024.08.058.
4. What Are "Biologics" Questions and Answers. United States Food and Drug Administration. February 6, 2018. Accessed 4 Feb 2024. https://www.fda.gov/about-fda/center-biologics-evaluation-and-research-cber/what-are-biologics-questions-and-answers.
5. Charrow A, Santiago-Soltero K, Porter M. Biologics in hidradenitis suppurativa: progress and new directions. J Am Acad Dermatol. 2024;91(6S):S27–30. https://doi.org/10.1016/j.jaad.2024.09.027.
6. FDA Purple book Bimekizumab-bkzx – Label BLA 761151. United States Food and Drug Administration. November 19, 2024. Accessed 4 Feb 2024. https://www.accessdata.fda.gov/drugsatfda_docs/label/2024/761151s010lbl.pdf.
7. UCB USA. UCB Receives U.S. FDA approval for BIMZELX® (bimekizumab-bkzx) as the first IL-17A and IL-17F inhibitor for adults with moderate-to-severe hidradenitis Suppurativa November 20, 2024. Accessed 4 Feb 2024. https://www.ucb-usa.com/stories-media/UCB-U-S-News/detail/article/ucb-receives-us-fda-approval-for-bimzelxr-bimekizumab-bkzx-as-the-first-il-17a-and-il-17f-inhibitor-for-adults-with-moderate-to-severe-hidradenitis-suppurativa.
8. Kimball AB, Jemec GBE, Sayed CJ, et al. Efficacy and safety of bimekizumab in patients with moderate-to-severe hidradenitis suppurativa (BE HEARD I and BE HEARD II): two 48-week, randomised, double-blind, placebo-controlled, multicentre phase 3 trials. Lancet. 2024;403(10443):2504–19. https://doi.org/10.1016/S0140-6736(24)00101-6.
9. Glatt S, Jemec GBE, Forman S, et al. Efficacy and safety of Bimekizumab in moderate to severe hidradenitis Suppurativa: a phase 2, double-blind, placebo-controlled randomized clinical trial [published correction appears in JAMA Dermatol. 2021 Nov 1;157(11):1384. https://doi.org/10.1001/jamadermatol.2021.4442.]. JAMA Dermatol. 2021;157(11):1279–88. https://doi.org/10.1001/jamadermatol.2021.2905.
10. Gordon KB, Foley P, Krueger JG, et al. Bimekizumab efficacy and safety in moderate to severe plaque psoriasis (BE READY): a multicentre, double-blind, placebo-controlled, randomised withdrawal phase 3 trial [published correction appears in Lancet. 2021 Mar 27;397(10280):1182. https://doi.org/10.1016/S0140-6736(21)00669-3.]. Lancet. 2021;397(10273):475–86. https://doi.org/10.1016/S0140-6736(21)00126-4.
11. Reich K, Papp KA, Blauvelt A, et al. Bimekizumab versus ustekinumab for the treatment of moderate to severe plaque psoriasis (BE VIVID): efficacy and safety from a 52-week, multicentre, double-blind, active comparator and placebo controlled phase 3 trial [published correction appears in lancet. 2021 Feb 20;397(10275):670. https://doi.org/10.1016/S0140-6736(21)00387-1.]. Lancet. 2021;397(10273):487–98. https://doi.org/10.1016/S0140-6736(21)00125-2.

12. Lebwohl M, Merola JF, Strober B, Armstrong A, Yoshizaki A, Gisondi P, Szilagyi B, Peterson L, de Cuyper D, Cross N, Davies O, Gottlieb AB. Bimekizumab safety in moderate to severe plaque psoriasis: rates of hepatic events and changes in liver parameters over 2 years in randomized phase 3/3b trials. J Am Acad Dermatol. 2024;91:281.
13. Mease PJ, Merola JF, Tanaka Y, et al. Safety and efficacy of Bimekizumab in patients with psoriatic arthritis: 2-year results from two phase 3 studies. Rheumatol Ther. 2024;11(5):1363–82. https://doi.org/10.1007/s40744-024-00708-8.
14. Coates LC, Landewé R, McInnes IB, et al. Bimekizumab treatment in patients with active psoriatic arthritis and prior inadequate response to tumour necrosis factor inhibitors: 52-week safety and efficacy from the phase III BE COMPLETE study and its open-label extension BE VITAL. RMD Open. 2024;10(1):e003855. Published 2024 Feb 22. https://doi.org/10.1136/rmdopen-2023-003855.
15. Sood S, Rimke A, Rankin BD, et al. Real-world experience of bimekizumab for plaque psoriasis in adult patients with prior exposure to interleukin-17 inhibitors: a 16-week multicenter retrospective review. J Am Acad Dermatol. 2024;91(6):1265–7. https://doi.org/10.1016/j.jaad.2024.07.1515.
16. Baraliakos X, Deodhar A, van der Heijde D, et al. Long-term safety and efficacy of Bimekizumab in axial Spondyloarthritis: 2-year results from two phase 3 studies. Rheumatology (Oxford). Published online January 11. 2025; https://doi.org/10.1093/rheumatology/keaf009.
17. Merola JF, Landewé R, McInnes IB, et al. Bimekizumab in patients with active psoriatic arthritis and previous inadequate response or intolerance to tumour necrosis factor-α inhibitors: a randomised, double-blind, placebo-controlled, phase 3 trial (BE COMPLETE). Lancet. 2023;401(10370):38–48. https://doi.org/10.1016/S0140-6736(22)02303-0.
18. Warren RB, Blauvelt A, Bagel J, et al. Bimekizumab versus Adalimumab in Plaque Psoriasis. N Engl J Med. 2021;385(2):130–41. https://doi.org/10.1056/NEJMoa2102388.
19. Kokolakis G, Warren RB, Strober B, Blauvelt A, Puig L, Morita A, Gooderham M, Körber A, Vanvoorden V, Wang M, de Cuyper D, Madden C, Nunez Gomez N, Lebwohl M. Bimekizumab efficacy and safety in patients with moderate-to-severe plaque psoriasis who switched from adalimumab, ustekinumab or secukinumab: results from phase III/IIIb trials. Br J Dermatol. 2023;188(3):330–40. https://doi.org/10.1093/bjd/ljac089.
20. Battista T, Gallo L, Martora F, et al. Biological therapy for psoriasis in cancer patients: an 8-year retrospective real-life study. J Clin Med. 2024;13(7):1940. https://doi.org/10.3390/jcm13071940. PMID: 38610706; PMCID: PMC11012886
21. FDA Purple book Adalimumab – Label BLA 125057. United States Food and Drug Administration. November 03, 2023. Accessed 4 Feb 2024. https://www.accessdata.fda.gov/drugsatfda_docs/label/2023/125057s423lbl.pdf#page=57.

Chapter 14
Surgical Treatment of HS: Deroofing

Cory Kosche and Drew K. Saylor

Case Title A 34-Year-Old Male with Draining Nodules in the Axilla

Case
A 34-year-old male presents with bilateral axillary involvement due to his hidradenitis suppurativa (HS). His history includes 1 year of adalimumab therapy (40 mg weekly), which significantly improved his pain and drainage. While he no longer develops new lesions in new locations, he continues to experience intermittent flares with tenderness and drainage in persistent areas. The patient is satisfied with his current medication regimen and does not wish to make changes to his adalimumab.

Board Review Question
On examination of the above patient, erythematous, scarred plaques with rope-like subcutaneous tunnels and 2–3 patent epidermal tunnel openings are noted. What is the best next step in treatment?

A. Switch adalimumab to infliximab
B. Recommend deroofing procedure
C. Start clindamycin and rifampin
D. Start spironolactone

C. Kosche · D. K. Saylor (✉)
Department of Dermatology, University of California, San Francisco,
San Francisco, CA, USA

N. Brownstone (ed.), *Clinical Cases in Hidradenitis Suppurativa*, Clinical Cases in Dermatology, https://doi.org/10.1007/978-3-032-15200-8_14

Surgical Treatment of Hidradenitis Suppurativa: The Deroofing Procedure

Introduction

The surgical management of hidradenitis suppurativa (HS) encompasses a spectrum of approaches, including simple incision and drainage, deroofing, and excisional techniques. Excision, including both lesional and regional excision, remains a mainstay of treatment but may be associated with significant morbidity [1]. Surgical deroofing offers a minimally invasive, office-based intervention that spares significant morbidity while effectively targeting localized disease. This procedure is particularly well-suited for patients with persistent lesions refractory to optimal medical therapy or those with minimal, localized disease.

Rationale for Deroofing

Many patients with HS report persistent, recurrent flares within involved anatomic areas. These flares, characterized by pain, swelling, drainage, erythema, and odor, can persist despite optimal medical therapy. This could be explained by the persistence of the inflammatory content within the subcutaneous nodules and tunnels that define HS [2].

As HS lesions progress from inflammatory nodules to interconnected subcutaneous tunnels or sinus tracts, they fill with a mixture of keratin debris, neutrophils and other inflammatory cells, biofilm producing bacteria, and numerous inflammatory mediators, termed the ‘infiltrative proliferative gelatinous mass’ [2]. Though medical therapies have improved to better target the inflammatory pathogenesis of HS, without the removal of these inflammatory contents, the lesions of HS likely remain unable to heal spontaneously.

The technique of HS deroofing was first described in the literature in 2010 by van der Zee et al. [3]. Deroofing is a technique that surgically exposes and debrides the tunnels within HS lesions, allowing the removal of IPGM while preserving the base of the tunnel. This creates a favorable environment for second-intent healing, ultimately removing the driver of inflammation and recurrence.

Candidate Selection

Deroofing is most effective for patients meeting the following criteria:

- *Disease Stability*: Patients optimized on medical therapy who are no longer forming new lesions in previously uninvolved areas.

- *Localized Disease*: Persistent lesions in confined areas suitable for outpatient treatment.
- *Patient Preference*: A willingness to undergo the awake procedure under local anesthesia and participate in post-operative care.

Notably, medical therapy, including biologics, should be continued perioperatively, as recommended by the North American Clinical Management Guidelines for HS [4].

Special Considerations

Deroofing can be performed in various anatomic locations. However, areas such as the vulva and perianal region may require additional expertise.

Technique

Deroofing is typically performed in an outpatient clinic setting under local anesthesia. Key steps include:

1. *Anesthesia*: Local or tumescent anesthesia is used for adequate numbing of the planned treatment area.
2. *Tunnel Identification*: A blunt-tipped probe is inserted into a visible opening and advanced into subcutaneous tunnels. Moderate pressure helps identify tunnel connections while avoiding false openings.

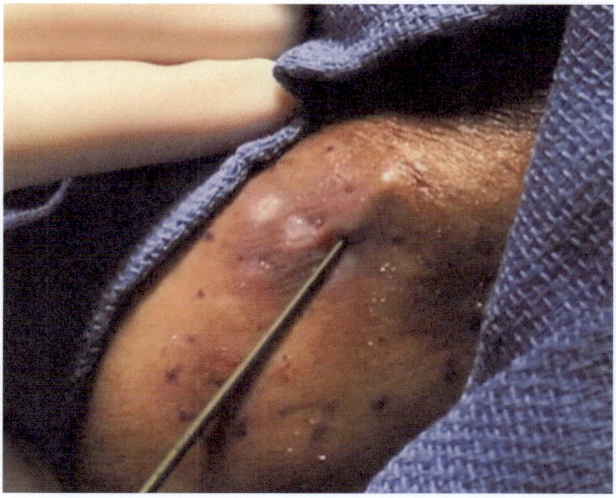

3. *Incision*: The overlying skin is incised along the length of the probe using a scalpel, scissors, electrosurgery, or CO_2 laser.

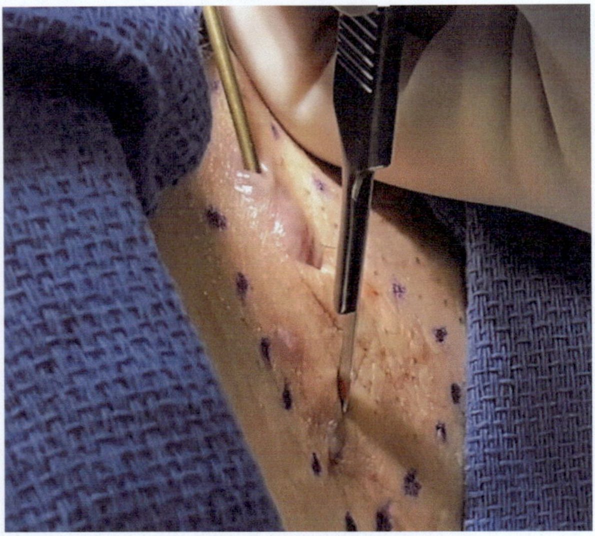

4. *Tissue Removal*: Overlying tissue is excised until flush with the wound edges.
5. *Debridement*: The IPGM is removed using a 4x4 woven gauze with rough debridement or a curette.
6. *Additional Tunnel Identification*: The edges of the tunnels are carefully explored with the probe to identify any additional tunnels. Manual palpation for areas of fluctuance may be helpful. The deroofing procedure is repeated for any additional tunnels.
7. *Wound Management*: The wound is dressed and left to heal by second intent, leading to scar contracture (Fig. 14.1).

Variations on the Deroofing Technique

- Some providers utilize extensive electrodessication of the wound edges to prevent early re-epithelialization.
- Preoperative ultrasound may be used to map subcutaneous tunnel location [5].
- More extensive resection of tunnels may be performed as pictured below [6] (Fig. 14.2).

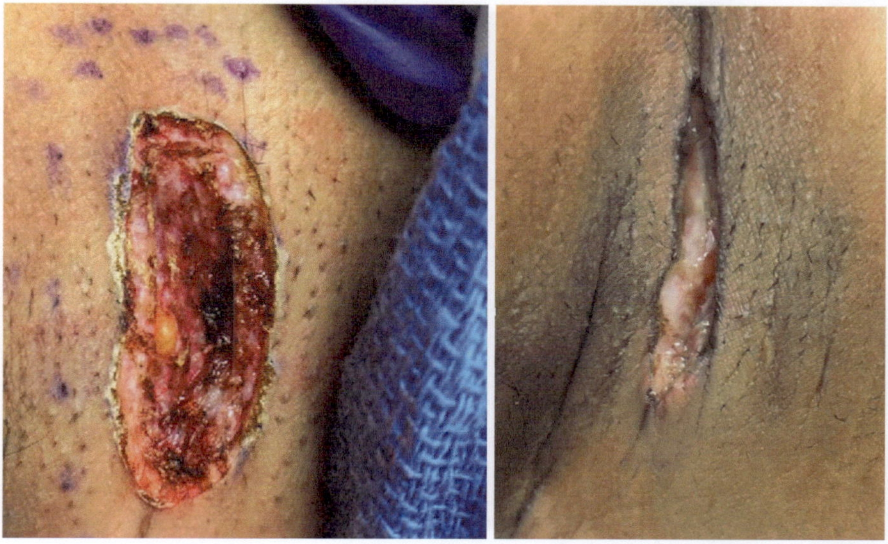

Fig. 14.1 Wound contraction tends to occur quickly during second intention healing of even larger areas, as evidenced by this wound pictured immediately post-operatively on the left and after only 2 days of healing on the right

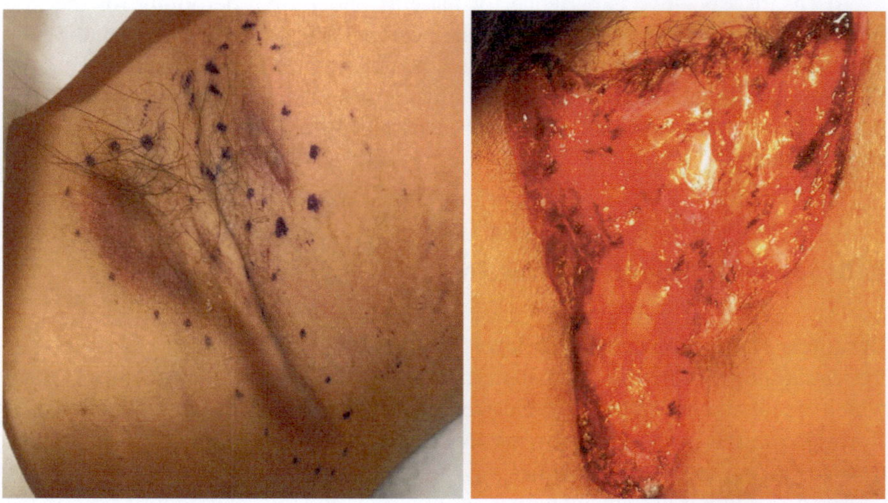

Fig. 14.2 Regional deroofing of the axillary vault due to extensive interconnected subcutaneous tunnels

Post-procedural Care and Recovery

Surgical sites post-deroofing are typically left to heal by second intent, meaning no primary closure, skin graft, or suturing is performed to close the surgical wound [3, 5]. The rationale for avoiding wound closure is that fewer complications and lower recurrence rates have been noted with second intention healing. Patients are advised to maintain a moist wound environment, which is commonly achieved using petroleum jelly and non-stick gauze. Regular wound cleansing is strongly encouraged to promote optimal healing and prevent complications.

Patients should be counseled that swelling, mild bleeding, mild pain, and itch are expected in the immediate postoperative period [3, 5]. However, in the authors' experience, patients often report that the discomfort associated with healing wounds is notably less than the pain experienced during active HS flares. Additionally, second-intent healing sites frequently require similar or even less care compared to managing active HS lesions.

Healing times vary widely and depend on factors such as the size and depth of the treated tunnels and their anatomic location. A 2024 prospective study by Krajewski et al. reported a mean healing time of 4.4 weeks, with deeper tunnels and lesions on the buttocks being associated with longer recovery periods [5]. Over time, patients can expect significant contracture of the wound with the formation of cosmetically acceptable scars [3].

To ensure a positive experience for patients undergoing deroofing for the first time, it is imperative to thoroughly discuss postoperative expectations, including the appearance of wounds during healing and the anticipated degree of scar formation. Sharing photographs of healed surgical sites or using cartoon illustrations for those uncomfortable with medical imagery can be highly beneficial in setting realistic expectations.

Efficacy and Patient Satisfaction

Deroofing has demonstrated high levels of efficacy, although most evidence comes from small retrospective studies. Recurrence rates of 14.5–20% have been reported, which are favorable compared to the average recurrence rate of 30% following excision [1]. Variability in accompanying medical management could contribute to differences in outcomes across studies.

The procedure is associated with a low complication rate, averaging 12.5% in the literature [1]. Reported complications include minor issues such as postoperative bleeding, excess granulation tissue, and localized infection. Notably, one recent study documented zero complications in their patient cohort [5].

Patient satisfaction with deroofing is exceptionally high, earning an average of 9.9/10 in one study [5]. In the original study by van der Zee et al., 90% of patients stated they would recommend the procedure to others with HS [3]. This aligns with subsequent findings, underscoring deroofing as a safe, effective, and well-tolerated intervention that provides long-term relief for localized disease.

Board Review Question Explanation

On examination of the above patient, erythematous, scarred plaques with rope-like subcutaneous tunnels and 2–3 patent epidermal tunnel openings are noted. What is the best next step in treatment?

A. Switch adalimumab to infliximab
B. Recommend deroofing procedure (Correct)
C. Start clindamycin and rifampin
D. Start spironolactone

Answer Explanation

The patient in the case example is an excellent candidate for deroofing. He has localized disease, Hurley 2–3 based on exam, without significant disease activity. He is well controlled on medication and, most importantly, is not forming new lesions in new places. Depending on patient and provider preference, he could consider undergoing deroofing of one axilla and then the other once healed from the first procedure. He should be counseled to continue his adalimumab throughout the process. Antibiotics are not indicated at this time, as he is not currently experiencing a disease flare. Spironolactone would not be an appropriate choice for this patient as he is not experiencing hormonal triggers of his disease.

Key Takeaways

- Deroofing is a long-lasting treatment for localized HS lesions, offering high satisfaction and cosmetically acceptable scars.
- The procedure is best performed during quiescent disease, with medical therapy optimized.
- Post-operative recovery is generally well-tolerated, with manageable wound care.

References

1. Klufas DM, Saylor DK. Surgical management of hidradenitis suppurativa: a review of techniques, data, and future directions. Dermatol Rev. 2022;3(2):111–7.
2. Kidacki M, et al. Invasive proliferative gelatinous mass of hidradenitis suppurativa. Br J Dermatol. 2019;181(1):192–3.
3. van der Zee HH, et al. Deroofing: a tissue-saving surgical technique for mild to moderate hidradenitis suppurativa lesions. J Am Acad Dermatol. 2010;63(3):475–80.
4. Alikhan A, et al. North American clinical management guidelines for hidradenitis suppurativa. J Am Acad Dermatol. 2019;81(1):76–90.
5. Krajewski PK, et al. Deroofing: a safe, effective, and well-tolerated procedure in HS. J Eur Acad Dermatol Venereol. 2024;38(5):931–6.
6. Dahmen RA, et al. Deroofing followed by thorough sinus tract excision: a modified surgical approach for hidradenitis suppurativa. JDDG J Dtsch Dermatol Ges. 2019;17(7):698–702.

Chapter 15
Surgical Treatment of HS: Plastic Surgery

Alexander H. Chang, Marion W. Tapp, Lauren E. Blaha, Christian A. Kauffman, Adam C. Walchak, Kyle E. Robinson, and Sameer A. Patel

Case Title What Medicine Cannot Heal, the Knife Will: Management of Hidradenitis Suppurativa with Plastic Surgery

Case

A 48-year-old woman with a 20-year history of hidradenitis suppurativa (HS) presented with chronic, draining sinus tracts and fibrosis of the left axilla and infra-abdominal fold. Four years earlier, the patient underwent gastric bypass surgery, resulting in a 110-pound weight loss. The patient was managed by her dermatologist with long-term antibiotics. Physical examination revealed a follicular scarring pattern consistent with Hurley Stage III HS of the lower abdomen and bilateral axillae. She had a BMI of 31 and did not smoke. Initially, she was scheduled for a panniculectomy, which successfully treated her abdominal HS. However, she continued to experience left axillary symptoms paired with excessive skin and subcutaneous tissue of the left upper extremity. Due to the excess tissue in the left arm, she was deemed an excellent candidate for excision of her left axillary HS disease and reconstruction with a left posterior arm flap. Figure 15.1 shows the preoperative presentation of hidradenitis suppurativa with axillary involvement.

A. H. Chang (✉) · A. C. Walchak · S. A. Patel
Division of Plastic and Reconstructive Surgery, Lewis Katz School of Medicine Temple University Hospital/Fox Chase Cancer Center, Philadelphia, PA, USA
e-mail: chalexa@sas.upenn.edu

M. W. Tapp · K. E. Robinson
Department of Plastic and Reconstructive Surgery, Wake Forest University, Winston-Salem, NC, USA

L. E. Blaha · C. A. Kauffman
Department of Plastic and Reconstructive Surgery, Geisinger Medical Center, Danville, PA, USA

N. Brownstone (ed.), *Clinical Cases in Hidradenitis Suppurativa*, Clinical Cases in Dermatology, https://doi.org/10.1007/978-3-032-15200-8_15

Board Review Questions

Question 1

A 28-year-old woman presents with chronic, painful nodules and draining sinuses in both axillae. She has failed multiple courses of antibiotics and is currently on adalimumab with partial response. She reports recurrent abscess formation despite medical therapy. Examination reveals extensive scarring and sinus tracts. What is the next best step in management?

A. Continue adalimumab and add intralesional steroids
B. Incision and drainage of active nodules
C. Wide local excision of affected tissue
D. Carbon dioxide laser therapy
E. Oral clindamycin and rifampin for 10 weeks

Question 2

A 36-year-old man with recurrent hidradenitis suppurativa involving the groin and buttocks has undergone multiple courses of antibiotics and recently underwent deroofing of several sinus tracts. He now presents with disease recurrence in the same area. Which of the following is the primary advantage of wide local excision over deroofing in this patient?

A. Faster healing time
B. Reduced cost
C. Less postoperative pain
D. Lower recurrence rate
E. Preserves more tissue

Question 3

A 32-year-old woman presents with painful, recurrent nodules and draining sinuses in the axillae and groin. She has a 5-year history of hidradenitis suppurativa (HS) and has tried multiple topical and oral antibiotics. On physical exam, she has bilateral sinus tracts with scarring but no diffuse interconnected tracts across

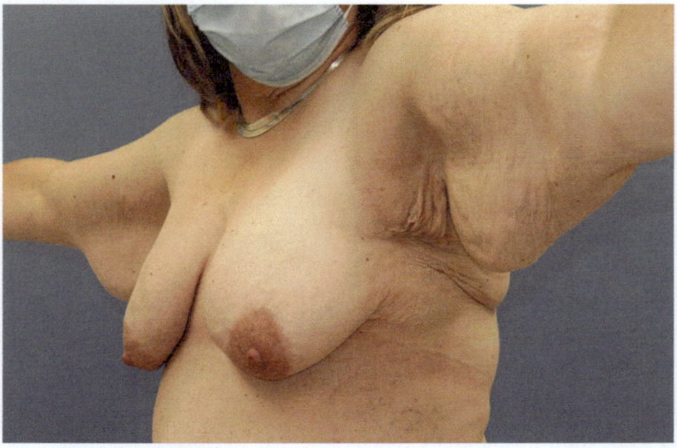

Fig. 15.1 The preoperative presentation of hidradenitis suppurativa with axillary involvement

large surface areas. The surgical team is evaluating her for potential deroofing versus wide local excision. To guide treatment, which validated clinical staging system is the most commonly used in determining the appropriate surgical management of HS?

A. The Koo-Brownstone System
B. The Hurley Staging System
C. The Marsh Classification
D. The Hinchey Classification System

After the induction of general anesthesia, the patient was positioned on an arm board with the operating table turned 90°. The left axillary disease was outlined with a marking pen and injected circumferentially with 60 mL of a tumescent solution of 1:100,000 epinephrine and injectable normal saline. Markings for a left posterior arm flap were drawn from the olecranon to the junction of the long head of the triceps and the latissimus dorsi muscle. A pencil Doppler was used to identify the dominant perforator, located 4 cm distal to the muscular intersection and 2 cm anterior to the drawn flap axis. A pinch test was performed to determine the maximum width of the flap. The left upper extremity and chest were prepped and draped in the standard fashion.

A #10 blade was used to make a circumferential incision around the marked area of disease in the left axilla. Electrocautery was used to deepen the excision to the level of the superficial axillary fascia, carefully preserving lymphatics and critical neurovascular structures. Figure 15.2 shows the extirpation of diseased tissue. The diseased tissue was sent for pathological examination. The wound was cleaned with a chlorhexidine scrub brush and irrigated with 3 liters of normal saline. Hemostasis was achieved with electrocautery.

The surgical team began raising the flap on the left arm. A Doppler was used to verify the location of a perforator. A #10 blade was used to make a curvilinear incision on the posterior arm, beginning 4 cm from the posterior axillary line and extending from proximal to distal. The incision was deepened with electrocautery

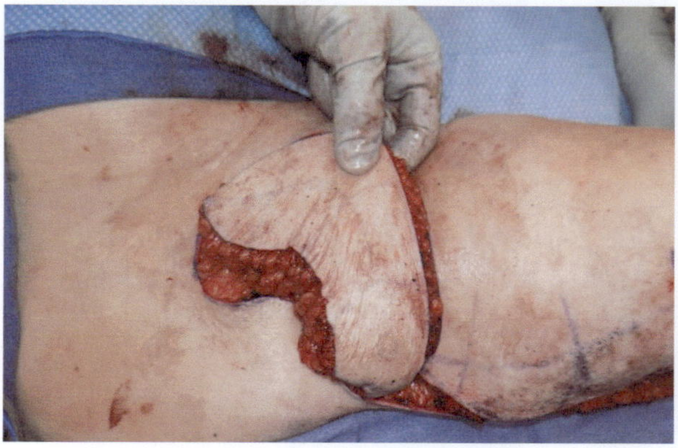

Fig. 15.2 Intraoperative view demonstrating wide surgical excision of hidradenitis suppurativa–affected tissue, allowing for optimal exposure and clear margin control

through the subcutaneous tissue to the fascia of the triceps muscle, which was then incised. The flap was raised from distal to proximal, deep to the posterior arm fascia and just superficial to the triceps muscle. A large perforator from the profunda brachii was identified at the site of the Doppler signal and was islandized. Figure 15.3 shows the flap that will be used for reconstruction.

The flap was elevated to the level of the perforator and rotated 180° into the axillary wound. Excess skin and subcutaneous tissue were removed from the flap to fit the defect. The donor site wound was connected to the recipient wound to allow for tension-free closure, and the flap was inset circumferentially using 2–0 PDS suture. Two 19-French JP drains were placed—one in the arm and one in the axilla—and tunneled out through the anterior chest wall, then secured with 2–0 silk, Biopatches®, and Tegaderm®.

Closure was performed in layers. The donor site was closed primarily. The deep dermal layer was closed with buried interrupted 3–0 Monocryl sutures, and the skin was closed with a running subcuticular 3–0 Monocryl suture. Finally, a Dermabond® Prineo® closure system was applied over the incisions. Figure 15.4 shows the inset of the flap.

On postoperative day 1, the flap was viable with no signs of venous congestion or ischemia. The patient tolerated the procedure well and was discharged with drain care and a short course of antibiotics (2 weeks of clindamycin and rifampin). A shoulder sling was worn for the first week, and gentle range of motion was initiated at 2 weeks. The patient was instructed not to engage in any heavy lifting for 6 weeks. At the 8-week follow-up, the flap had fully healed with excellent contour and restoration of mobility. Figure 15.5 shows the 8-week post-operative result demonstrating excellent coverage and color match.

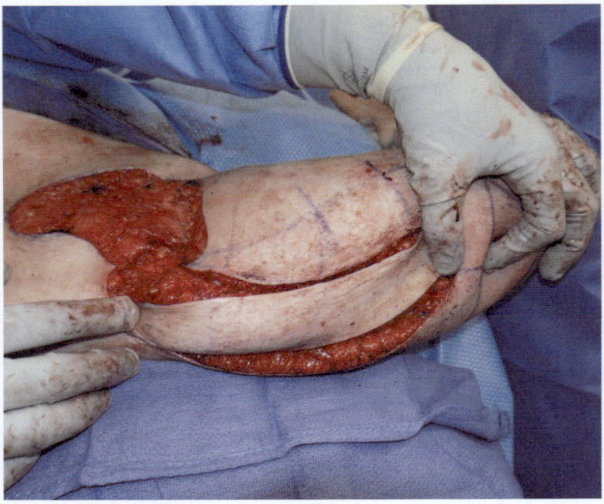

Fig. 15.3 Intraoperative view of a pedicled perforator propeller flap based on a profunda brachii artery perforator, mobilized to reconstruct the axillary defect following wide excision of hidradenitis suppurativa

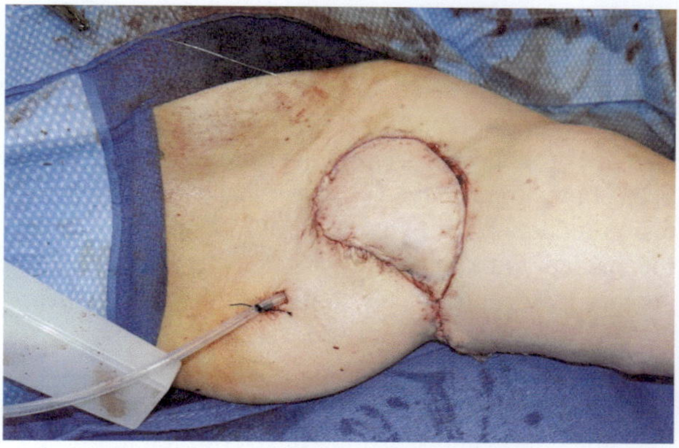

Fig. 15.4 Immediate postoperative view showing the inset perforator propeller flap with closed donor site and drain placement in the axillary region

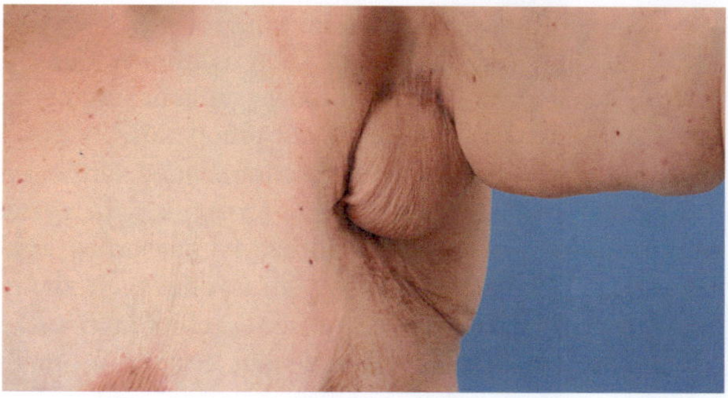

Fig. 15.5 8-week postoperative view demonstrating healed axillary region

Introduction

> What medicine cannot fix, the knife will.
> —Hippocrates, *Aphorisms* [1].

Hidradenitis suppurativa (HS), also referred to as acne inversa, is a chronic, inflammatory skin condition that affects the folliculosebaceous units [2, 3]. This disease disproportionately impacts women, particularly those of African descent, and usually manifests in the third or fourth decade of life [4]. Clinically, HS presents with recurrent painful nodules, abscesses, sinus tracts, and scarring, predominantly in intertriginous areas such as the axillae, groin, perineum, inframammary folds, and buttocks [5]. These lesions are not only physically painful but also socially stigmatizing due to malodor and drainage, often resulting in profound psychosocial impairment, social withdrawal, and reduced quality of life [6, 7]. Many patients experience difficulties with maintaining employment, relationships, and daily physical activity due to the disease burden.

The pathogenesis of HS begins with follicular occlusion that leads to rupture of the pilosebaceous unit, triggering inflammation [8]. Various immune and genetic components are implicated, including alterations in the Notch signaling pathway, increased expression of cytokines like TNF-α and IL-17A, and dysregulation of

T-helper cells [9, 10]. Elevated markers such as CRP and ESR further support the inflammatory nature of the disease [11]. HS is commonly associated with obesity—present in up to 75% of patients—and related comorbidities such as polycystic ovarian syndrome, diabetes, metabolic syndrome, inflammatory bowel disease, and psychiatric conditions including depression and anxiety [12, 13]. Weight loss has been shown to improve HS severity, and bariatric surgery has resulted in significant lesion reduction for many patients [12]. Some studies suggest that the reduction in mechanical friction, hormonal changes, and inflammatory load post-weight loss surgery may contribute to clinical improvement [14].

The Hurley staging system remains the most widely accepted framework for classifying HS severity [15]. Stage I is characterized by recurrent nodules or abscesses without significant scarring. Stage II includes recurrent lesions with limited sinus tracts and scarring. Stage III, seen in Fig. 15.6, represents the most severe form, involving diffuse interconnected sinus tracts and widespread scarring. This staging not only assists in determining severity but also guides therapeutic planning. Advanced imaging modalities, such as high-frequency ultrasound and MRI, have recently been utilized to supplement clinical staging, helping to delineate subclinical sinus tracts and disease extent preoperatively [16, 17]. Table 15.1 reviews the Hurley staging system and the recommended surgical procedures at each stage.

Medical management typically begins with systemic antibiotics, which are employed for their anti-inflammatory properties rather than their antimicrobial action [18–20]. Agents such as tetracyclines, clindamycin, and rifampin are commonly used [19]. In more severe cases, combinations like rifampin with moxifloxacin and metronidazole or intravenous ertapenem may be administered. Hormonal therapies such as oral contraceptives and spironolactone are effective in some female patients, particularly those with Stage I disease [21]. Steroids, both intralesional and oral, are valuable for acute flares and localized inflammation [18].

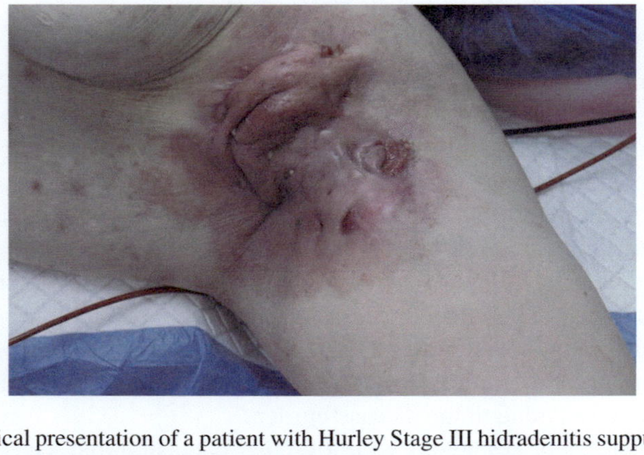

Fig. 15.6 Clinical presentation of a patient with Hurley Stage III hidradenitis suppurativa, demonstrating extensive interconnected sinus tracts, scarring, and chronic inflammatory lesions. The severity of the disease made this patient a good surgical candidate; subsequently, a wide local excision was performed with a split-thickness skin graft

Table 15.1 Hurley Staging is a three-stage classification system used to assess the severity of Hidradenitis Suppurativa (HS)

Hurley stage	Clinical description	Recommended surgical management
Stage I	Single or multiple abscesses without sinus tracts or scarring	Deroofing, punch debridement, laser therapy (CO_2); consider early intervention
Stage II	Recurrent abscesses with sinus tracts and scarring; widely separated lesions	Deroofing, limited local excision; staged procedures may be used
Stage III	Diffuse involvement with multiple interconnected sinus tracts and extensive scarring	Wide local excision; may require flap/graft reconstruction or healing by secondary intention

Biologic agents are used for moderate to severe disease [22]. These targeted therapies aim to modulate the inflammatory milieu in HS and may be especially helpful in patients with concomitant autoimmune or inflammatory comorbidities [23].

Surgical treatment plays a pivotal role in managing chronic or refractory HS [24]. Surgical deroofing is a conservative technique used in Stage I and some Stage II cases [25]. It involves removing the superficial aspect of sinus tracts to allow healing by secondary intention [26]. While it can provide temporary relief, deroofing is less effective in deep or extensive disease and has a higher recurrence rate [27]. Carbon dioxide lasers have also been used to achieve similar effects by ablating the superficial tissue [28]. These techniques are often performed in outpatient settings and offer the advantage of tissue preservation, although they may require multiple sessions and diligent postoperative wound care.

Wide local excision (WLE) is considered the definitive treatment for Hurley Stage III HS [29]. This surgical approach involves the complete removal of all affected skin and underlying sinus tracts, extending into healthy tissue to achieve adequate margins [30]. The goal is to eradicate chronic inflammation, sinus formation, and recurrent abscesses that are hallmarks of Hurley Stage III disease. Unlike more conservative interventions, WLE addresses both the superficial and deeper dermal components of HS, significantly reducing the risk of recurrence. Surgical margins are carefully planned based on clinical judgement to ensure complete excision of subclinical disease.

Post-excision, the resulting defect can be managed with a range of reconstructive options depending on size and location. It is essential for practitioners to understand that the reconstructive ladder (Fig. 15.7) serves as a conceptual framework in plastic and reconstructive surgery, guiding the selection of optimal techniques for wound closure and tissue reconstruction based on the complexity and size of the defect [31]. Table 15.2 summarizes the various options from the Reconstructive Ladder.

Starting with the simplest technique, secondary intention healing allows wounds to granulate and epithelialize without intervention [31]. If the defect is small and clean, primary intention closure using sutures is employed for quick healing [32]. For larger defects that cannot be closed primarily, skin grafting provides coverage by transferring epidermal and dermal layers from a donor site [33]. If additional tissue volume and blood supply are needed, local flaps are mobilized from adjacent

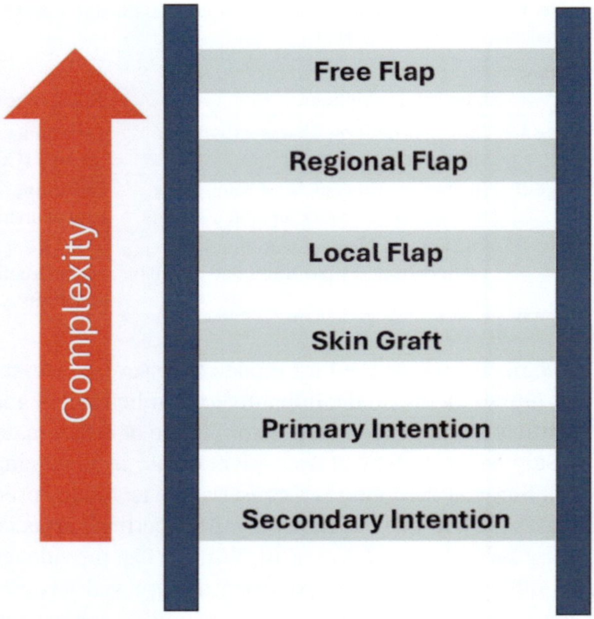

Fig. 15.7 The reconstructive ladder is a hierarchical framework for wound closure

tissue with preserved vascular connections. For more extensive defects or areas lacking local options, regional flaps are transferred from nearby regions with a known blood supply. At the highest level of complexity, free flaps involve the complete detachment and microvascular anastomosis of tissue to a distant site, allowing for large, well-vascularized reconstructions. The ladder progresses stepwise from less invasive to more complex techniques, balancing surgical complexity, healing time, and functional and aesthetic outcomes.

Surgeons often utilize tumescent anesthesia for better visualization and hemostasis. Zigzag or W-plasty incisions are preferred over traditional ellipsoid designs because they preserve a greater amount of healthy tissue and reduce the risk of contracture [34]. Tissues excised during WLE are routinely sent for pathology due to the rare occurrence of squamous cell carcinoma in chronic lesions. With wide excisions, it is important to communicate to patients that healing may take weeks to months and that complications such as wound dehiscence or infection are not uncommon. Preoperative counseling should include a discussion of expectations, wound care requirements, and the possibility of staged procedures in the setting of extensive disease.

Reconstruction following excision depends on the size of the defect, its location, and the degree of contamination [35]. Healing by secondary intention is acceptable for small or acutely inflamed wounds but often results in prolonged recovery and possible contractures. Primary closure is used in clean, small wounds and offers faster recovery, though it carries a risk of wound breakdown due to high tension or shearing forces from excessive movement. Negative pressure wound therapy

Table 15.2 Summary notes of the Reconstructive Ladder for HS

Technique	Description	Indication	Notes
Free flap	Complete detachment and reattachment of tissue with microvascular anastomosis	Large or complex defects requiring significant tissue coverage after HS excision	Allows for large tissue transfers; customizable for defect type; requires microvascular surgery; higher failure rates; longer operative time
Regional flap	Tissue transferred from a nearby region with a known vascular supply	Larger defects or where local flaps are insufficient	Greater reach than local flaps; reliable vascular supply; may require microvascular anastomosis; increased risk of failure
Local flap	Mobilization of tissue adjacent to the wound while maintaining its blood supply	Moderate-sized defects after HS excision where local tissue is available	Good color and texture match; maintains vascular supply; limited reach; donor site morbidity; risk of necrosis
Skin graft	Transfer of skin (split or full-thickness) from a donor site to cover a wound	Large defects after wide excision in Hurley Stage II/III HS, especially when primary closure is not feasible	Requires well-vascularized wound bed; risk of graft failure; may have poor aesthetic match; immobilization needed post-op
Primary intention closure	Closure of wound edges using sutures, staples, or adhesives for fast healing with minimal scarring	Clean, small wounds after limited HS excision with well-approximated edges and low infection risk	Fast healing; minimal scarring; aesthetically pleasing if well-aligned; straight-line scars can develop contracture; may require revisions
Secondary intention healing	Wound is left open to heal by granulation, contraction, and epithelialization from the base	Large, contaminated, or inflamed wounds unsuitable for closure; wounds with high infection risk	Simple; avoids tension on wound edges; good for contaminated wounds; requires long-term wound care; higher risk of contractures

Surgical management of HS follows a Reconstructive Ladder for closing a wide local excision, progressing from simple wound healing by secondary intention to complex free flap transfers, offering a stepwise approach to address tissue defects based on severity and anatomical requirements

(NPWT), including internal vacuum-assisted closure devices, has transformed post-operative care by enhancing granulation tissue formation, reducing bacterial burden, and supporting delayed primary closure [36]. This method has shown particularly favorable outcomes in large wounds, with lower recurrence and complication rates [36]. NPWT can be combined with dermal substitutes to facilitate eventual grafting or flap placement [37].

Skin grafting is another cornerstone of HS reconstruction, especially for large defects [33]. Split-thickness skin grafts (STSGs) are frequently used and often meshed to allow for better drainage and adherence to irregular surfaces [33]. An innovative technique involves harvesting a reused skin graft from the affected area itself—removing a superficial graft above the folliculopilosebaceous units before excising the diseased tissue [38]. This method minimizes donor site morbidity and has demonstrated durable results [38]. Dermal scaffolds may be used in conjunction with grafts to improve cosmesis, though these add cost and complexity.

Flap-based reconstruction is essential for defects requiring robust tissue coverage (Table 15.3). Local tissue advancement via V-Y flaps, perforator-based flaps (such as the thoracodorsal and gluteal artery flaps), and posterior thigh flaps can provide well-vascularized coverage [34]. The choice depends on the anatomical site, extent of disease, and patient-specific factors. For example, thoracodorsal artery perforator flaps are effective in the axilla, while gluteal and perineal defects may benefit from gluteal artery flaps [39]. In post-bariatric patients or those with redundant skin, body contouring procedures can be coordinated with HS excision, improving both disease management and body image.

Anatomical considerations play a central role in surgical planning [40]. Axillary lesions may be closed by primary intention, with skin grafts, or with perforator flaps especially in post-bariatric patients with excess tissue [41]. Inguinal and perineal HS requires meticulous dissection to avoid injuring vital structures and may necessitate staged closure or grafting [42]. Scrotal disease can be addressed using meshed skin grafts or reused scrotal skin, avoiding secondary donor sites [40]. Gluteal disease often includes deep tunneling and requires thorough excision and robust reconstruction. For inframammary and abdominal HS, surgical options such as breast reduction or panniculectomy may be incorporated into the treatment plan [40].

Table 15.3 Common flaps used by plastic surgeons to close defects

Flap	Anatomic region	Key features
V-Y advancement	Axilla, groin, perineum	Local flap that advances tissue forward while preserving blood supply; great for medium-sized defects; tissue-sparing and versatile
Posterior arm fasciocutaneous	Axilla	Based on brachial or profunda brachii perforators; rotational flap ideal for post-excisional axillary defects, especially in Hurley Stage III HS
Thoracodorsal Artery Perforator (TDAP)	Axilla, lateral chest	Perforator-based flap with minimal donor site morbidity; provides robust coverage, especially in recurrent or scarred fields
Gracilis myocutaneous	Perineum, ischiorectal fossa	Provides bulk and excellent vascularity for deep, contaminated wounds; useful when simpler flaps are inadequate
Posterior thigh	Gluteal, perineal, sacral regions	Reliable and bulky fasciocutaneous flap; ideal for large defects requiring durable, sensate coverage
Superior/Inferior Gluteal Artery Perforator (SGAP/IGAP Flaps)	Gluteal, sacral HS	Muscle-sparing alternatives provide durable coverage for complex or recurrent disease; require perforator dissection expertise

These combined procedures offer functional improvement and facilitate hygiene and wound care.

Postoperative care emphasizes continued multimodal management. Biologics are sometimes paused perioperatively and resumed once wound healing is stable; however, institutional protocols may vary [43]. Antibiotics may be administered intravenously initially, then transitioned to oral forms guided by intraoperative cultures. NPWT is crucial for maintaining wound hygiene and optimizing graft or flap take. In anatomically challenging areas like the perineum, urinary catheters may be used to protect dressings. Patients should receive long-term follow-up and counseling on hygiene, smoking cessation, weight control, and stress management—all of which influence recurrence risk [44].

Complications include infection, bleeding, non-healing wounds, dehiscence, contractures, and disease recurrence [45]. Risk factors for poor healing include malnutrition, smoking, and obesity [46]. Recurrence rates differ depending on the procedure: Incision and drainage approaches have near 100% recurrence, while wide excision with skin grafting has recurrence rates as low as 6% [26, 45]. The highest recurrence rates are seen in the genital region, followed by the inguinal and axillary areas. Pain management also plays a key role in recovery; multimodal regimens including acetaminophen, NSAIDs, and local anesthetics are preferred to minimize opioid dependence [47].

HS significantly impairs quality of life, limiting personal and professional functioning. Wide excision with thoughtful reconstruction has been shown to substantially improve both physical symptoms and emotional well-being. In retrospective analyses, most patients reported satisfaction with surgical outcomes and indicated they would recommend surgery to others [6]. The comprehensive care model, involving dermatologists, plastic surgeons, infectious disease specialists, and wound care teams, is essential to deliver optimal, patient-centered care.

Effective management of hidradenitis suppurativa requires a comprehensive, multidisciplinary approach [48]. Surgery—particularly wide local excision with appropriate reconstruction—remains the cornerstone of treatment for advanced disease. With coordinated care, targeted medical therapy, and innovative surgical strategies, patients with HS can achieve meaningful relief from this physically and emotionally burdensome condition. As the field evolves, continued research into biologics, surgical techniques, and integrated care pathways will be essential to improve outcomes and reduce disparities in HS care.

Board Review Question Explanations

Question 1

A 28-year-old woman presents with chronic, painful nodules and draining sinuses in both axillae. She has failed multiple courses of antibiotics and is currently on adalimumab with partial response. She reports recurrent abscess formation despite medical therapy. Examination reveals extensive scarring and sinus tracts. What is the next best step in management?

A. Continue adalimumab and add intralesional steroids
B. Incision and drainage of active nodules

C. Wide local excision of affected tissue (Correct)
D. Carbon dioxide laser therapy
E. Oral clindamycin and rifampin for 10 weeks

Question 2
A 36-year-old man with recurrent hidradenitis suppurativa involving the groin and buttocks has undergone multiple courses of antibiotics and recently underwent deroofing of several sinus tracts. He now presents with disease recurrence in the same area. Which of the following is the primary advantage of wide local excision over deroofing in this patient?

A. Faster healing time
B. Reduced cost
C. Less postoperative pain
D. Lower recurrence rate (Correct)
E. Preserves more tissue

Question 3
A 32-year-old woman presents with painful, recurrent nodules and draining sinuses in the axillae and groin. She has a 5-year history of hidradenitis suppurativa (HS) and has tried multiple topical and oral antibiotics. On physical exam, she has bilateral sinus tracts with scarring but no diffuse interconnected tracts across large surface areas. The surgical team is evaluating her for potential deroofing versus wide local excision. To guide treatment, which validated clinical staging system is the most commonly used in determining the appropriate surgical management of HS?

A. The Koo-Brownstone System
B. The Hurley Staging System (Correct)
C. The Marsh Classification
D. The Hinchey Classification System

Answer Explanation
1. Once HS has progressed to Hurley Stage III with extensive scarring and sinus tract formation and has failed medical therapy (e.g., antibiotics, biologics), definitive surgical excision is the treatment of choice. Incision and drainage is discouraged long-term because it does not prevent recurrence. CO_2 laser is useful but less definitive than excision.
2. Wide local excision offers the lowest recurrence rate of all surgical treatments for HS, though at the expense of greater tissue removal and longer healing. Deroofing is useful for localized disease or for patients unfit for wide excision, but recurrence is higher. Healing time is longer with excision, not shorter.
3. The Hurley staging system is the most widely accepted and clinically useful classification for hidradenitis suppurativa (HS), particularly in guiding surgical decision-making. It categorizes HS into three stages based on the extent of disease: Stage I includes isolated abscesses without scarring or sinus tracts; Stage II involves recurrent abscesses with sinus tract formation and scarring but with lesions that are still widely separated; and Stage III represents diffuse or

near-complete involvement of a region with interconnected sinus tracts and significant fibrosis. This staging system helps surgeons determine the most appropriate intervention, such as deroofing for limited disease (Stage I–II) or wide local excision for more extensive disease (Stage III).

The other options are incorrect. The Koo-Brownstone System is a classification system for delusional parasitosis. The Marsh Classification is used in celiac disease to stage histological damage in the small intestine. The Hinchey Classification is relevant to diverticulitis, not HS, and categorizes disease severity based on the presence and extent of abscess or perforation. Only the Hurley system directly applies to HS and is essential knowledge for both board exams and surgical management.

Key Takeaway Points

- Surgical deroofing is a tissue-sparing technique appropriate for limited, superficial disease (Hurley Stage I/II) and has lower morbidity but higher recurrence than WLE
- Wide local excision (WLE) is the definitive treatment for severe (Hurley Stage III) HS, offering the lowest recurrence rates among surgical options
- Primary closure is suitable for small, clean wounds but carries a risk of dehiscence in tension-prone areas
- Secondary intention healing is useful in contaminated or high-risk wounds but has longer healing time and higher risk of contracture
- Negative pressure wound therapy (NPWT) supports wound granulation, reduces bacterial load, and can bridge to definitive closure or skin grafting
- Split-Thickness Skin Grafting (STSG) is a reliable method for covering large defects, especially when flaps are not feasible
- Flap-based reconstruction, including local tissue advancement and perforator flaps (e.g., TDAP, SGAP), provides durable coverage for large or functionally sensitive areas like the axilla or groin
- Site-specific planning is critical—different anatomical areas (e.g., axilla, perineum, gluteal region) require tailored reconstructive strategies
- Biologic therapy can be used in conjunction with surgery
- Multidisciplinary care involving dermatology, plastic surgery, wound care, and infectious disease teams leads to optimal outcomes
- Patient education and postoperative care (e.g., hygiene, smoking cessation, weight control) are essential in reducing complications and recurrence

References

1. Lloyd GER, editor. Hippocratic writings. Penguin Classics; 1983.
2. Castelli E, Orlando E, Porcasi R, et al. Histopathological progression of hidradenitis suppurativa/acne inversa: a morphological study with a closer look on the early changes of the folliculosebaceous apocrine apparatus. Wien Med Wochenschr. 2022;172(5–6):126–34. https://doi.org/10.1007/s10354-021-00859-1.
3. Van Straalen KR, Prens EP, Gudjonsson JE. Insights into hidradenitis suppurativa. J Allergy Clin Immunol. 2022;149(4):1150–61. https://doi.org/10.1016/j.jaci.2022.02.003.

4. Goldburg SR, Strober BE, Payette MJ. Hidradenitis suppurativa epidemiology, clinical presentation, and pathogenesis. J Am Acad Dermatol. 2020;82(5):1045–58. https://doi.org/10.1016/j.jaad.2019.08.090.
5. Saunte DML, Jemec GBE. Hidradenitis suppurativa: advances in diagnosis and treatment. JAMA. 2017;318(20):2019–32. https://doi.org/10.1001/jama.2017.16691.
6. Kohorst JJ, Baum CL, Otley CC, et al. Patient satisfaction and quality of life following surgery for hidradenitis suppurativa. Dermatologic Surg. 2017;43(1):125–33. https://doi.org/10.1097/DSS.0000000000000942.
7. Schneider-Burrus S, Kalus S, Fritz B, Wolk K, Gomis-Kleindienst S, Sabat R. The impact of hidradenitis suppurativa on professional life. Br J Dermatol. 2023;188(1):122–30. https://doi.org/10.1093/bjd/ljac027.
8. Wolk K, Join-Lambert O, Sabat R. Aetiology and pathogenesis of hidradenitis suppurativa. Br J Dermatol. 2020;183(6):999–1010. https://doi.org/10.1111/bjd.19556.
9. Preda-Naumescu A, Ahmed HN, Mayo TT, Yusuf N. Hidradenitis suppurativa: pathogenesis, clinical presentation, epidemiology, and comorbid associations. Int J Dermatol. 2021;60(11):e449–58. https://doi.org/10.1111/ijd.15579.
10. Yao Y, Thomsen SF. The role of interleukin-17 in the pathogenesis of hidradenitis suppurativa. Dermatol Online J. 2017;23(7):13030. https://doi.org/10.5070/d3237035729.
11. Jiménez-Gallo D, de la Varga-Martínez R, Ossorio-García L, Albarrán-Planelles C, Rodríguez C, Linares-Barrios M. The clinical significance of increased serum proinflammatory cytokines, C-reactive protein, and erythrocyte sedimentation rate in patients with hidradenitis suppurativa. Mediat Inflamm. 2017;2017(1):2450401. https://doi.org/10.1155/2017/2450401.
12. Kromann C, Ibler KS, Kristiansen V, Jemec GBE. The influence of body weight on the prevalence and severity of hidradenitis suppurativa. Acta Derm Venereol. 2014;94(5):553–7. https://doi.org/10.2340/00015555-1800.
13. Tzellos T, Zouboulis CC. Review of comorbidities of hidradenitis suppurativa: implications for daily clinical practice. Dermatol Ther (Heidelb). 2020;10(1):63–71. https://doi.org/10.1007/s13555-020-00354-2.
14. Sivanand A, Gulliver WP, Josan CK, Alhusayen R, Fleming PJ. Weight loss and dietary interventions for hidradenitis suppurativa: a systematic review. J Cutan Med Surg. 2020;24(1):64–72. https://doi.org/10.1177/1203475419874412.
15. Hurley HJ, Hurley HJ. Axillary hyperhidrosis, apocrine bromhidrosis, hidradenitis suppurativa, and familial benign pemphigus: surgical approach. In: Roenigk & Roenigk's dermatologic surgery: principles and practice. 2nd ed. Marcel Dekker; 1996. p. 623–45.
16. Wortsman X. Imaging of hidradenitis suppurativa. Dermatol Clin. 2016;34(1):59–68. https://doi.org/10.1016/j.det.2015.08.003.
17. Elkin K, Daveluy S, Avanaki K. Review of imaging technologies used in hidradenitis suppurativa. Skin Res Technol. 2020;26(1):3–10. https://doi.org/10.1111/srt.12772.
18. Johnston LA, Alhusayen R, Bourcier M, et al. Practical guidelines for managing patients with hidradenitis suppurativa: an update. J Cutan Med Surg. 2022;26(2_suppl):2S–24S. https://doi.org/10.1177/12034754221116115.
19. Molinelli E, De Simoni E, Candelora M, et al. Systemic antibiotic therapy in hidradenitis suppurativa: a review on treatment landscape and current issues. Antibiotics. 2023;12(6):978. https://doi.org/10.3390/antibiotics12060978.
20. Robert E, Bodin F, Paul C, et al. Non-surgical treatments for hidradenitis suppurativa: a systematic review. Ann Chir Plast Esthet. 2017;62(4):274–94. https://doi.org/10.1016/j.anplas.2017.03.012.
21. Clark AK, Quinonez RL, Saric S, Sivamani RK. Hormonal therapies for hidradenitis suppurativa: review. Dermatol Online J. 2017;23(10):13030/qt6383k0n4. https://doi.org/10.5070/d32310036990.
22. Maronese CA, Moltrasio C, Genovese G, Marzano AV. Biologics for hidradenitis suppurativa: evolution of the treatment paradigm. Expert Rev Clin Immunol. 2024;20(5):525–45. https://doi.org/10.1080/1744666X.2023.2298356.

23. Krueger JG, Frew J, Jemec GBE, et al. Hidradenitis suppurativa: new insights into disease mechanisms and an evolving treatment landscape. Br J Dermatol. 2024;190(2):149–62. https://doi.org/10.1093/bjd/ljad345.
24. Menderes A, Sunay O, Vayvada H, Yilmaz M. Surgical management of hidradenitis suppurativa. Int J Med Sci. 2010;7(4):240–7. https://doi.org/10.7150/ijms.7.240.
25. van der Zee HH, Prens EP, Boer J. Deroofing: a tissue-saving surgical technique for the treatment of mild to moderate hidradenitis suppurativa lesions. J Am Acad Dermatol. 2010;63(3):475–80. https://doi.org/10.1016/j.jaad.2009.12.018.
26. Allison. Surgical deroofing for hidradenitis suppurativa. Cutis. 2022;110(3):147–9. https://doi.org/10.12788/cutis.0597.
27. van Hattem S, Spoo JR, Horváth B, Jonkman MF, Leeman FWJ. Surgical treatment of sinuses by deroofing in hidradenitis suppurativa. Dermatologic Surg. 2012;38(3):494. https://doi.org/10.1111/j.1524-4725.2011.02255.x.
28. Clark SR, Soti V. Effectiveness of surgical deroofing and carbon dioxide laser in moderate-to-severe hidradenitis suppurativa patients. Cureus. 2024;16:e56959. Published online March 26. https://doi.org/10.7759/cureus.56959.
29. Shukla R, Karagaiah P, Patil A, et al. Surgical treatment in hidradenitis suppurativa. J Clin Med. 2022;11(9):2311. https://doi.org/10.3390/jcm11092311.
30. Alharbi Z, Kauczok J, Pallua N. A review of wide surgical excision of hidradenitis suppurativa. BMC Dermatol. 2012;12(1):9. https://doi.org/10.1186/1471-5945-12-9.
31. Janis JE, Kwon RK, Attinger CE. The new reconstructive ladder: modifications to the traditional model. Plast Reconstr Surg. 2011;127:205S–12S. https://doi.org/10.1097/prs.0b013e318201271c.
32. Mathes S, Nahai F. Reconstructive surgery: principles, anatomy & technique. Quality Medical Publishing; 1997.
33. Chen E, Friedman HI. Management of regional hidradenitis suppurativa with vacuum-assisted closure and split thickness skin grafts. Ann Plast Surg. 2011;67(4):397–401. https://doi.org/10.1097/sap.0b013e3181f77bd6.
34. Janis J. Essentials of plastic surgery. Thieme; 2023.
35. Burney RE. 35-Year experience with surgical treatment of hidradenitis suppurativa. World J Surg. 2017;41(11):1. https://doi.org/10.1007/s00268-017-4091-7.
36. Orgill DP, Bayer LR. Negative pressure wound therapy: past, present and future. Int Wound J. 2013;10(s1):15–9. https://doi.org/10.1111/iwj.12170.
37. Lalezari S, Lee CJ, Borovikova AA, et al. Deconstructing negative pressure wound therapy. Int Wound J. 2017;14(4):649–57. https://doi.org/10.1111/iwj.12658.
38. Maeda T, Kimura C, Murao N, Takahashi K. Promising long-term outcomes of the reused skin-graft technique for chronic gluteal hidradenitis suppurativa. J Plast Reconstr Aesthet Surg. 2015;68(9):1268–75. https://doi.org/10.1016/j.bjps.2015.05.025.
39. Unal C, Yirmibesoglu OA, Ozdemir J, Hasdemir M. Superior and inferior gluteal artery perforator flaps in reconstruction of gluteal and perianal/perineal hidradenitis suppurativa lesions. Microsurgery. 2011;31(7):539–44. https://doi.org/10.1002/micr.20918.
40. Taylor EM, Hamaguchi R, Kramer KM, Kimball AB, Orgill DP. Plastic surgical management of hidradenitis suppurativa. Plast Reconstr Surg. 2021;147(3):479–91. https://doi.org/10.1097/prs.0000000000007677.
41. Vellaichamy G, Braunberger TL, Nahhas AF, Hamzavi IH. Surgical procedures for hidradenitis suppurativa. Cutis. 2018;102(1):13–6.
42. Balik E, Eren T, Bulut T, Büyükuncu Y, Bugra D, Yamaner S. Surgical approach to extensive hidradenitis suppurativa in the perineal/perianal and gluteal regions. World J Surg. 2009;33(3):481–7. https://doi.org/10.1007/s00268-008-9845-9.
43. Issa CJ, Hong AC, Lio PA. Combined biologic and surgical interventions for hidradenitis suppurativa: a systematic review. Dermatol Ther. 2024;2024(1):6637006. https://doi.org/10.1155/2024/6637006.

44. Ravi S, Miles JA, Steele C, Christiansen MK, Sayed CJ. Patient impressions and outcomes after clinic-based hidradenitis suppurativa surgery. JAMA Dermatol. 2022;158(2):132–41. https://doi.org/10.1001/jamadermatol.2021.4741.
45. Bouazzi D, Chafranska L, Saunte DML, Jemec GBE. Systematic review of complications and recurrences after surgical interventions in hidradenitis suppurativa. Dermatologic Surg. 2020;46(7):914–21. https://doi.org/10.1097/dss.0000000000002323.
46. Worden A, Yoho DJ, Houin H, et al. Factors affecting healing in the treatment of hidradenitis suppurativa. Ann Plast Surg. 2020;84(4):436–40. https://doi.org/10.1097/sap.0000000000002105.
47. Horváth B, Janse IC, Sibbald GR. Pain management in patients with hidradenitis suppurativa. J Am Acad Dermatol. 2015;73(5):S47–51. https://doi.org/10.1016/j.jaad.2015.07.046.
48. Chiricozzi A, Micali G, Veraldi S. The patient journey: a voyage from diagnosis to hidradenitis suppurativa multidisciplinary unit. J Eur Acad Dermatol Venereol. 2019;33(S6):15–20. https://doi.org/10.1111/jdv.15850.

Chapter 16
Surgical Treatment of HS: Energy-Based Devices

Connor Sheehan and Saira Agarwala

Case Title A 33-Year-Old Female with Recurring Boils in the Axilla and Groin

Case

A 33-year-old woman presents to clinic with a 7-year history of painful, recurring "boils" in her axillae and groin. She reports multiple courses of antibiotics with temporary relief, but the lesions recur. On examination, she has several open comedones, inflamed nodules, and sinus tracts in both axillae and along the groin folds. She has tried topical clindamycin, oral doxycycline, and a biologic agent (adalimumab), with only partial improvement. She expresses interest in procedural treatment options.

Board-Review Question

A 33-year-old woman with Hurley stage II hidradenitis suppurativa presents with recurrent nodules and sinus tracts in the axillae and groin. She has failed multiple systemic therapies. Which of the following energy-based devices has the strongest evidence base for improving lesion counts in HS?

A. 755 nm Alexandrite laser
B. Intense pulsed light (IPL)
C. Long-pulsed Nd:YAG laser
D. Photodynamic therapy (PDT)
E. Radiofrequency (RF) therapy

C. Sheehan (✉) · S. Agarwala
Temple University Hospital, Department of Dermatology, Philadelphia, PA, USA
e-mail: connor.sheehan@temple.edu; saira.agarwala@tuhs.temple.edu

N. Brownstone (ed.), *Clinical Cases in Hidradenitis Suppurativa*, Clinical Cases in Dermatology, https://doi.org/10.1007/978-3-032-15200-8_16

Introduction

Hidradenitis suppurativa (HS) is a chronic, relapsing inflammatory skin condition involving the pilosebaceous unit, particularly in apocrine gland-rich intertriginous areas. The pilosebaceous unit consists of the hair follicle, sebaceous glands, apocrine sweat glands, arrector pili muscle, and the surrounding connective tissue. These structures are especially concentrated in intertriginous regions such as the axillae, groin, inframammary folds, and perianal area. Thus, these are the common sites for HS lesions [1].

In HS, follicular occlusion is believed to be the initiating event. This leads to follicular rupture and a cascade of immune dysregulation, bacterial colonization, and chronic inflammation [1]. This manifests clinically as nodules, abscesses, sinus tracts, and scarring. Understanding the pilosebaceous unit's role in HS helps explain why many energy-based devices (e.g., lasers targeting hair follicles) are beneficial in HS treatment.

The mainstay of treatment includes topical and systemic agents, but these often yield incomplete responses. Energy-based devices (EBDs) have emerged as promising adjuncts for refractory cases. This chapter explores the role of various EBDs in HS management.

There are two main treatment paradigms for the application of EBDs in the treatment of HS. First, by targeting the hair follicle, the structure primarily implicated in HS is destroyed. Secondly, EBDs can be used as a surgical approach. Surgical management remains a cornerstone of treatment for moderate-to-severe HS, especially in cases with sinus tract formation, scarring, or failure of medical therapy. Surgical options range from deroofing of sinus tracts to wide local excision of affected areas. Surgery offers low recurrence rates in appropriate patients. Energy-based devices such as CO_2 lasers can serve as precise surgical tools for deroofing or excision, with the advantage of reduced bleeding and postoperative discomfort. Table 16.1 summarizes the EBDs used in the treatment of HS.

Table 16.1 Summary of energy-based devices used in HS

Energy-based device	Evidence strength	Clinical outcomes	Indications	Notes
Nd:YAG laser	Strong	HS-LASI ↓ up to 72.7%	Mild-moderate HS	Safe across skin types
IPL	Moderate	DLQI & HS-LASI ↓	Early disease	Often paired with RF
Alexandrite laser	Weak	Case report only	Experimental	Not recommended
CO_2 laser	Moderate	Excision success 70–97%	Chronic localized HS	Surgical option
Diode laser	Weak	Minimal data	Investigational	Low availability
RF devices	Moderate	IHS4, DLQI, HiSCR improved	Mild-moderate HS	Used with IPL
PDT	Weak	Limited efficacy	Investigational	Rarely used

Long-Pulsed Nd:YAG Laser (1064 nm)

Mechanism of Action

The 1064 nm Nd:YAG laser targets melanin within the hair follicle, inducing selective photothermolysis of follicular and perifollicular structures implicated in HS pathogenesis [2].

Clinical Evidence

A 2020 systematic review and meta-analysis involving five RCTs and 11 case series ($n = 211$) showed that Nd:YAG laser treatment resulted in up to 72.7% reduction in HS-LASI scores at 6 months post-treatment. It is considered safe across all Fitzpatrick skin types and demonstrates high patient tolerability [2].

Indications

- Mild to moderate HS
- Follicular-dominant lesions
- Adjuvant for patients with an incomplete response to systemic therapy

Considerations

- Requires 4–6 treatment sessions.
- Minimal downtime.
- Long-term efficacy is maintained with maintenance sessions.
- *Darker skin tones*: Safe for Fitzpatrick IV–VI; lower melanin absorption reduces risk of dyspigmentation compared to shorter-wavelength lasers. Use caution with higher fluences to minimize post-inflammatory hyperpigmentation (PIH).

Carbon Dioxide (CO_2) Laser

Mechanism of Action

CO_2 lasers allow surgical excision or deroofing of sinus tracts with precision, reducing disease burden in localized areas.

Clinical Evidence

A review of 17 studies indicated success rates ranging from 70.7% to 96.7% for CO_2 laser excision [3]. This modality is especially useful in chronic, localized disease.

Considerations

- May require anesthesia.
- Healing time varies (1–4 weeks).
- Can result in scarring.
- *Darker skin tones*: Risk of PIH and hypertrophic or keloidal scarring is higher. Postoperative wound care and pigment modulation (e.g., topical hydroquinone) may be beneficial.

Intense Pulsed Light (IPL)

Mechanism of Action

IPL is not a laser as it emits non-coherent, broad-spectrum light. It can reduce inflammation and bacterial colonization while targeting vascular and pigmented lesions.

Clinical Evidence

Two small RCTs found improvement in HS-LASI and DLQI scores [4, 5]. While promising, IPL requires more robust data to define its role definitively. Furthermore, it is typically not safe in darker skin tones. Many patients with HS have Fitzpatrick type III+ and therefore are not good candidates for IPL.

Indications

- Early inflammatory lesions.
- Adjunct for superficial disease.

Considerations

- Operator-dependent.
- Often combined with RF devices (e.g., LAight®).
- *Darker skin tones*: Higher risk of PIH and burns.

Alexandrite Laser (755 nm)

Mechanism of Action

The Alexandrite laser delivers energy at 755 nm, which is highly absorbed by melanin in the hair follicle. This selective photothermolysis leads to destruction of the follicular unit, aiming to reduce HS lesion formation.

Clinical Evidence

Limited to single case reports. One study suggested clinical improvement, but broader adoption is not advised due to insufficient evidence [6].

Considerations

- Not routinely recommended.
- Should only be used in investigational settings.
- *Darker skin tones*: Increased melanin absorption makes this laser higher risk for thermal injury and hyperpigmentation in Fitzpatrick IV–VI. Generally avoided.

Diode Laser

Clinical Evidence

Sparse data exists. A small retrospective study suggested a possible benefit, but high-quality trials are lacking [7].

Considerations

- Not routinely recommended.
- Lacks consistent evidence in HS.
- *Darker skin tones*: Intermediate melanin absorption—more caution needed than Nd:YAG, especially with high fluences. Start with conservative parameters.

Radiofrequency (RF) Devices

Mechanism of Action

RF delivers thermal energy to the dermis, promoting glandular destruction and anti-inflammatory effects.

Clinical Evidence

A 2024 systematic review showed significant improvements in IHS4, DLQI, and HiSCR scores for mild-to-moderate HS [8]. Monotherapy appears insufficient in severe disease.

Considerations

- Non-invasive with minimal downtime.
- Requires regular treatments (biweekly to monthly).
- Effective as part of multimodal therapy.
- *Darker skin tones*: Generally safe due to non-chromophore-dependent mechanism. Still monitor for rare PIH or irritation when combined with IPL.

Photodynamic Therapy (PDT)

Mechanism of Action

Photosensitizers (e.g., ALA) accumulate in pilosebaceous units, activated by specific light wavelengths to induce localized destruction.

Clinical Evidence

Limited to case series and small studies. PDT's use in HS remains experimental.

Considerations

- Risk of phototoxicity.
- Limited access and training.
- Often used off-label.
- *Darker skin tones*: Risk of PIH post-treatment. Patients should be counseled regarding sun avoidance and pigmentary side effects.

Board-Review Question Explanation

A 33-year-old woman with Hurley stage II hidradenitis suppurativa presents with recurrent nodules and sinus tracts in the axillae and groin. She has failed multiple systemic therapies. Which of the following energy-based devices has the strongest evidence base for improving lesion counts in HS?

A. 755 nm Alexandrite laser
B. Intense pulsed light (IPL)
C. Long-pulsed Nd:YAG laser (Correct)
D. Photodynamic therapy (PDT)
E. Radiofrequency (RF) therapy

Answer Explanation

Correct Answer: *C. Long-pulsed Nd:YAG laser*

This device has the most robust clinical data supporting its use in HS, with multiple randomized controlled trials and a meta-analysis showing significant improvements in disease severity and quality of life [1, 2].

Key Takeaway Points

- Long-pulsed Nd:YAG laser has the strongest evidence among EBDs for HS treatment
- CO_2 lasers are effective for localized, chronic lesions requiring excision
- RF therapy, especially when combined with IPL, benefits mild-to-moderate HS
- Other devices like Alexandrite, diode lasers, and PDT lack sufficient evidence
- EBDs serve as valuable adjuncts when systemic therapies alone are inadequate

References

1. Goldburg SR, Strober BE, Payette MJ. Hidradenitis suppurativa: epidemiology, clinical presentation, and pathogenesis. J Am Acad Dermatol. 2020;82(5):1045–58. https://doi.org/10.1016/j.jaad.2019.08.090.
2. Jfri A, Saxena A, Rouette J, et al. The efficacy and effectiveness of non-ablative light-based devices in hidradenitis suppurativa: a systematic review and meta-analysis. Front Med (Lausanne). 2020;7:591580. https://doi.org/10.3389/fmed.2020.591580.
3. Saunte DML, Jemec GBE. Laser and intense pulsed light in the treatment of hidradenitis suppurativa. Clin Dermatol. 2023;41(5):628–38. https://doi.org/10.1016/j.clindermatol.2023.08.024.
4. Highton L, Chan WY, Khwaja N, Laitung JKG. Treatment of hidradenitis suppurativa with intense pulsed light: a prospective study. Plast Reconstr Surg. 2011;128(2):459–66. https://doi.org/10.1097/PRS.0b013e31821e6fb5.
5. Wilden S, Friis M, Tuettenberg A, et al. Combined treatment of hidradenitis suppurativa with intense pulsed light (IPL) and radiofrequency (RF). J Dermatolog Treat. 2021;32(5):530–7. https://doi.org/10.1080/09546634.2019.1677842.
6. Tsai YC, Wang SH, Lu P-H, Tsai T-H. Hidradenitis suppurativa treated with a long-pulsed alexandrite laser. Dermatol Sin. 2014;32(2):115–7. https://doi.org/10.1016/j.dsi.2013.04.007.
7. Özdemir AK, Tamer E. 808 nm diode laser in the treatment of hidradenitis suppurativa: a retrospective study. Arch Dermatol Res. 2024;316(10):708. https://doi.org/10.1007/s00403-024-03472-5.
8. Nilforoushzadeh MA, Heidari N, Heidari A, et al. Efficacy and safety of radiofrequency in the treatment of hidradenitis suppurativa; a systematic review. Lasers Med Sci. 2024;39(1):139. https://doi.org/10.1007/s10103-024-04077-0.

Chapter 17
Treatment of Pediatric HS

Sahithi Talasila and Sherry Yang

Case Title A 15-year-old girl presents with recurrent painful nodules in axillae and groin, worsening around menstrual periods

Case

A 15-year-old female presents with a 6-month history of recurrent, painful nodules and abscesses in her axillae and groin. The lesions worsen around her menstrual periods. She reports significant pain and embarrassment, which have led to her avoiding social activities. Physical examination reveals multiple erythematous, tender nodules and sinus tracts with purulent drainage. Some areas show scarring from previous lesions. You diagnose her with hidradenitis suppurativa (HS). What is your approach to this patient's plan of care?

Board Review Question

A 15-year-old female presents with a 6-month history of recurrent, painful nodules and abscesses in the axillae and groin, which worsen around her menstrual periods. On physical examination, there are multiple erythematous, tender nodules, and sinus tracts with purulent drainage, along with scarring from previous lesions. The patient has not previously seen a dermatologist and has not received any prior treatments. She reports using over-the-counter antibacterial washes with minimal relief. Which of the following is the best initial management approach to treat her acute flare at this point?

S. Talasila
Thomas Jefferson University Sidney Kimmel Medical College, Philadelphia, PA, USA

S. Yang (✉)
Department of Dermatology & Cutaneous Biology, Thomas Jefferson University, Philadelphia, PA, USA
e-mail: sherry.yang@jefferson.edu

N. Brownstone (ed.), *Clinical Cases in Hidradenitis Suppurativa*, Clinical Cases in Dermatology, https://doi.org/10.1007/978-3-032-15200-8_17

A. Secukinumab
B. Oral isotretinoin
C. Combination of oral clindamycin and rifampin
D. Adalimumab
E. Surgical excision of affected areas

Clinical Presentation of Hidradenitis Suppurativa in Pediatric Patients

Hidradenitis suppurativa in the pediatric population typically presents during adolescence, with mean symptom onset around 12.5 years of age and diagnostic delay occurring 2–3 years later [1]. Characteristic lesions are painful, deep-seated nodules and abscesses located in intertriginous areas such as the axillae and groin [1]. These lesions can progress to form sinus tracts and scarring, leading to significant physical discomfort and potential complications like anemia and lymphedema [1].

Atypical presentations of pediatric HS can occur when the disease manifests before puberty, which is rare but possible [2]. Especially in younger children, the condition is often misdiagnosed as folliculitis or comedonal acne before an accurate diagnosis of HS is made [2]. Less than 2% of cases present before age 11, often in the setting of positive family history and genetic susceptibility. Early onset, prepubertal HS occurs more often in males, and post-pubescent onset is significantly more common in females than males [3]. This shift in sex distribution between pre- and post-pubescent onset is unexplained, but it is hypothesized that ovarian hormones may play a less important role in prepubescent HS compared to adult-onset disease [3]. Pediatric HS has not been shown to be significantly associated with precocious puberty or hormonal/endocrine pathologies, aside from polycystic ovarian syndrome (PCOS). However, pediatric HS patients should be screened for precocious puberty and hormonal disorders for comprehensive care.

The distribution of lesions in pediatric HS is similar to that in adults, primarily affecting apocrine gland-rich intertriginous areas like the axillae and groin [4]. Children may also experience lesions in the inframammary area, buttocks, and pubic region [4]. The spectrum of clinical manifestations of pediatric HS, from early to late disease, is shown in Fig. 17.1.

While both pediatric and adult patients experience similar lesion distribution, pediatric patients tend to have a higher female predominance (approximately 85% female) compared to adults (77% female) [4]. The typical onset of pediatric HS occurs earlier in females than males, contributing to a higher overall prevalence among adolescent girls [1]. Pediatric patients often utilize high-cost emergency department care more frequently than adults, likely due to challenges in diagnosis

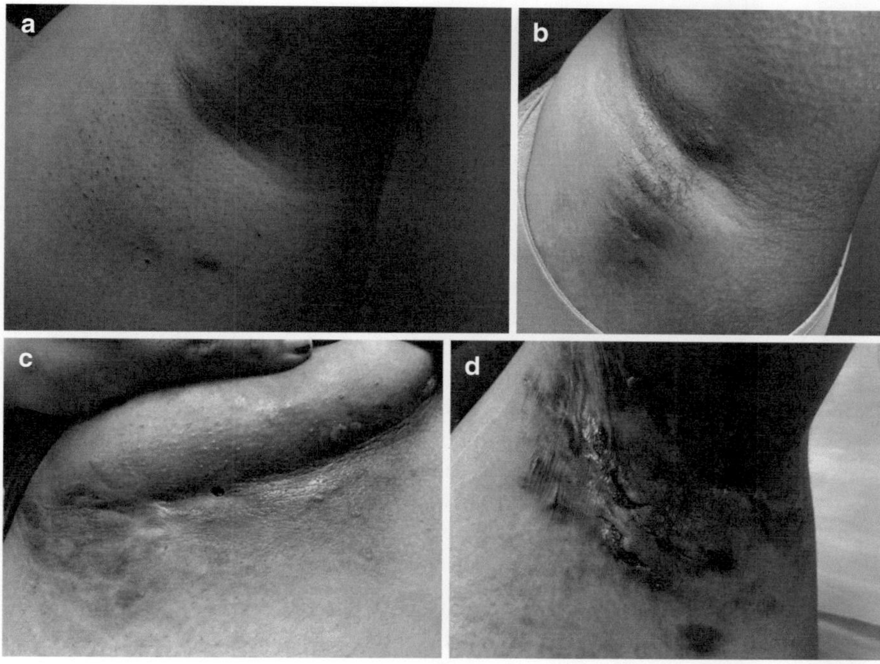

Fig. 17.1 Clinical spectrum of pediatric hidradenitis suppurativa in the axillary and inframammary regions: Early to late manifestations. Early manifestations: (**a**) multiple open comedones with subtle atrophic scar in inferolateral axilla; (**b**) multiple subcutaneous nodules of the axilla. Late manifestations: (**c**) open draining sinus tract and scar in inframammary fold; (**d**) multiple connecting sinus tracts and bridging fibrosis of the axilla. (Reproduced with permission from Patel et al. [5]. © Wolters Kluwer Health, Inc. License Number: 5883740327950)

and management in outpatient settings [4]. However, adults are more likely to experience inpatient stays compared to pediatric patients [4]. Additionally, children with HS have a higher tendency to display comorbid conditions such as obesity, acne vulgaris, and endocrinologic abnormalities than their adult counterparts [1, 2, 4]. These comorbidities are significant as they can complicate the clinical picture and affect treatment outcomes.

The physical impact of HS includes chronic pain, recurrent infections, and restricted movement due to lesion location and scarring [2]. Mentally, pediatric patients may suffer from low self-esteem and social withdrawal due to visible skin changes and the stigma associated with the condition [2]. These combined effects highlight the importance of early recognition and management to improve outcomes for affected children.

Challenges in Diagnosis of Hidradenitis Suppurativa in Pediatric Patients

The diagnosis of pediatric HS, as in adults, is based on patient history and the recognition of characteristic clinical manifestations. Pediatric HS may initially present with more subtle features, such as double-headed open comedones and tender subcutaneous nodules, which may drain malodorous discharge [5–7]. However, due to diagnostic delays, pronounced tunneling and fibrotic scarring are often visible by the time of dermatologic assessment [6]. One study reported that 48% of pediatric patients exhibited advanced scarring at their first dermatologic visit, despite initial symptoms like papules, pustules, or cysts/abscesses [1]. The axillae are the most commonly affected site in pediatric HS, with involvement in 75–85% of cases [6, 7]. Other common sites include the groin or inguinal folds (47–58%) and buttocks (6–27%), similar to adults, but often with fewer body sites involved [7]. The disease course in children may be less predictable due to the subtler presentation, leading to misdiagnosis or delayed diagnosis [6]. The Hurley staging system for hidradenitis suppurativa is a widely used tool to assess disease severity, but its application in pediatric patients presents some differences and challenges:

- Stage I: Characterized by single or multiple abscesses without sinus tracts or scarring. In pediatric HS, this stage is common, with many patients presenting initially with these milder symptoms [7].
- Stage II: Involves recurrent abscesses with discrete sinus tract formation and scarring. Pediatric patients often progress to this stage, but the presentation may be less pronounced compared to adults.
- Stage III: Describes diffuse involvement with interconnected tracts and abscesses across large areas. While less common in pediatric patients, those who do reach this stage may experience rapid progression due to delayed diagnosis [7].

A thorough history can reveal onset during adolescence or young adulthood, recurrent or persistent disease, and family history of HS. Full skin examination helps assess disease extent and severity [8]. While skin biopsy is not usually necessary, it can exclude other disorders if diagnosis is uncertain. Bacterial cultures and serologic studies are not routinely helpful in the diagnosis of HS. Imaging like ultrasound may be used to assess subclinical disease extent and to help guide surgical planning [8].

HS can be mistaken for several conditions due to overlapping symptoms:

- Folliculitis/furunculosis: Unlike HS, these infections are transient and respond quickly to antibiotics. They do not cause comedones, atrophic scarring, or persistent tunnels in the skin [9].
- Acne Vulgaris: This primarily affects the face, chest, and back, whereas HS involves deeper lesions in axillae and groin [10].
- Pilonidal Disease: This occurs in the superior gluteal cleft, may coexist with HS, and is considered a phenotypic variant in the follicular occlusion spectrum [11].

- Crohn's Disease: This can present with similar perianal and genital manifestations, including perianal fistulas and lymphedema; however, the presence of gastrointestinal symptoms can help differentiate the two [12]. Patients with HS are notably 2–3 times more likely to develop Crohn's colitis, so simultaneous occurrence of both conditions should also be considered [13, 14].

Pediatric HS is often under-recognized because its presentation can differ from adults. Many pediatric patients do not meet standard diagnostic criteria due to atypical lesion frequency or location. Primary care providers may not suspect HS initially, leading to diagnostic delays [15]. Delayed diagnosis can lead to disease progression and increased severity, impacting quality of life [1]. Complications include physical discomfort, psychological distress, social impairment, and difficulty managing comorbidities like obesity [1]. Long-standing HS may lead to strictures, lymphedema, depression, anemia, and squamous cell carcinoma [1]. Management is complicated by limited data on long-term treatment outcomes in children. Common treatments include antibiotics and lifestyle changes. More targeted therapies are needed for pediatric patients. Increasing awareness among healthcare providers is essential to reduce diagnostic delays and improve management strategies. Addressing these challenges requires improved diagnostic criteria tailored for pediatric patients, increased awareness among healthcare providers, and more research into effective treatments for this age group.

Current Management Strategies for Hidradenitis Suppurativa in Pediatric Patients

Management of hidradenitis suppurativa in the pediatric population is largely adapted from adult treatment guidelines, as there are no specific pediatric guidelines. Many systemic treatments are used off-label, highlighting the need for further research in this area [16].

Topical treatments are often first-line for mild, Hurley Stage 1 HS. Chlorhexidine and benzoyl peroxide washes reduce bacterial load and are applied daily to affected areas [1]. Clindamycin 1% is the preferred topical antibiotic and is available in solution, lotion, and gel formulations for use one or two times daily [1]. Resorcinol, a keratolytic agent, can be applied to active lesions during flares [17].

Systemic antibiotics like doxycycline, clindamycin, and rifampin are effective in managing pediatric HS, particularly in acute flares or as a bridge to long-term therapies. Doxycycline should be avoided in children less than 8 years of age due to its potential for permanent staining of teeth [16]. Clindamycin and rifampin combination therapy is effective across all Hurley stages but should be used cautiously due to resistance concerns [16]. Azithromycin is another option with a favorable safety profile in pediatrics [1]. Weight-based dosing of these medications should be considered for individuals weighing less than 40 kg [18].

Hormonal therapies can be beneficial, especially in adolescents. Finasteride can be considered in female pediatric patients, particularly post-pubertal females, to reduce HS flare frequency. It has shown efficacy in reducing lesion frequency and severity, especially when other treatments have failed [19]. Monitoring should include ensuring effective contraception due to its teratogenic potential and counseling on hormonal side effects such as breast tenderness and menstrual irregularities [19]. Finasteride should be avoided in males until after puberty due to concerns about its effects on sexual development and potential impacts on prostate size and function [17]. The long-term effects on pubertal development are not fully understood, necessitating caution [17]. Spironolactone and estrogen-containing oral contraceptive pills can be utilized for their anti-androgenic effects for females, preferably in patients over 14 years of age due to hormonal stability post-menarche [16]. Before this age, hormonal fluctuations may lead to unpredictable side effects and efficacy issues [16]. These treatments require careful consideration of age, hormonal status, and potential side effects to ensure safe and effective use in pediatric patients. Metformin may also be useful in patients with metabolic comorbidities such as obesity, PCOS, or insulin resistance [16].

Systemic retinoids are generally considered second- or third-line treatments due to inconsistent efficacy data [16, 17]. Isotretinoin may be beneficial for patients with follicular-type HS and widespread comedones or nodulocystic acne. Regular monitoring should involve monthly pregnancy tests, as mandated by the iPledge program for isotretinoin, along with laboratory evaluations such as liver function tests and lipid panels at treatment initiation and with dosage increases [16]. Acitretin is typically avoided in patients of childbearing potential. Systemic retinoids are not recommended in pre-pubertal children due to risk of premature epiphyseal plate closure and subsequent short stature [20].

Adalimumab is currently the only FDA-approved biologic for moderate-to-severe HS in pediatric patients 12 years and older. Dosing depends on weight:

- 30–60 kg: Start with 80 mg on day 1, followed by 40 mg on day 8, and then 40 mg every other week [21].
- ≥60 kg: Follow the adult regimen with an initial dose of 160 mg on day 1, 80 mg on day 15, and then 40 mg weekly [21].

Common adverse effects include injection site reactions and increased infection risk [21]. Monitoring includes initial and annual TB screening, and a hepatitis-B serology panel at initiation [21]. While biosimilars offer a cost-effective alternative, their efficacy in HS compared to adalimumab requires further study, as retrospective studies show varying outcomes. Infliximab can be considered for severe or recalcitrant disease and has shown positive outcomes in adolescents, though it is only FDA-approved for pediatric patients with other conditions such as Crohn's disease [22]. Secukinumab and ustekinumab are currently approved down to 6 years of age for other conditions and may be considered based on their efficacy in adult HS studies [23].

Oral small molecule inhibitors like apremilast, a phosphodiesterase 4 (PDE-4) inhibitor, and upadacitinib, a Janus kinase (JAK) inhibitor, offer alternatives for children who cannot tolerate injections [24]. Although not specifically approved for pediatric HS, they have shown promise in adult studies and other pediatric conditions [24]. Apremilast does not typically require any routine lab monitoring. Suggested screening tests for upadacitinib include baseline CBC, LFTs, lipid panel, TB screening, and hepatitis panel checks. Ongoing monitoring includes CBC and LFTs at 4–8 weeks after initiation, lipid panel at 12 weeks after initiation and then as clinically indicated, and annual TB screening [24].

A recent systematic review and meta-analysis demonstrated significant improvement in HS disease severity across various laser modalities, particularly long-pulsed Nd:YAG [25]. The 1064 nm Nd:YAG laser is thought to work by targeting and destroying hair follicles, which are central to HS pathogenesis, or by disrupting inflammatory infiltrates through dermal heating [26, 27]. For pediatric patients, Nd:YAG laser treatment offers several advantages. It is minimally invasive compared to surgical interventions, potentially reducing scarring and recovery time. This is particularly beneficial for younger patients who may be more sensitive to invasive procedures. Additionally, the treatment can be performed in-office with topical anesthesia, making it well-tolerated by older children and adolescents. However, it is important to note that while promising, long-term data on the efficacy and safety of Nd:YAG laser treatment specifically in pediatric HS patients is limited. As with any treatment for pediatric HS, the decision to use Nd:YAG laser should be made on a case-by-case basis, considering the patient's age, disease severity, and overall health status. Further research is needed to fully establish the long-term outcomes and optimal treatment protocols for Nd:YAG laser in pediatric HS patients.

Surgical interventions can be considered for moderate to severe cases of hidradenitis suppurativa in pediatric patients when conservative treatments have not provided sufficient relief [15]. Deroofing is a minimally invasive technique that removes the "roof" of sinus tracts while preserving surrounding healthy tissue. This procedure is typically used for Hurley stage II or III disease with recurrent lesions and sinus tract formation [16]. Deroofing may offer shorter healing times and lower recurrence rates compared to wide excision [16]. However, it carries potential risks such as bleeding, infection, scarring, and recurrence. Wide excision surgery may be necessary for extensive disease or cases with significant scarring and sinus tract formation. While more invasive, it allows for removal of all affected tissue, potentially reducing recurrence likelihood [16]. Recovery times for wide excision are generally longer, and more noticeable scarring may result. The choice between deroofing and wide excision depends on factors such as disease severity, affected sites, and individual patient characteristics [16]. Surgical management of hidradenitis suppurativa in pediatric patients requires careful consideration due to ongoing growth and development [4]. While the principles of deroofing and wide excision remain similar to adult procedures, there may be a greater emphasis on tissue-sparing techniques in children to minimize long-term functional and cosmetic impacts [4]. Additionally, the timing of surgical interventions in pediatric patients may be influenced by factors such as pubertal stage and the potential for disease progression during adolescence [4].

Effective pain management is crucial for the surgical management of pediatric HS. Child life specialists play a vital role in pediatric hidradenitis suppurativa procedures by providing age-appropriate education and emotional support, helping children understand what to expect. They also teach coping strategies and use distraction techniques to reduce anxiety and pain during the procedures, enhancing the overall experience for young patients [28]. Vibrational devices, such as the Buzzy device, have shown promise in reducing pain during needle-related procedures in children. The Buzzy device combines cold and vibration to provide pain relief, and studies have demonstrated its effectiveness in reducing pain scores during intravenous injections and other needle-based interventions [29]. Additionally, EMLA (eutectic mixture of local anesthetics) cream, containing 2.5% lidocaine and 2.5% prilocaine, and lidocaine-based topical anesthetics have been shown to provide effective pain relief when applied to intact skin before procedures [30]. Cryotherapy, in the form of ice packs or cooling sprays, can also be employed to reduce pain and inflammation. When used in combination with other pain management techniques, cold therapy can enhance overall pain relief and improve patient comfort [31]. These techniques can be useful to manage pain in pediatric patients for minor in-office procedures, or to manage pain prior to administration of local or regional anesthesia for larger procedures. For more invasive procedures, regional anesthesia techniques should be considered. While evidence for specific hidradenitis suppurativa procedures is limited, studies have shown that regional anesthesia can provide effective pain control for various pediatric surgeries [32]. General anesthesia is also considered for larger or more invasive procedures, especially in patients who require extensive debridement or wide excision of sinus tracts. For pediatric patients, the need for general anesthesia may be influenced by the psychological distress that comes with repeated painful procedures or the necessity of prolonged surgical time [33]. The choice between local, regional, or general anesthesia depends on factors such as the extent of the procedure, patient age, and individual characteristics.

Practical tips for clinicians managing pediatric HS include the following:

- For Acute Symptomatic Flares: Weight-based dosing for doxycycline in children 8 years and older or combination clindamycin with rifampin can be used for acute management [16]. Older children who can tolerate procedural intervention may be candidates for intralesional corticosteroid injections [32]. Large fluctuant abscesses may require incision and drainage (I&D) for immediate relief of pressure and pain [34].
- Early Intervention: Initiating treatment early can prevent complications like scarring.
- Combination Therapy: A multimodal approach combining pharmacological treatments with lifestyle changes often yields the best results.
- Monitoring and Safety: Regular monitoring for side effects is crucial when using systemic treatments.
- Patient and Family Education: Educating families about HS's chronic nature and treatment adherence is vital.

While pediatric HS management relies heavily on adult treatment data, emerging studies highlight the potential of both pharmacological and non-pharmacological interventions. Further research is essential to optimize these strategies for safety and efficacy in children.

Comorbidities and Psychosocial Impact of Pediatric Hidradenitis Suppurativa

Obesity and metabolic syndrome are common comorbidities in pediatric patients with HS linked by shared inflammatory pathways [35]. Obesity contributes to HS through physical, microbial, immunological, and metabolic mechanisms [35]. Physically, excess weight leads to skin folds that promote friction and moisture [35]. Microbial changes in skin folds further exacerbate HS by altering the skin microbiome [35]. Hypertrophic adipose tissue in obesity secretes pro-inflammatory mediators like cytokines and chemokines, fostering systemic inflammation [36, 37]. This low-grade inflammation is a hallmark of both obesity and HS, driven by immune cells such as neutrophils and macrophages infiltrating adipose tissue [36, 37]. These cells release inflammatory signals, exacerbating HS symptoms and contributing to insulin resistance [36, 37]. In HS, adipokines—hormones from adipose tissue—are dysregulated [35]. Leptin levels increase while anti-inflammatory adiponectin decreases, promoting inflammation and obesity [35]. This imbalance affects immune cell function, creating a pathogenic immune-metabolic circuit that worsens HS [35]. Studies show that individuals with HS often exhibit adverse metabolic characteristics even when classified as metabolically healthy [38]. The presence of metabolic syndrome significantly increases the risk of developing HS, highlighting the importance of metabolic risk assessment in managing HS [38]. Understanding the interconnected pathways between obesity, metabolic syndrome, and HS is crucial for effective management. Targeted interventions addressing both metabolic health and inflammation can mitigate the severity of HS in pediatric patients.

Pediatric patients with HS often experience a range of comorbidities beyond obesity and metabolic syndrome. The most common cutaneous comorbidities include acne vulgaris, pilonidal cysts, acne conglobata, dissecting cellulitis, and psoriasis [1, 7, 39]. The most common systemic comorbidities include PCOS, diabetes, hyperlipidemia, hypertension, inflammatory bowel disease (IBD), arthritis or arthropathy, Down syndrome, and thyroid disease [1, 7, 35, 39]. Hidradenitis suppurativa (HS) is associated with an increased risk of developing inflammatory arthropathies, particularly seronegative arthropathies like spondyloarthritis (SpA). While HS itself is not directly linked to HLA-B27, patients with HS who develop spondyloarthritis may have a higher prevalence of HLA-B27, as this gene is commonly associated with SpA rather than HS alone [40]. Screening for symptoms like peripheral joint pain or morning stiffness can help detect early arthritis, which often manifests after the onset of HS skin lesions and can result in permanent joint destruction if left untreated. Additionally, HS can present as a part of PASH (pyoderma gangrenosum, acne, and suppurative hidradenitis) syndrome or PAPASH (pyogenic arthritis, pyoderma gangrenosum, acne, and suppurative hidradenitis) syndrome. PASH syndrome typically presents with severe acne, often of the nodulocystic or conglobata type, followed by the development of HS lesions and later pyoderma gangrenosum, presenting as inflammatory nodules, abscesses, and ulcers [7, 41]. PAPASH syndrome additionally includes pyogenic arthritis as part of its clinical manifestations [42, 43]. In pediatric cases, arthritis may be the initial and predominant symptom, while skin manifestations like pyoderma gangrenosum and acne may develop later [42, 43]. However, it is important to note that the clinical presentation can be highly variable, and not all patients will exhibit all four cardinal features simultaneously. Both PASH and PAPASH are rare autoinflammatory conditions and represent more severe and complex syndromic presentations of HS when present in the pediatric population, often requiring aggressive multidisciplinary management approaches.

Psychiatric conditions, including anxiety and depression, are also significant comorbidities that affect approximately 29% of pediatric HS patients [15]. This is notably higher compared to rates of depression and anxiety found in adult HS counterparts, which are reported at 16.9% and 4.9%, respectively [44]. Visible skin lesions and malodorous drainage can lead to low self-esteem and body image issues, affecting academic performance and social interactions. The chronic pain and social stigma associated with HS contribute to these mental health challenges. Children with HS may face bullying or social isolation, which can further deteriorate their mental health. The persistent nature of HS symptoms can lead to feelings of hopelessness and frustration, necessitating comprehensive mental health support. Addressing the comorbidities and psychological impacts of HS in pediatric patients requires a multidisciplinary approach [39]. Effective management should include medical treatment for HS symptoms, lifestyle interventions for comorbid conditions like obesity, and psychological support to improve mental health outcomes. Early intervention is crucial to mitigate these impacts and improve the quality of life for affected children.

Preventive Strategies and Lifestyle Modifications in the Management of Pediatric Hidradenitis Suppurativa

Preventive and lifestyle measures are crucial in managing HS, minimizing flare-ups, and slowing disease progression. Key strategies include weight management, smoking avoidance, and consistent use of preventative topicals.

Weight management is crucial for pediatric HS patients due to the strong association with metabolic disease [5]. Maintaining a healthy weight through diet and exercise reduces inflammatory mediators, potentially decreasing the severity and frequency of flare-ups. Early intervention in weight management can prevent the development of more severe forms of HS [5].

While direct evidence linking childhood tobacco exposure to HS is limited, smoking is known to exacerbate HS symptoms in adults [5]. Smoking induces systemic inflammation and impairs immune function, potentially worsening HS lesions [5]. Avoiding tobacco use can reduce this inflammatory burden and improve disease outcomes. Educating children about the dangers of smoking and creating smoke-free environments are essential preventive measures. Secondhand smoke exposure has been linked with respiratory infections and asthma attacks in children, contributing to an inflammatory state that can similarly aggravate HS symptoms [45].

Proper hygiene is vital in managing HS by reducing bacterial colonization of the skin and hair follicles. Regular cleansing with antiseptic washes can decrease bacterial load on the skin and minimize flare-ups [5]. Teaching children effective hygiene practices early on helps prevent secondary infections that can exacerbate HS symptoms. By addressing these lifestyle factors, pediatric patients can experience fewer flare-ups and slower disease progression. Pediatricians, primary care physicians, and pediatric dermatologists play a pivotal role in implementing these preventive measures by providing tailored advice during regular check-ups.

Board Review Question Explanation

A 15-year-old female presents with a 6-month history of recurrent, painful nodules and abscesses in the axillae and groin, which worsen around her menstrual periods. On physical examination, there are multiple erythematous, tender nodules and sinus tracts with purulent drainage, along with scarring from previous lesions. The patient has not previously seen a dermatologist and has not received any prior treatments. She reports using over-the-counter antibacterial washes with minimal relief. Which of the following is the best initial management approach to treat her acute flare at this point?

A. Secukinumab
B. Oral isotretinoin
C. Combination of oral clindamycin and rifampin (Correct)
D. Adalimumab
E. Surgical excision of affected areas

Answer Explanation

The combination of oral clindamycin and rifampicin (option C) is the most appropriate initial management strategy for an acute flare in this adolescent with hidradenitis suppurativa. Scheinfeld reported good results using clindamycin (300 mg, twice daily) and rifampin (300 mg, twice daily) in four cases of pediatric HS, supporting its efficacy in this population [46].

Secukinumab (Cosentyx) (A) is incorrect as this medication is only FDA approved for the treatment of moderate to severe HS in adults over 18 years of age [7, 47]. Its use in pediatric HS patients remains off-label, and is not recommended for use as a first-line treatment in this population [7, 47]. For a 15-year-old patient with no prior treatments, the initial management should focus on treatments that have been more extensively studied and approved for use in pediatric patients with HS. Oral isotretinoin (B) is not considered first-line therapy for HS in adolescents due to limited evidence of efficacy and potential side effects [48]. Adalimumab (D) is approved for children over 12 years of age with moderate-to-severe HS who have failed other treatments; however, response typically does not occur until several months later, so utility during acute flares is limited [48]. Surgical excision (E) is too aggressive as an initial approach for moderate HS in an adolescent, being more appropriate for severe, refractory cases [48]. The clindamycin-rifampicin combination offers a balance of efficacy and safety for pediatric patients, addressing both the inflammatory and potential infectious components of HS without resorting to more invasive or potent treatments prematurely.

Key Take Away Points

- Pediatric HS typically presents during adolescence, with a mean age of symptom onset around 12.5 years and formal diagnosis at 14.4 years.
- Pediatric HS is commonly associated with comorbidities such as obesity, metabolic syndrome, acne vulgaris, PCOS, hyperlipidemia, hypertension, asthma, acanthosis nigricans, and psychiatric conditions like anxiety and depression.
- Although pediatric HS is rarely a harbinger of precocious puberty or hormonal/endocrine disorders, all patients should undergo a comprehensive review of systems upon initial evaluation.
- The axillae are the most commonly affected site in pediatric HS, with involvement occurring in 75–85% of cases.
- Diagnosis of HS in pediatrics is often delayed due to atypical presentations and overlap with other conditions like folliculitis or comedonal acne.
- The Hurley staging system is used in pediatric HS, but presentation may be less pronounced compared to adults.
- First-line treatments of pediatric HS include topical antibacterial washes, topical antibiotics, and systemic antibiotics.
- Adalimumab, a TNF-alpha inhibitor, is FDA-approved for moderate-to-severe HS in patients 12 years and older, with weight-based dosing.
- Obesity is a common comorbidity linked to HS through shared inflammatory pathways, contributing to disease progression and complicating management.
- HS has a greater psychosocial impact on pediatric patients compared to adults, affecting self-esteem, social interactions, and quality of life.

References

1. Liy-Wong C, Kim M, Kirkorian AY, et al. Hidradenitis suppurativa in the pediatric population: an international, multicenter, retrospective, cross-sectional study of 481 pediatric patients. JAMA Dermatol. 2021;157(4):385. https://doi.org/10.1001/jamadermatol.2020.5435.
2. Vaiopoulos AG, Nikolakis G, Zouboulis CC. Hidradenitis suppurativa in paediatric patients: a retrospective monocentric study in Germany and review of the literature. J Eur Acad Dermatol Venereol. 2020;34(9):2140–6. https://doi.org/10.1111/jdv.16520.

3. Braunberger TL, Nicholson CL, Gold L, et al. Hidradenitis suppurativa in children: The Henry Ford experience. Pediatr Dermatol. 2018;35(3):370–3. https://doi.org/10.1111/pde.13466.
4. Hallock KK, Mizerak MR, Dempsey A, Maczuga S, Kirby JS. Differences between children and adults with hidradenitis suppurativa. JAMA Dermatol. 2021;157(9):1095. https://doi.org/10.1001/jamadermatol.2021.2865.
5. Patel K, Leszczynska M, Peña-Robichaux V, Diaz LZ. Caring for pediatric hidradenitis suppurativa patients in the emergency department. Pediatr Emerg Care. 2021;37(6):312–7. https://doi.org/10.1097/PEC.0000000000002448.
6. Lambert RA, Stein SL. Pediatric hidradenitis suppurativa: describing care patterns in the emergency department. Pediatr Dermatol. 2023;40(3):434–9. https://doi.org/10.1111/pde.15231.
7. Cotton CH, Chen SX, Hussain SH, Lara-Corrales I, Zaenglein AL. Hidradenitis suppurativa in pediatric patients. Pediatrics. 2023;151(5):e2022061049. https://doi.org/10.1542/peds.2022-061049.
8. Perelman School of Medicine at the University of Pennsylvania Philadelphia, Pennsylvania, Micheletti MRG. Natural history, presentation, and diagnosis of hidradenitis suppurativa. Semin Cutan Med Surg. 2014;33(3S):S51–3. https://doi.org/10.12788/j.sder.0092.
9. Raff AB, Kroshinsky D. Cellulitis: a review. JAMA. 2016;316(3):325. https://doi.org/10.1001/jama.2016.8825.
10. Jordan KM, Famisan DO, Myer SN, Fine J, Ren Y, Tartar DM. Acne vulgaris in black pediatric patients: clinical presentation, treatment patterns, and unique needs. Dermatol Online J. 2024;30(3). https://doi.org/10.5070/D330363861.
11. Khanna A, Rombeau J. Pilonidal disease. Clin Colon Rectal Surg. 2011;24(01):046–53. https://doi.org/10.1055/s-0031-1272823.
12. Roussomoustakaki M, Dimoulios P, Chatzicostas C, et al. Hidradenitis suppurativa associated with Crohn's disease and spondyloarthropathy: response to anti-TNF therapy. J Gastroenterol. 2003;38(10):1000–14. https://doi.org/10.1007/s00535-003-1185-9.
13. Chen WT, Chi CC. Association of hidradenitis suppurativa with inflammatory bowel disease: a systematic review and meta-analysis. JAMA Dermatol. 2019;155(9):1022. https://doi.org/10.1001/jamadermatol.2019.0891.
14. Garg A, Hundal J, Strunk A. Overall and subgroup prevalence of Crohn disease among patients with hidradenitis suppurativa: a population-based analysis in the United States. JAMA Dermatol. 2018;154(7):814. https://doi.org/10.1001/jamadermatol.2018.0878.
15. Seivright JR, Collier E, Grogan T, et al. Management landscape of pediatric hidradenitis suppurativa. Skin Appendage Disord. 2022;8(2):118–21. https://doi.org/10.1159/000519135.
16. Masson R, Ma E, Parvathala N, et al. Efficacy of medical treatments for pediatric hidradenitis suppurativa: a systematic review. Pediatr Dermatol. 2023;40(5):775–88. https://doi.org/10.1111/pde.15404.
17. Choi E, Ooi XT, Chandran NS. Hidradenitis suppurativa in pediatric patients. J Am Acad Dermatol. 2022;86(1):140–7. https://doi.org/10.1016/j.jaad.2020.08.045.
18. Matson KL, Horton ER, Capino AC, On behalf of the advocacy Committee for the Pediatric Pharmacy Advocacy Group. Medication dosage in overweight and obese children. J Pediatr Pharmacol Ther. 2017;22(1):81–3. https://doi.org/10.5863/1551-6776-22.1.81.
19. Randhawa HK, Hamilton J, Pope E. Finasteride for the treatment of hidradenitis suppurativa in children and adolescents. JAMA Dermatol. 2013;149(6):732. https://doi.org/10.1001/jamadermatol.2013.2874.
20. David M, Hodak E, Lowe NJ. Adverse effects of retinoids. Med Toxicol. 1988;3(4):273–88. https://doi.org/10.1007/BF03259940.
21. Kimball AB, Okun MM, Williams DA, et al. Two phase 3 trials of Adalimumab for hidradenitis suppurativa. N Engl J Med. 2016;375(5):422–34. https://doi.org/10.1056/NEJMoa1504370.
22. Sachdeva M, Kim P, Mufti A, Maliyar K, Sibbald C, Alavi A. Biologic use in pediatric patients with hidradenitis suppurativa: a systematic review. J Cutan Med Surg. 2022;26(2):176–80. https://doi.org/10.1177/12034754211049711.

23. Martora F, Megna M, Battista T, et al. Adalimumab, ustekinumab, and secukinumab in the management of hidradenitis suppurativa: a review of the real-life experience. Clin Cosmet Investig Dermatol. 2023;16:135–48. https://doi.org/10.2147/CCID.S391356.
24. Alikhan A, Sayed C, Alavi A, et al. North American clinical management guidelines for hidradenitis suppurativa: a publication from the United States and Canadian hidradenitis suppurativa foundations: part I: diagnosis, evaluation, and the use of complementary and procedural management. J Am Acad Dermatol. 2019;81(1):76–90. https://doi.org/10.1016/j.jaad.2019.02.067.
25. Shipman WD, Williams MN, Suozzi KC, Eisenstein AS, Dover JS. Efficacy of laser hair removal in hidradenitis suppurativa: a systematic review and meta-analysis. Lasers Surg Med. 2024;56(5):425–36. https://doi.org/10.1002/lsm.23796.
26. Jfri A, Saxena A, Rouette J, et al. The efficacy and effectiveness of non-ablative light-based devices in hidradenitis suppurativa: a systematic review and meta-analysis. Front Med. 2020;7:591580. https://doi.org/10.3389/fmed.2020.591580.
27. Xu LY, Wright DR, Mahmoud BH, Ozog DM, Mehregan DA, Hamzavi IH. Histopathologic study of hidradenitis suppurativa following long-pulsed 1064-nm Nd:YAG laser treatment. Arch Dermatol. 2010;147(1):21. https://doi.org/10.1001/archdermatol.2010.245.
28. Child Life Council, Committee on Hospital Care. Child life services. Pediatrics. 2006;118(4):1757–63. https://doi.org/10.1542/peds.2006-1941.
29. Cho YH, Chiang YC, Chu TL, Chang CW, Chang CC, Tsai HM. The effectiveness of the buzzy device for pain relief in children during intravenous injection: quasirandomized study. JMIR Pediatr Parent. 2022;5(2):e15757. https://doi.org/10.2196/15757.
30. Zaki HA, Elarref MA, Iftikhar H, et al. Efficacy of Emla (eutectic mixture of local anaesthetics) and let (Lidocaine, Epinephrine, Tetracaine) for topical use in wound management for children: a systematic review and meta-analysis. Cureus. Published online November 13. 2022. https://doi.org/10.7759/cureus.31447.
31. Ravindran V, Lakshmanan L. Efficacy of cryotherapy application on the pain perception during intraoral injection: a randomized controlled trial. Int J Clin Pediatr Dent. 2021;14(5):616–20. https://doi.org/10.5005/jp-journals-10005-2032.
32. Walker SM. Pain after surgery in children: clinical recommendations. Curr Opin Anaesthesiol. 2015;28(5):570–6. https://doi.org/10.1097/ACO.0000000000000227.
33. Eijlers R, Staals LM, Legerstee JS, et al. Predicting intense levels of child anxiety during anesthesia induction at hospital arrival. J Clin Psychol Med Settings. 2021;28(2):313–22. https://doi.org/10.1007/s10880-020-09716-6.
34. Kohorst JJ, Baum CL, Otley CC, et al. Surgical management of hidradenitis suppurativa: outcomes of 590 consecutive patients. Dermatologic Surg. 2016;42(9):1030–40. https://doi.org/10.1097/DSS.0000000000000806.
35. Witte K, Wolk K, Witte-Händel E, Krause T, Kokolakis G, Sabat R. Targeting metabolic syndrome in hidradenitis suppurativa by phytochemicals as a potential complementary therapeutic strategy. Nutrients. 2023;15(17):3797. https://doi.org/10.3390/nu15173797.
36. Saltiel AR, Olefsky JM. Inflammatory mechanisms linking obesity and metabolic disease. J Clin Invest. 2017;127(1):1–4. https://doi.org/10.1172/JCI92035.
37. Wu H, Ballantyne CM. Metabolic inflammation and insulin resistance in obesity. Circ Res. 2020;126(11):1549–64. https://doi.org/10.1161/CIRCRESAHA.119.315896.
38. Mintoff D, Agius R, Fava S, Pace NP. Investigating adiposity-related metabolic health phenotypes in patients with hidradenitis suppurativa: a cross-sectional study. J Clin Med. 2023;12(14):4847. https://doi.org/10.3390/jcm12144847.
39. Seivright JR, Collier E, Grogan T, Hogeling M, Shi VY, Hsiao JL. Physical and psychosocial comorbidities of pediatric hidradenitis suppurativa: a retrospective analysis. Pediatr Dermatol. 2021;38(5):1132–6. https://doi.org/10.1111/pde.14765.
40. Almuhanna N, Finstad A, Alhusayen R. Association between hidradenitis suppurativa and inflammatory arthritis: a systematic review and meta-analysis. Dermatology. 2021;237(5):740–7. https://doi.org/10.1159/000514582.

41. Yan A, Gallardo M, Savu A, Kaffenberger B. Pyoderma gangrenosum, acne, and suppurative hidradenitis (PASH) syndrome: a single-institution case series with a focus on management. Arch Dermatol Res. 2024;316(7):397. https://doi.org/10.1007/s00403-024-03125-7.
42. Cugno M, Borghi A, Marzano AV. PAPA, PASH and PAPASH syndromes: pathophysiology, presentation and treatment. Am J Clin Dermatol. 2017;18(4):555–62. https://doi.org/10.1007/s40257-017-0265-1.
43. Dejenie R, Wong M, Love N, He Y, Fung MA, Tartar DM. Granulomatosis with polyangiitis with pyoderma gangrenosum, acne, hidradenitis suppurativa-like features. JAAD Case Rep. 2024;51:30–3. https://doi.org/10.1016/j.jdcr.2024.05.040.
44. Machado MO, Stergiopoulos V, Maes M, et al. Depression and anxiety in adults with hidradenitis suppurativa: a systematic review and meta-analysis. JAMA Dermatol. 2019;155(8):939. https://doi.org/10.1001/jamadermatol.2019.0759.
45. Matt GE, Bernert JT, Hovell MF. Measuring secondhand smoke exposure in children: an ecological measurement approach. J Pediatr Psychol. 2007;33(2):156–75. https://doi.org/10.1093/jpepsy/jsm123.
46. Scheinfeld N. Hidradenitis suppurativa in prepubescent and pubescent children. Clin Dermatol. 2015;33(3):316–9. https://doi.org/10.1016/j.clindermatol.2014.12.007.
47. Cosentyx (secukinumab). Package insert. Novartis Pharmaceuticals Corporation; 2015. Updated August 2025. https://www.novartis.com/us-en/sites/novartis_us/files/cosentyx.pdf.
48. Nesbitt E, Clements S, Driscoll M. A concise clinician's guide to therapy for hidradenitis suppurativa. Int J Women's Dermatol. 2020;6(2):80–4. https://doi.org/10.1016/j.ijwd.2019.11.004.

Chapter 18
Treatment of HS in Female Patients

Sahithi Talasila and Sherry Yang

Case Title A 28-year-old woman with polycystic ovary syndrome presents with recurrent painful nodules in axillae and groin and plans to conceive within a year

Case

A 28-year-old woman with a history of polycystic ovary syndrome and Hurley stage 2 hidradenitis suppurativa presents due to an acute flare under breasts and in her groin. During her pregnancy, she stopped taking adalimumab (Humira) in her third trimester and has not restarted the medication. She is currently only using topical clindamycin, benzoyl peroxide wash, and metformin. She is now 6 weeks postpartum, currently breastfeeding, and is experiencing a postpartum flare with painful nodules and abscesses under her breasts and in her groin. She asks you about the safety of treatments while breastfeeding and seeks guidance on managing her HS symptoms. What is your treatment approach for this patient?

Board Review Question

A 28-year-old woman with a history of polycystic ovary syndrome presents 6 weeks postpartum for evaluation of Hurley stage 2 hidradenitis suppurativa. She is experiencing an acute flare under her breasts and in her groin. She stopped adalimumab (Humira) during her third trimester and is currently breastfeeding. She is currently using topical clindamycin, benzoyl peroxide wash, and metformin. Which of the following is contraindicated as a potential treatment for this patient?

S. Talasila (✉)
Thomas Jefferson University Sidney Kimmel Medical College, Philadelphia, PA, USA
e-mail: sahithitalasila912@gmail.com

S. Yang
Department of Dermatology & Cutaneous Biology, Thomas Jefferson University, Philadelphia, PA, USA

N. Brownstone (ed.), *Clinical Cases in Hidradenitis Suppurativa*, Clinical Cases in Dermatology, https://doi.org/10.1007/978-3-032-15200-8_18

A. Re-starting adalimumab (Humira)
B. Oral doxycycline
C. Intralesional corticosteroids
D. Oral clindamycin and rifampin
E. Oral spironolactone

Clinical Features, Hormonal Influences, and Disease Course of Hidradenitis Suppurativa in Women of Reproductive Age

In epidemiological studies conducted in North America and Europe, hidradenitis suppurativa (HS) has been observed to disproportionately affect women of reproductive age [1–4]. Women of reproductive age with HS experience distinct challenges related to menstruation, hormonal changes, sexual health, pregnancy, childbirth, and breastfeeding.

One of the key challenges for women with HS is fertility, which has been studied with varying conclusions in recent research. While some studies suggest an association between HS and infertility, others do not support this finding. A population-based, cross-sectional, matched controlled study involving 4191 HS patients and 20,941 controls, found that HS was linked to infertility in both males and females across reproductive age groups, with the strongest association observed in individuals aged 36–45 years [5]. Notably, female HS patients demonstrated a higher risk of infertility, and this association remained significant even after adjusting for demographic and clinical factors [5]. However, other research indicates no significant difference in fertility between HS patients and control groups [6]. A cross-sectional study in Denmark found no statistically significant difference in infertility rates between HS patients, those with other dermatological diseases, and healthy controls [6].

The common manifestations of HS—such as pain, itching, unpleasant odor, and suppuration—can significantly disrupt patients' lives and may influence their desire for pregnancy [7]. Additionally, HS negatively affects sexual function, especially in women with active lesions in the groin and genital areas [8]. Poor self-esteem and body image, as well as a higher risk of anxiety and depression, may also contribute to reduced reproductive desire [9, 10]. Moreover, comorbidities associated with HS, such as obesity, polycystic ovary syndrome (PCOS), Crohn's disease, type 2 diabetes, and cardiovascular disease, further contribute to lower fertility rates [11].

In women of reproductive age, HS typically presents with painful, recurrent nodules, abscesses, and sinus tracts in intertriginous areas. The onset of HS in this population often occurs in the late teens or early twenties, with a mean age of disease onset around 23 years [12]. In women of reproductive age, HS lesions most commonly affect the following areas:

1. Axillae
2. Inguinal and genital regions
3. Inframammary folds
4. Buttocks and perianal area

Compared to men, women are more likely to have genitofemoral lesions and involvement of the sub- and intermammary folds [13].

The progression of HS in women of reproductive age is often characterized by periods of flare-ups and remissions. Hormonal factors play a significant role in the pathogenesis and clinical course of HS in women of reproductive age [14, 15]. Specifically, a comprehensive study of 283 women with HS revealed that 62.4% reported worsening of symptoms with menses, with 78.9% of those experiencing flares in the week preceding menstruation [16]. This high prevalence of perimenstrual flares suggests a strong hormonal influence on HS pathogenesis similar to that of hormonally induced acne vulgaris. The decline in estrogen and progesterone levels during the luteal phase is thought to trigger these flares, as progesterone suppresses the proliferation of CD4+ T cells and Th17 cells involved in the chronic inflammatory state of HS (Fig. 18.1) [13].

Pregnancy and postpartum periods also significantly impact HS disease activity. A meta-analysis of 672 cases across eight studies found that 24% of women experienced HS improvement during pregnancy, while 20% reported worsening of symptoms [17]. Notably, 60% of patients experienced postpartum flaring [17]. The pathophysiology behind these findings likely involves hormonal and weight fluctuations. During pregnancy, rising estrogen levels may shift the immune response from pro-inflammatory to anti-inflammatory cytokines, while progesterone suppresses interferon production and the activity of CD4+ T cells and T helper-17 cells [17]. The dramatic reduction in estrogen and high prolactin levels associated with the postpartum period may explain the high rate of postpartum flares (Fig. 18.1) [15].

The pathophysiology underlying hormonal influences on HS is multifaceted. While early studies suggested elevated testosterone levels in women with HS, recent research shows no significant difference in serum androgen levels between HS patients and controls, except in those with comorbid PCOS [18]. In non-PCOS HS patients, there may be increased end-organ receptor sensitivity to normal levels of circulating androgens rather than absolute elevations in androgen levels [18]. Estrogen and progesterone have sex-specific immune-modulating actions, either by directly acting on transcription factors and gene expression in inflammatory cells or indirectly via incompletely understood mechanisms [15]. These hormonal fluctuations can lead to TH1/TH17 polarization, which is recognized as an inflammatory contributor to HS (Fig. 18.1) [15].

Comorbid conditions associated with hormonal imbalances are also prevalent in women with HS. The prevalence of PCOS among HS patients is 9.0%, approximately twice the independent odds for patients without HS [2]. This association suggests shared pathophysiological mechanisms between HS and PCOS, such as hormonal dysregulation and metabolic dysfunction. Furthermore, the prevalence of metabolic syndrome in patients with HS is significantly higher than in the general population. A study published by Gold et al. found that 50.6% of HS patients met the criteria for metabolic syndrome compared to 30.2% of controls [19]. This higher prevalence suggests that patients with HS may be at increased risk for cardiovascular disease and other complications associated with metabolic syndrome.

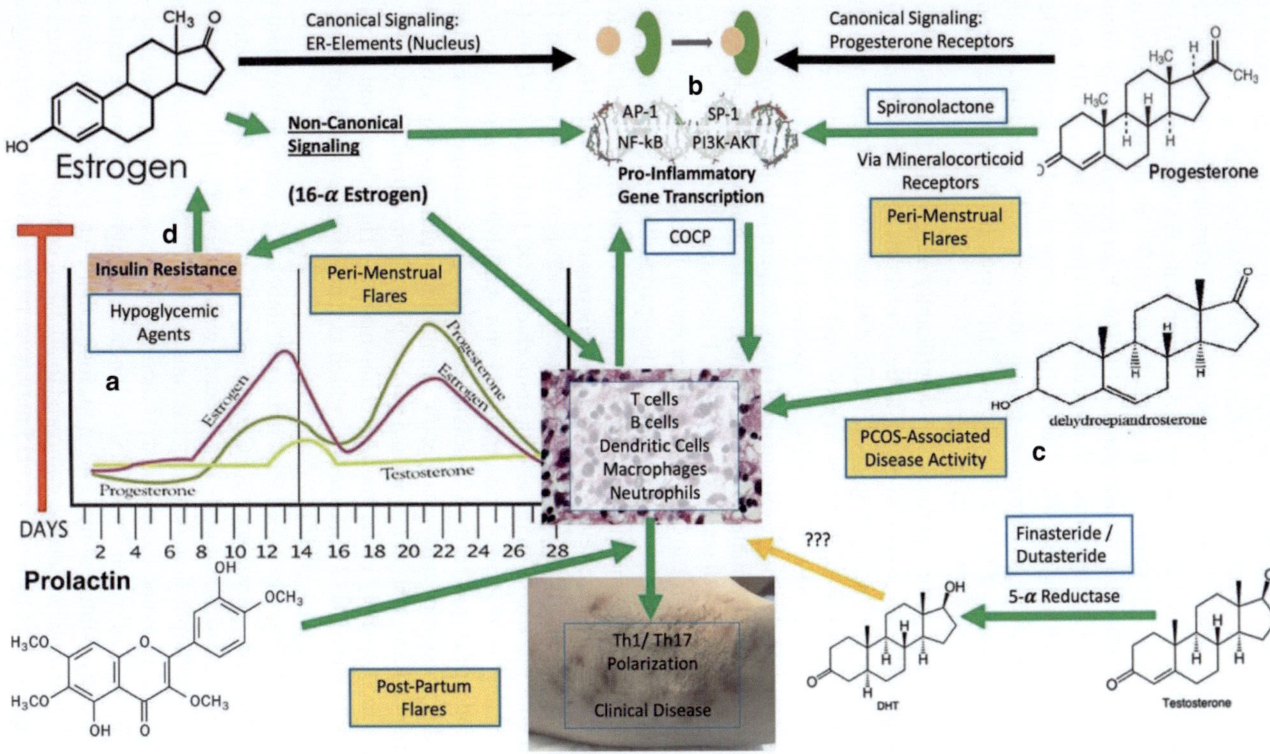

Fig. 18.1 Hormonal influences on the pathogenesis and flares of hidradenitis suppurativa in women of reproductive age. Red arrows indicate suppressive activity, yellow arrows indicate unknown activity, and green arrows indicate contributory activity. (Reproduced with permission from Kozera et al. [15], published by Elsevier, under the Creative Commons CC-BY license)

Preconception Counseling and Pregnancy Considerations for Women with Hidradenitis Suppurativa

Preconception counseling for women with HS should address several key areas:

- Fertility and Pregnancy Planning: Some studies report women with HS report higher rates of infertility compared to the general population [5]. This possibility should be discussed, along with potential contributing factors such as comorbid PCOS, which is more prevalent in HS patients [5].
- Impact of HS on Sexual Health: 73% of women with HS agree that the condition negatively impacts their sexual health [1]. This can lead to decreased sexual activity, which 24% of patients believe impedes their ability to become pregnant [1].
- Medication Review: 49% of HS patients believe pregnancy requires discontinuation of all HS medications [1]. It is crucial to review current medications and discuss which are safe to continue during pregnancy and which need to be discontinued or replaced.
- Disease Management During Pregnancy: Develop a plan for safe treatment options and potential flare management strategies. The goal is to achieve optimal disease control before conception, as HS has been associated with gestational hypertension [20], pre-eclampsia [20], lower odds of a live birth [21], and higher odds of a Cesarean delivery [21], gestational diabetes [22], and maternal morbidity [22].
- Genetic susceptibility: Recent research has shown that HS has a strong hereditary component, with a narrow-sense heritability of 77% [23]. Approximately 50% of individuals diagnosed with HS report a positive family history [24, 25]. Furthermore, sibling recurrence risk is 19.9 and parent-offspring risk is 18.6 [25].
- Despite these findings, genome-wide association studies have failed to consistently identify pathogenic mutations in HS patients. Mutations in the gamma-secretase complex have been implicated in very rare familial HS variants that account for less than 7% of HS cases [24]. Environmental factors also contribute to the susceptibility of HS, supporting a multifactorial cause [23]. It is crucial for patients to understand that having a genetic predisposition does not guarantee disease occurrence.
- Delivery: Address questions about childbirth difficulties, a common concern reported by women with HS involving the vulva and groin [1]. Reassure patients that while HS can make childbirth more challenging, many women with HS have successful vaginal deliveries. Discuss the slightly increased risk of complications such as wound breakdown or infection at HS sites during delivery, which can often be managed effectively with proper care and close monitoring during labor and postpartum [15]. Expectant mothers should be reassured that there is no evidence of HS transmission to the baby during childbirth [1].
- Breastfeeding: While HS on the breasts can make breastfeeding more challenging due to maternal pain or discomfort, many women with breast HS can still breastfeed successfully. Options include nursing from the unaffected breast if

lesions are unilateral, or using a breast pump to maintain milk supply if breastfeeding is not possible due to extensive disease [15]. Patients should be reassured that HS transmission does not occur through breast milk.

Managing teratogenic medications in women with HS planning to conceive should address:

- Hormonal Agents: Spironolactone has teratogenic effects, particularly on male fetuses, due to its anti-androgenic properties [26]. Animal studies have shown feminization of male fetuses and endocrine disruption in females exposed to spironolactone in utero [26]. The medication should be discontinued at least 1 month before attempting conception to ensure complete elimination of the drug and its metabolites from the body before pregnancy [27]. Spironolactone may also affect fertility by disrupting the menstrual cycle and potentially causing amenorrhea [28, 29]. After discontinuation, regular menstrual cycles and ovulation usually return within 3–4 weeks. However, it may take up to 2–3 months for cycles to fully normalize and for successful ovulation to occur consistently [28, 29]. Additionally, combined oral contraceptives (COCs) suppress ovulation as their primary mechanism of action [30]. After discontinuation in preparation for conception, it may take up to 3 months for regular ovulation and menstrual cycles to fully normalize after stopping hormonal contraceptives [30]. It is crucial for healthcare providers to have detailed discussions with patients about these medications, their potential risks, and the appropriate timing for discontinuation when planning pregnancy.
- Antibiotics: For women with HS planning pregnancy, the preferred, safe antibiotic choices are clindamycin, penicillins, cephalosporins, and macrolides [31–33]. Tetracyclines and fluoroquinolones should be avoided due to teratogenic effects [31–33]. The safety of specific antibiotics during pregnancy and breastfeeding will be discussed in more detail in the following section.
- Retinoids: Oral retinoids (isotretinoin, acitretin) are absolutely contraindicated during pregnancy due to their teratogenic effects. Guidelines recommend discontinuing isotretinoin at least 1 month before conception [34]. For acitretin, a washout period of at least 3 years is required due to its long half-life [35].
- Biologics: Current guidelines and research suggest that most biologic medications used to treat HS can be safely continued during the preconception period [31]. TNF-α inhibitors are considered safe to use while planning pregnancy, and women with HS who are planning pregnancy can generally remain on their biologic therapy during the preconception phase [31].
- Contraception During Washout: Emphasize the importance of effective contraception during the medication washout period to prevent unintended pregnancy while teratogenic drugs are still in the system. It's important to note that 83% of HS patients report not receiving counseling on how HS could impact pregnancy [1], highlighting the need for improved patient education and communication in this area. Healthcare providers should aim to address these topics comprehensively during preconception counseling sessions with women who have HS.

Management Considerations for Hidradenitis Suppurativa During Pregnancy, Breastfeeding, and the Postpartum Period

A large cohort study of over 1.3 million deliveries in Quebec, Canada, found that pregnant patients with HS had a 30–60% increased risk of adverse pregnancy complications, including gestational diabetes, hypertension, Cesarean delivery, postpartum hemorrhage, peripartum sepsis, and intensive care unit admission [22]. Neonates born to mothers with HS also had a higher risk of preterm birth and birth defects [22]. These associations persisted even after adjusting for factors such as maternal age, comorbidities, and socioeconomic status, although the study notably did not control for HS-specific treatments. Close monitoring by obstetricians and maternal-fetal medicine (MFM) specialists is helpful for early detection of hypertensive disorders, glucose intolerance, and infection risks that may arise or worsen during pregnancy. Furthermore, postnatal monitoring of both mother and infant may be indicated due to the risk of long-term health effects associated with HS. Ensuring ongoing care coordination between dermatology, obstetrics, and MFM throughout pregnancy can optimize outcomes, offering both preventive and targeted support tailored to the specific needs of patients with HS.

Hidradenitis suppurativa management during pregnancy and the postpartum period therefore requires careful consideration to balance maternal disease control with fetal and neonatal safety (Table 18.1), as described in the following discussion:

Table 18.1 Safety summary of hidradenitis suppurativa treatments during pregnancy and lactation

Treatment	Pregnancy	Lactation	Key considerations	FDA pregnancy categories[a]
Benzoyl peroxide wash	Safe during pregnancy	Safe during lactation		C
Chlorhexidine wash	Safe during pregnancy	Safe during lactation		B
Topical clindamycin 1%	Safe during pregnancy	Safe during lactation		B
Topical metronidazole 0.75%	Safe during pregnancy	Safe during lactation		B
Topical erythromycin 2%	Safe during pregnancy	Safe during lactation		B
Tetracyclines	Contraindicated during pregnancy	Contraindicated during lactation	Associated with teeth staining and poor bone growth	D

(continued)

Table 18.1 (continued)

Treatment	Pregnancy	Lactation	Key considerations	FDA pregnancy categories[a]
Dapsone	Safe during pregnancy but advised to stop in last month of pregnancy to minimize kernicterus risk	Safe during lactation, but avoid in neonates with G6PD deficiency due to risk of hemolytic anemia	Consider G6PD screening for neonates of mothers taking dapsone	C
Rifampin	Use with caution—should not be used during pregnancy unless the benefit outweighs the risk to the fetus	Safe during lactation—excreted into breast milk, but with no adverse effects	CYP450 inducer; potential for drug-drug interactions	C
Quinolones	Not recommended during pregnancy	Typically avoided during lactation—but recent studies show minimal risk to infant, provided there is monitoring for diarrhea or candidiasis, and breastfeeding is timed 4–6 h after dosing	Associated with cartilage toxicity	C
Systemic metronidazole	Safe during pregnancy	Typically safe during lactation, but some sources recommended to discontinue 12–24 h prior to breastfeeding		B
Systemic erythromycin	Safe during pregnancy	Use with caution—some studies suggested an association with pyloric stenosis in neonates breastfed at <2 weeks of age, but short term use is typically regarded as safe		B
Clindamycin	Safe during pregnancy	Safe during lactation		B
Cephalexin	Safe during pregnancy	Safe during lactation		B
Cefdinir	Safe during pregnancy	Safe during lactation		B
Amoxicillin/clavulanate	Safe during pregnancy	Safe during lactation		B

(continued)

Table 18.1 (continued)

Treatment	Pregnancy	Lactation	Key considerations	FDA pregnancy categories[a]
Adalimumab	Generally safe for first and second trimester, consider stopping in third trimester due to unknown safety of placental antibody transfer	Safe during lactation		B
Infliximab	Generally safe for first and second trimester, consider stopping in third trimester due to unknown safety of placental antibody transfer	Safe during lactation		B
Secukinumab	Safety uncertain due to limited data	Safety uncertain due to limited data, but likely safe		C
Spironolactone	Contraindicated during pregnancy	Minimal excretion into breast milk, safe during lactation	Causes feminization of male fetus during pregnancy	X
Oral contraceptive pills	Contraindicated during pregnancy	Safe during lactation (though combined hormonal contraceptives should be avoided for 3 weeks postpartum due to increased risk for venous thromboembolism)		X
Oral retinoids	Contraindicated during pregnancy	Safety uncertain due to limited data, but typically avoided	iPledge required for isotretinoin; 1 month wash out period for isotretinoin and 3 year wash out period prior to conception for acitretin advised	X
Metformin	Safe during pregnancy	Safe during lactation	Additionally useful for patients with gestational diabetes	B

(continued)

Table 18.1 (continued)

Treatment	Pregnancy	Lactation	Key considerations	FDA pregnancy categories[a]
Systemic steroids	Minor risk of cleft lip/palate	Safe during lactation	Some sources advise to wait 4 h after ingestion before breastfeeding	C
Topical or intralesional steroids	Safe during pregnancy	Safe during lactation		B
Small molecule inhibitor—Upadacitinib	Avoid use during pregnancy	Avoid use during lactation		N/A
Small molecule inhibitor—Apremilast	Avoid use during pregnancy	Avoid use during lactation		C
Methotrexate	Avoid use during pregnancy	Avoid use during lactation	Advised not to breastfeed for 1 week after taking last dose of methotrexate	X
Zinc	Safe during pregnancy	Safe during lactation		C

Footnotes: [a]Category A: Adequate and well-controlled studies have failed to demonstrate a risk to the fetus in the first trimester (and there is no evidence of risk in later trimesters). Category B: Animal reproduction studies have failed to demonstrate a risk to the fetus, and there are no adequate and well-controlled studies in pregnant women. Category C: Animal reproduction studies have shown an adverse effect on the fetus, and there are no adequate and well-controlled studies in humans, but potential benefits may warrant use of the drug in pregnant women despite potential risks. Category D: There is positive evidence of human fetal risk based on adverse reaction data, but potential benefits may warrant use of the drug in pregnant women despite potential risks. Category X: Studies in animals or humans have demonstrated fetal abnormalities, and the risk of using the drug in pregnant women clearly outweighs any possible benefit. These drugs are contraindicated in pregnancy

Topical Antibiotics and Antiseptics

Topical clindamycin 1% is considered safe during pregnancy (FDA Category B) and can be recommended for treating active HS lesions [32]. It provides localized antibiotic and anti-inflammatory effects with minimal systemic absorption. Antiseptic washes, including chlorhexidine and benzoyl peroxide, are safe to use in pregnancy. Benzoyl peroxide, while classified as FDA Pregnancy Category C, is generally considered safe for topical use during pregnancy due to its short contact time and minimal systemic absorption [32, 36].

Topical medications (chlorhexidine wash, benzoyl peroxide, clindamycin) are generally considered safe in the postpartum period and during breastfeeding as there is minimal systemic absorption and excretion into breast milk [13]. However, application of clindamycin to the nipple area immediately before nursing should be avoided or wiped off, as direct ingestion can theoretically result in thrush, antibiotic-associated colitis, or diarrhea due to effects on the gastrointestinal flora in susceptible neonates [37].

Systemic Antibiotics

Several systemic antibiotics are generally considered safe for use during pregnancy and are commonly prescribed by HS experts, including clindamycin, cephalexin, cefdinir, amoxicillin/clavulanate, and metronidazole [32]. However, amoxicillin should be avoided in the first trimester due to its potential association with cleft lip and palate, and its use is generally limited to the second and third trimesters [38]. While clindamycin is often paired with rifampin, monotherapy with clindamycin may offer similar efficacy [39].

Rifampin carries teratogenic risks observed in animal studies and has been linked to postnatal hemorrhage when used near delivery [40]. Nonetheless, tuberculosis guidelines suggest cautious use in pregnancy only when benefits outweigh risks and safer alternatives are not available [41]. Dapsone, though not linked to congenital defects, has been associated with dose-related neonatal hemolysis and hyperbilirubinemia and should be discontinued a month before birth to prevent kernicterus [42, 43]. Tetracyclines, including doxycycline, are typically avoided during pregnancy, especially after the first trimester, as they have been associated with potential staining of developing teeth in the fetus, possible effects on fetal bone growth, and rare cases of maternal hepatotoxicity [44]. Sulfamethoxazole-trimethoprim (SMX-TMP) should also be avoided during all stages of pregnancy. In early pregnancy, SMX-TMP use is associated with an increased risk of congenital malformations, particularly neural tube defects, due to its interference with folic acid metabolism [45]. Use after 32 weeks is associated with severe neonatal jaundice and kernicterus [45].

Most medications deemed safe during pregnancy are generally compatible with breastfeeding. Clindamycin appears in breast milk in small amounts and is considered acceptable for breastfeeding, although it carries a minor risk of affecting the infant's gut microbiome [46]. Metronidazole, which can reach high levels in breast milk, should be stopped 12–24 h before breastfeeding [47]. Rifampin is also excreted into breast milk and causes orange discoloration, but has not been linked to harmful effects in infants [48]. While short-term use of doxycycline (up to 21 days) during breastfeeding is generally considered acceptable due to low milk levels and inhibited infant absorption, it is not recommended as a first-line treatment for hidradenitis suppurativa in breastfeeding mothers. Instead, the first-line oral antibiotic combination recommended for moderate to severe HS during lactation is clindamycin and rifampin, rather than doxycycline [49, 50]. SMX-TMP appears safe during breastfeeding of healthy, full-term infants [51].

Hormonal Agents

Spironolactone and all forms of contraceptives are contraindicated during pregnancy due to their potential teratogenic effects and interference with normal fetal development, as discussed previously. In the post-partum period, the use of hormonal agents requires careful counseling. Spironolactone can potentially interfere with milk production and the return of regular menstrual cycles. Additionally, given the medication's teratogenic risk, proper contraception should be discussed when prescribing spironolactone to postpartum women, especially once breastfeeding ceases and menses resumes [26]. In the postpartum period, combined OCPs are generally not recommended during the first 6 weeks after delivery due to increased thrombosis risk [52]. Though progestin-only pills can be safely used as early as 3 weeks postpartum, these medications do not appear to have the same beneficial effects on HS disease control as estrogen-containing OCPs [53].

Corticosteroids

During pregnancy, the use of corticosteroids for HS should be carefully weighed against potential risks. Within this category, topical corticosteroids are the preferred first-line treatment due to their localized effect and minimal systemic absorption [54]. They can be applied directly to affected areas to reduce inflammation and alleviate symptoms. Studies have shown that topical corticosteroids are generally safe during pregnancy and breastfeeding when used appropriately [54]. Mild to moderate potency steroids such as hydrocortisone and triamcinolone are preferred, but for more severe cases, potent topical corticosteroids like clobetasol may be considered [54]. For topical applications, care should be taken to avoid direct contact between the treated area and the infant during nursing.

Intralesional injections are another safe and effective localized treatment for managing acute flares of HS during pregnancy and breastfeeding [49]. Similar to non-pregnant patients, triamcinolone at a concentration of 10 mg/mL is the most commonly used corticosteroid [49]. While specific data on the maximum intralesional steroid dose per session in pregnant patients is limited, current recommendations for dermatologic indications in the general population suggest a maximum of 40 mg per session to limit the risk of systemic absorption [55]. While intralesional administration offers the safety benefit of skin-directed therapy, this method may not be feasible in patients with more severe disease or widespread involvement. Such cases often require short-term systemic pulse steroid therapy for adequate disease control, ideally as a bridge to other therapies [56]. Hydrocortisone, cortisone, prednisolone, and methylprednisolone are metabolized by the placenta, protecting the fetus from excessive maternal glucocorticoids [57]. However, before 12 weeks of gestation, the placenta is not fully developed and there may be more passive diffusion of these drugs to the fetus [58]. Further, though prednisone at standard therapeutic doses is not linked to teratogenic effects in humans, high doses (1–2 mg/kg) should be avoided in the first trimester to reduce the risk of cleft palate [57]. Daily doses exceeding 20 mg prednisone equivalent may lead to fetal adrenal hypoplasia, potentially resulting in transient adrenal insufficiency post-delivery [57]. Prednisone doses above 5–10 mg/day are associated with an increased risk of gestational diabetes, hypertension, and premature membrane rupture [57]. Corticosteroids are generally safe during breastfeeding, though it is advised to wait

4 h after dosing, especially when doses exceed 20 mg of prednisone daily, to limit infant exposure [57]. Prednisolone is preferred over prednisone during breastfeeding, as it has lower transfer to breast milk [59, 60].

Biologics and Small Molecule Medications
Adalimumab and infliximab have not been linked to pregnancy or neonatal complications based on decades of safety data from the inflammatory bowel disease and rheumatology literature [61]. It is generally agreed that these drugs are safe to use during the first two trimesters of pregnancy. However, due to increased active transfer of IgG antibodies across the placenta in the third trimester, shared decision making is recommended to discuss whether treatment should be continued at this point in pregnancy [62]. Weighing the risks of fetal drug exposure against the potential for poorly controlled disease after medication cessation is crucial, as HS itself carries an increased risk of adverse maternal and neonatal outcomes [22]. Furthermore, prolonged use of systemic corticosteroids and/or antibiotics are not necessarily safer alternatives to biologic continuation. If TNF-alpha inhibitors are continued up to the time of delivery, live vaccines should be avoided for the newborn for at least the first 6 months of life [62]. In the United States, the only live vaccine routinely administered within this time period is the rotavirus vaccine series.

There is currently insufficient safety data to recommend using IL-17 inhibitors like secukinumab during pregnancy. In 238 reported exposures, the Novartis Global Safety Database found no increased risk of spontaneous abortion, congenital malformations, or other safety concerns. Data on pregnancy outcomes in the second and third trimesters is limited, as most patients discontinued the drug in the first trimester [63]. Ustekinumab, an IL-12/23 antagonist, also has limited pregnancy data. In 47 reported exposures, the Pregnancy Inflammatory Bowel Disease and Neonatal Outcomes registry found no increased risk of spontaneous abortion or congenital malformations [64, 65]. Due to the overall lack of safety data, it is recommended that secukinumab and ustekinumab be considered only if a patient cannot use or has contraindications to TNF-alpha inhibitors. Additionally, small molecule medications, such as JAK inhibitors and apremilast, also lack sufficient safety data to support their use during pregnancy.

Both adalimumab and infliximab are excreted in very small amounts in breast milk and are poorly absorbed through the infant's gut, making them generally safe for use during lactation with no adverse effects reported [66]. While data on secukinumab and ustekinumab use during breastfeeding are limited, these drugs are expected to be present in breast milk at low levels [67, 68]. Apremilast and JAK inhibitors should be avoided during breastfeeding due to a lack of sufficient human data [57].

Adjunctive Therapies
Metformin can be used as an adjunct therapy for HS in pregnancy, especially in patients with gestational diabetes [32]. Zinc gluconate supplementation may have

therapeutic effects on HS and is generally considered safe during pregnancy, though safety data is limited [32]. Chronic zinc supplementation can impair copper absorption, potentially leading to copper deficiency [69, 70]. This risk may be more pronounced during pregnancy due to increased nutritional demands. Therefore, patients taking zinc supplementation should be counseled to take a copper-containing multivitamin concurrently to avoid iatrogenic deficits [69, 70]. Major surgical procedures that require sedation should be postponed until after delivery [32]. However, in-office procedures such as intralesional steroid injections and incision and drainage performed with local anesthesia are safe options for managing HS flares during pregnancy [32].

Metformin is only minimally excreted into breast milk and is considered safe for breastfeeding patients with HS [71]. Zinc does not pass into breast milk and is therefore safe to use [31].

Pain Management

Pain control is another aspect of HS management that must be considered thoughtfully during pregnancy. Although controlling the underlying disease state is key, severe cases may require additional methods of analgesia. Non-pharmacologic options include warm compresses and Epsom salt soaks. For pharmacological pain management, acetaminophen is the safest option throughout gestation [72]. Non-steroidal anti-inflammatories (NSAIDs) such as ibuprofen and naproxen are contraindicated after 20 weeks gestational age due to potential effects on fetal kidney development and premature closure of the ductus arteriosus [73]. For cases where additional analgesia is required, topical lidocaine (FDA category B), applied at the lowest effective concentration and within recommended usage limits, can be utilized [74]. In severe cases unresponsive to other pharmacologic and non-pharmacologic methods, opioids may be considered as a last resort. However, caution is warranted. A cohort study of 48,202 opioid-exposed pregnancies found that strong agonists and long half-life prescription opioids were associated with a higher risk of neonatal opioid withdrawal syndrome (NOWS) compared to weak agonists and short half-life products [75]. Additionally, a case-control study of 251,087 pregnant patients found a continuous positive association between total opioid exposure and the odds of spontaneous preterm birth, with each doubling of opioid morphine milligram equivalents (MME) associated with a 4% increase in the odds of spontaneous preterm birth compared with no opioid exposure [76]. These findings support guidance to minimize opioid exposure during pregnancy and prescribe the lowest dose necessary when opioids are required.

In the postpartum period and during breastfeeding, acetaminophen and NSAIDs can be safely used [77, 78]. Ibuprofen is the preferred analgesic agent for breastfeeding mothers due to its extremely low levels in breastmilk, short half-life, and safe use in infants [77]. Topical lidocaine is considered safe for use while breastfeeding, as it is only likely to pass into breast milk in tiny amounts [79]. However, care should be taken to avoid applying it directly to the breast or nipple area if nursing. Opioids should be used with caution, as they can pass into breast milk and potentially affect the infant [80]. If necessary, short-acting opioids like morphine or hydromorphone are preferred over long-acting ones [80].

Surgical and Procedural Interventions
Major surgical procedures that require sedation should be postponed until after delivery [32]. However, in-office procedures such as intralesional steroid injections and incision and drainage performed with local anesthesia are safe options for managing HS flares during pregnancy and the postpartum period [32].

Hidradenitis Suppurativa Associated with Polycystic Ovary Syndrome and Tailored Treatment Approaches

HS and PCOS have been shown to have a significant association, with several shared pathophysiological factors contributing to their relationship [2]. One study reports HS patients are 2.14 times more likely to develop PCOS [2], while another study reports HS patients have a 2.64-fold greater risk of PCOS [81].

Both HS and PCOS are characterized by hyperandrogenism, which plays a crucial role in their pathogenesis. In PCOS, hyperandrogenemia leads to virilization and LH dominance [81]. For HS patients, the influence of androgens is evident in the disease's typical onset during puberty and its tendency to improve during pregnancy or menopause [14].

Insulin resistance is a key pathophysiological factor shared by both conditions. In HS, insulin resistance is significantly more common than in healthy patients, regardless of BMI, age, and gender [82]. PCOS is characterized by insulin resistance, which leads to increased androgen synthesis by IGF-1 in the ovary [81]. The presence of insulin resistance in both conditions contributes to an increased risk of cardiovascular disease [14].

Obesity is a common feature in both HS and PCOS. In HS, obesity is associated with a dysregulated adipokine release that is shifted towards pro-inflammatory adipokines [83]. One study found that obesity had an odds ratio of 3.93 for association with PCOS [84]. Obesity-induced inflammation in HS has been shown to impact insulin signaling [85].

Both conditions are associated with an imbalance in adipokines. In HS, there is a decrease in the anti-inflammatory adipokine adiponectin and an increase in pro-inflammatory adipokines such as visfatin, resistin, omentin-1, and RBP4 [14]. This adipokine imbalance could lead to impairment in the regulation of fat storage, glucose tolerance, and insulin release [14].

Hormonal therapies play an important role in managing HS symptoms in women with PCOS. Combined oral contraceptives containing low-dose estrogen and progesterone have shown benefit in managing perimenstrual HS flares, as they help regulate hormonal fluctuations that can trigger HS symptoms [15]. However, not all progestins have the same effects on androgens. Among available progestins, drospirenone stands out as the only one with antiandrogenic properties, making it a favorable option for patients with PCOS-related HS [86]. Combined with ethinyl estradiol, this COC is marketed as Yasmin® and Yaz® in the United States. Other progestins, such as levonorgestrel and norgestrel, have high androgenic effects, while norethindrone has a medium androgenic effect, and ethynodiol has a low androgenic effect [86]. Norgestimate and desogestrel have no androgenic activity [86]. Therefore, drospirenone-containing OCPs are preferred for their ability to reduce androgen levels and manage associated symptoms like acne and hirsutism [86]. Additionally, evidence indicates that progestogen-only contraceptives can exacerbate HS and should be avoided [87]. One retrospective cohort study demonstrated patients using combination estrogen-progesterone contraceptives were 3.14 times more likely to experience stable or improved HS compared to those using progesterone-only contraceptives [53]. Further, women using progesterone-only contraceptives were 2.97 times more likely to experience worsening of HS [53].

Antiandrogen medications like spironolactone, finasteride, and cyproterone acetate have demonstrated clinical improvement in female HS patients [87]. Metformin, commonly used to treat insulin resistance in PCOS, can also have beneficial effects on HS in normoglycemic individuals [88]. One study found that metformin use in HS patients was associated with improved cardiovascular risk biomarkers and insulin resistance [88]. When prescribing hormonal treatments, clinicians should consider both HS symptom control and reproductive health implications such as teratogenicity and fertility. The North American HS guidelines recommend using hormonal agents in appropriate patients with mild to moderate HS [87].

Lifestyle modifications targeting weight loss and metabolic control are crucial for improving outcomes in HS patients with PCOS. Obesity and insulin resistance are highly prevalent in HS patients [88], highlighting the need for metabolic screening and management. While high-quality evidence is limited, expert consensus supports weight loss efforts to improve HS severity, and obesity is associated with worsening HS symptoms [33]. Therefore, dietary modifications and exercise are likely beneficial.

Psychosocial Impact of Hidradenitis Suppurativa and Integrated Care Approaches

The prevalence of depression in HS patients is 16.9% and anxiety is 4.9% [10]. The odds ratio for depression among people with HS was 1.84 compared to controls [10]. Women with HS are at a greater risk for suicide than men in a nationwide registry study [89]. A multicenter cross-sectional study found that sexual health and quality of life are significantly impaired in HS patients [90]. Women with HS reported higher levels of sexual distress compared to men [91]. Risk factors for sexual dysfunction in HS patients include disease severity, symptoms, and lack of a stable relationship [92]. Further, HS patients tend to have lower body image quality of life scores compared to patients with other skin conditions [90]. Qualitative studies have found HS has a major emotional impact on patients, promoting isolation due to fear of stigmatization [93]. Shame, irritation, and low self-worth are common [93]. The chronic nature of HS and its effects on intimate areas contribute to psychological distress [10]. Screening for and addressing these psychosocial effects is an important part of comprehensive care for female HS patients.

Referrals to mental health professionals should be considered as part of the care team [1]. Collaboration between dermatologists and gynecologists is particularly important for female patients with anogenital HS lesions, as HS can be mistaken for other vulvar diseases [1]. Patient education and counseling should cover HS etiology, treatment options, self-care practices, and coping strategies [94]. An integrated care model involving dermatologists, surgeons, mental health professionals, and other specialists is recommended to develop personalized treatment plans and address comorbidities [95]. Quality of life assessments using validated instruments like the Dermatology Life Quality Index (DLQI) should be incorporated to address factors such as pain, odor, stigmatization, and sleep disturbances [96]. Additionally, encouraging participation in support groups or online communities can help patients connect with others experiencing similar challenges [94]. By implementing these comprehensive recommendations, healthcare providers can offer more patient-centered care that addresses both the physical and psychosocial aspects of HS, ultimately improving outcomes and quality of life for those affected by this challenging condition [95, 97].

Board Review Question Explanation

A 28-year-old woman with a history of polycystic ovary syndrome presents 6 weeks postpartum for evaluation of Hurley stage 2 hidradenitis suppurativa. She is experiencing an acute flare under her breasts and in her groin. She stopped adalimumab (Humira) during her third trimester and is currently breastfeeding. She is currently using topical clindamycin, benzoyl peroxide wash, and metformin. Which of the following is contraindicated as a potential treatment for this patient?

A. Re-starting adalimumab (Humira)
B. Oral doxycycline (Correct)
C. Intralesional corticosteroids
D. Oral clindamycin and rifampin
E. Oral spironolactone

Answer Explanation

Oral doxycycline is generally not recommended as a first-line treatment for hidradenitis suppurativa in breastfeeding mothers due to potential risks to infant teeth and bone development. Short-term use (up to 21 days) may be acceptable in some cases when safer alternatives are not available [49, 50].

A. Re-starting adalimumab (Humira)—Not contraindicated. Adalimumab is considered safe during breastfeeding. Studies have shown that it is excreted in breast milk in negligible concentrations and is not well-absorbed through the infant's gut. No adverse effects have been reported in breastfed infants [66].

B. Oral doxycycline—Contraindicated. Tetracyclines, including doxycycline, are generally contraindicated during breastfeeding due to potential staining of infants' dental enamel or bone deposition. While short-term use may be considered in some cases, it is not recommended as a first-line treatment for breastfeeding mothers [49, 50].
C. Intralesional corticosteroids—Not contraindicated. Topical and intralesional steroids are considered safe during lactation [98].
D. Oral clindamycin and rifampin—Not contraindicated. Both clindamycin and rifampin are considered safe for use in breastfeeding mothers. Clindamycin is excreted into breast milk in small quantities, and rifampin, while excreted into breast milk, has no reported adverse effects on infants [46, 48].
E. Oral spironolactone—Not contraindicated, and spironolactone can be used safely in breastfeeding mothers for acne or HS. However, it's advisable to delay its use until milk supply is well established, typically 1–2 months postpartum, to avoid any potential risk of decreased milk production due to its mild diuretic effect [56, 99, 100].

Key Take Away Points

- HS typically affects women in their late teens or early twenties, with common sites of involvement being the axillae, inguinal, and inframammary areas.
- Over 60% of women report worsening HS symptoms around the time of menses, which may correspond with decreasing estrogen and progesterone levels during the late luteal phase. Combination estrogen and progesterone contraceptives and spironolactone can be particularly helpful in mitigating hormonally-driven HS flares.
- Women with HS who are planning pregnancy require preconception counseling to address fertility, medication safety, and hereditary aspects of HS. Some studies suggest higher infertility rates in HS patients, and 68% of women with HS express concern about passing the condition to their children.
- Pregnancy affects HS in various ways, with around 24% of women experiencing symptom improvement during pregnancy, while 60% suffer from flares postpartum. Hormonal changes during pregnancy, such as increased estrogen and progesterone, can reduce inflammation. However, the sharp drop in estrogen and rise in prolactin after delivery often trigger postpartum flares.
- HS patients demonstrate higher rates of pregnancy complications compared to non-HS controls, most notably gestational diabetes, hypertension, Cesarean delivery, postpartum hemorrhage, peripartum sepsis, and preterm labor.
- Safe HS treatments during pregnancy include topical clindamycin, antiseptic washes, and certain antibiotics. Biologics like adalimumab and infliximab may be continued during the first two trimesters; however, dose de-escalation or discontinuation during late pregnancy should be considered when possible to decrease fetal exposure and immunosuppression.
- Postpartum HS management focuses on selecting safe treatments for breastfeeding mothers. Topical antibiotics (e.g., clindamycin), intralesional corticosteroids, and certain systemic antibiotics are considered safe, while oral doxycycline is generally avoided.

- HS is frequently associated with PCOS, with women with HS being twice as likely to have PCOS. Both conditions share common factors like insulin resistance, hyperandrogenism, and obesity, which complicate management and fertility outcomes. Metformin may be a suitable treatment for HS patients with comorbid PCOS.
- Obesity is a major comorbidity in HS, often aggravating the condition. Women with HS frequently have metabolic syndrome, increasing the risk of cardiovascular complications and complicating disease management.
- HS severely affects women's quality of life, sexual health, and mental well-being. Depression, anxiety, and sexual dysfunction are common, often exacerbated by the chronic and intimate nature of HS lesions. Integrated care involving dermatologists, mental health professionals, and gynecologists is critical for providing comprehensive care.

References

1. Adelekun AA, Villa NM, Hsiao JL, Micheletti RG. Pregnancy in hidradenitis suppurativa—patient perspectives and practice gaps. JAMA Dermatol. 2021;157(2):227. https://doi.org/10.1001/jamadermatol.2020.5162.
2. Garg A, Malviya N, Strunk A, et al. Comorbidity screening in hidradenitis suppurativa: evidence-based recommendations from the US and Canadian Hidradenitis Suppurativa Foundations. J Am Acad Dermatol. 2022;86(5):1092–101. https://doi.org/10.1016/j.jaad.2021.01.059.
3. Miller IM, Ahlehoff O, Ibler K, et al. Hidradenitis suppurativa may not be associated with venous thromboembolia: results from a large Danish cross-sectional study. J Dermatol Sci. 2016;81(1):61–3. https://doi.org/10.1016/j.jdermsci.2015.10.007.
4. Ding J, Zhou Y, Khan MS, Sy RN, Khosa F. Representation of sex, race, and ethnicity in pivotal clinical trials for dermatological drugs. Int J Women's Dermatol. 2021;7(4):428–34. https://doi.org/10.1016/j.ijwd.2021.02.007.
5. Tzur Bitan D, Kridin K, Hodak E, Cohen A, Sherman S. The association between hidradenitis suppurativa and male and female infertility: a population-based study. Aust J Dermatol. 2021;62(2). https://doi.org/10.1111/ajd.13529.
6. Medianfar CE, Kursawe Larsen C, Saunte SK, Saunte DML, Jemec GBE, Andersen RK. Hidradenitis suppurativa and female infertility: a pilot study conducted amongst 110 dermatological patients. Arch Dermatol Res. 2024;316(9):649. https://doi.org/10.1007/s00403-024-03390-6.
7. Zouboulis CC, Desai N, Emtestam L, et al. European S1 guideline for the treatment of hidradenitis suppurativa/acne inversa. J Eur Acad Dermatol Venereol. 2015;29(4):619–44. https://doi.org/10.1111/jdv.12966.
8. Cuenca-Barrales C, Ruiz-Villaverde R, Molina-Leyva A. Sexual distress in patients with hidradenitis suppurativa: a cross-sectional study. J Clin Med. 2019;8(4):532. https://doi.org/10.3390/jcm8040532.
9. Schneider-Burrus S, Jost A, Peters EMJ, Witte-Haendel E, Sterry W, Sabat R. Association of hidradenitis suppurativa with body image. JAMA Dermatol. 2018;154(4):447. https://doi.org/10.1001/jamadermatol.2017.6058.
10. Machado MO, Stergiopoulos V, Maes M, et al. Depression and anxiety in adults with hidradenitis suppurativa: a systematic review and meta-analysis. JAMA Dermatol. 2019;155(8):939. https://doi.org/10.1001/jamadermatol.2019.0759.

11. Zouboulis CC, Bechara FG, Dickinson-Blok JL, et al. Hidradenitis suppurativa/acne inversa: a practical framework for treatment optimization – systematic review and recommendations from the HS ALLIANCE working group. J Eur Acad Dermatol Venereol. 2019;33(1):19–31. https://doi.org/10.1111/jdv.15233.
12. Naik HB, Paul M, Cohen SR, Alavi A, Suàrez-Fariñas M, Lowes MA. Distribution of self-reported hidradenitis suppurativa age at onset. JAMA Dermatol. 2019;155(8):971. https://doi.org/10.1001/jamadermatol.2019.0478.
13. Collier EK, Parvataneni RK, Lowes MA, et al. Diagnosis and management of hidradenitis suppurativa in women. Am J Obstet Gynecol. 2021;224(1):54–61. https://doi.org/10.1016/j.ajog.2020.09.036.
14. Abu Rached N, Gambichler T, Dietrich JW, et al. The role of hormones in hidradenitis suppurativa: a systematic review. Int J Mol Sci. 2022;23(23):15250. https://doi.org/10.3390/ijms232315250.
15. Kozera EK, Lowes MA, Hsiao JL, Frew JW. Clinical considerations in the management of hidradenitis suppurativa in women. Int J Women's Dermatol. 2021;7(5):664–71. https://doi.org/10.1016/j.ijwd.2021.10.012.
16. Collier EK, Price KN, Grogan TR, Naik HB, Shi VY, Hsiao JL. Characterizing perimenstrual flares of hidradenitis suppurativa. Int J Women's Dermatol. 2020;6(5):372–6. https://doi.org/10.1016/j.ijwd.2020.09.002.
17. Seivright JR, Villa NM, Grogan T, et al. Impact of pregnancy on hidradenitis suppurativa disease course: a systematic review and meta-analysis. Dermatology. 2022;238(2):260–6. https://doi.org/10.1159/000517283.
18. Riis PT, Ring HC, Themstrup L, Jemec GB. The role of androgens and estrogens in hidradenitis suppurativa - a systematic review. Acta Dermatovenerol Croat. 2016;24(4):239–49.
19. Gold DA, Reeder VJ, Mahan MG, Hamzavi IH. The prevalence of metabolic syndrome in patients with hidradenitis suppurativa. J Am Acad Dermatol. 2014;70(4):699–703. https://doi.org/10.1016/j.jaad.2013.11.014.
20. Lyons AB, Peacock A, McKenzie SA, et al. Retrospective cohort study of pregnancy outcomes in hidradenitis suppurativa. Br J Dermatol. 2020;183(5):945–7. https://doi.org/10.1111/bjd.19155.
21. Sakya SM, Hallan DR, Maczuga SA, Kirby JS. Outcomes of pregnancy and childbirth in women with hidradenitis suppurativa. J Am Acad Dermatol. 2022;86(1):61–7. https://doi.org/10.1016/j.jaad.2021.05.059.
22. Li K, Piguet V, Croitoru D, et al. Hidradenitis suppurativa and maternal and offspring outcomes. JAMA Dermatol. Published online October 16. 2024. https://doi.org/10.1001/jamadermatol.2024.3584.
23. Van Straalen KR, Prens EP, Willemsen G, Boomsma DI, Van Der Zee HH. Contribution of genetics to the susceptibility to hidradenitis suppurativa in a large, cross-sectional Dutch twin cohort. JAMA Dermatol. 2020;156(12):1359. https://doi.org/10.1001/jamadermatol.2020.3630.
24. Eble SM, Wisco OJ, Boccuto L, et al. Genetic factors associated with hidradenitis suppurativa, a literature review. Int J Women's Dermatol. 2024;10(2):e158. https://doi.org/10.1097/JW9.0000000000000158.
25. Bruinsma RL, Fajgenbaum K, Yang Y, et al. Assessment of familial risk in patients with hidradenitis suppurativa. Br J Dermatol. 2021;184(4):753–4. https://doi.org/10.1111/bjd.19664.
26. Pfizer Medical. ALDACTONE® (spironolactone) [package insert]. Published online June 15, 2022. Accessed November 10, 2024. https://labeling.pfizer.com/ShowLabeling.aspx?id=12861%20.
27. Ly S, Kamal K, Manjaly P, Barbieri JS, Mostaghimi A. Treatment of acne vulgaris during pregnancy and lactation: a narrative review. Dermatol Ther (Heidelb). 2023;13(1):115–30. https://doi.org/10.1007/s13555-022-00854-3.

28. Levitt JI. Spironolactone therapy and amenorrhea. JAMA. 1970;211(12):2014. https://doi.org/10.1001/jama.1970.03170120058015.
29. Kim GK, Del Rosso JQ. Oral spironolactone in post-teenage female patients with acne vulgaris: practical considerations for the clinician based on current data and clinical experience. J Clin Aesthet Dermatol. 2012;5(3):37–50.
30. Nassaralla CL, Stanford JB, Daly KD, Schneider M, Schliep KC, Fehring RJ. Characteristics of the menstrual cycle after discontinuation of oral contraceptives. J Womens Health (Larchmt). 2011;20(2):169–77. https://doi.org/10.1089/jwh.2010.2001.
31. Perng P, Zampella JG, Okoye GA. Management of hidradenitis suppurativa in pregnancy. J Am Acad Dermatol. 2017;76(5):979–89. https://doi.org/10.1016/j.jaad.2016.10.032.
32. Chung CS, Park SE, Hsiao JL, Lee KH. A review of hidradenitis suppurativa in special populations: considerations in children, pregnant and breastfeeding women, and the elderly. Dermatol Ther (Heidelb). 2024;14(9):2407–25. https://doi.org/10.1007/s13555-024-01249-2.
33. Sayed CJ, Hsiao JL, Okun MM. For the hidradenitis suppurativa foundation women's health subcommittee. Clinical epidemiology and management of hidradenitis suppurativa. Obstet Gynecol. 2021;137(4):731–46. https://doi.org/10.1097/AOG.0000000000004321.
34. Jajoria H, Mysore V. Washout period for pregnancy post isotretinoin therapy. Indian Dermatol Online J. 2020;11(2):239. https://doi.org/10.4103/idoj.IDOJ_101_19.
35. Stiefel Laboratories. ACITRETIN Capsules, USP [package insert]. Published online September 1, 2017. Accessed November 10, 2024. https://www.accessdata.fda.gov/drugsatfda_docs/label/2017/019821s028lbl.pdf.
36. Chien AL, Qi J, Rainer B, Sachs DL, Helfrich YR. Treatment of acne in pregnancy. J Am Board Fam Med. 2016;29(2):254–62. https://doi.org/10.3122/jabfm.2016.02.150165.
37. Clindamycin. In: Drugs and lactation database (LactMed®). National Institute of Child Health and Human Development; 2006. Accessed 2 Nov 2024. http://www.ncbi.nlm.nih.gov/books/NBK501208/.
38. Lin KJ, Mitchell AA, Yau WP, Louik C, Hernández-Díaz S. Maternal exposure to amoxicillin and the risk of oral clefts. Epidemiology. 2012;23(5):699–705. https://doi.org/10.1097/EDE.0b013e318258cb05.
39. Caposiena Caro RD, Cannizzaro MV, Botti E, et al. Clindamycin versus clindamycin plus rifampicin in hidradenitis suppurativa treatment: clinical and ultrasound observations. J Am Acad Dermatol. 2019;80(5):1314–21. https://doi.org/10.1016/j.jaad.2018.11.035.
40. Sanofi-Aventis U.S. LLC. RIFADIN® (rifampin) Capsules USP [package insert]. Published online February 1, 2019. Accessed November 10, 2024.
41. API Consensus Expert Committee. API TB consensus guidelines 2006: management of pulmonary tuberculosis, extra-pulmonary tuberculosis and tuberculosis in special situations. J Assoc Physicians India. 2006;54:219–34.
42. Hocking DR. Neonatal haemolytic disease due to dapsone. Med J Aust. 1968;1(26):1130–1. https://doi.org/10.5694/j.1326-5377.1968.tb29209.x.
43. Thornton YS, Bowe ET. Neonatal hyperbilirubinemia after treatment of maternal leprosy. South Med J. 1989;82(5):668. https://doi.org/10.1097/00007611-198905000-00037.
44. Cross R, Ling C, Day NPJ, McGready R, Paris DH. Revisiting doxycycline in pregnancy and early childhood – time to rebuild its reputation? Expert Opin Drug Saf. 2016;15(3):367–82. https://doi.org/10.1517/14740338.2016.1133584.
45. Sulfamethoxazole/Trimethoprim (Bactrim® or Septra®). In: Mother to baby | fact sheets. Organization of Teratology Information Specialists (OTIS); 1994. Accessed 2 Nov 2024. http://www.ncbi.nlm.nih.gov/books/NBK582966/.
46. Stéen B, Rane A. Clindamycin passage into human milk. Br J Clin Pharmacol. 1982;13(5):661–4. https://doi.org/10.1111/j.1365-2125.1982.tb01433.x.
47. Metronidazole. In: Drugs and lactation database (LactMed®). National Institute of Child Health and Human Development; 2006. Accessed 2 Nov 2024. http://www.ncbi.nlm.nih.gov/books/NBK501315/.

48. Chellappan. Dermatologic management of hidradenitis suppurativa and impact on pregnancy and breastfeeding. Cutis. 2022;109(3). https://doi.org/10.12788/cutis.0480.
49. Nesbitt E, Clements S, Driscoll M. A concise clinician's guide to therapy for hidradenitis suppurativa. Int J Women's Dermatol. 2020;6(2):80–4. https://doi.org/10.1016/j.ijwd.2019.11.004.
50. Doxycycline. In: Drugs and lactation database (LactMed®). National Institute of Child Health and Human Development; 2006. Accessed 2 Nov 2024. http://www.ncbi.nlm.nih.gov/books/NBK500561/.
51. Trimethoprim-sulfamethoxazole. In: Drugs and lactation database (LactMed®). National Institute of Child Health and Human Development; 2006. Accessed 2 Nov 2024. http://www.ncbi.nlm.nih.gov/books/NBK501289/.
52. Randel A. CDC updates recommendations for contraceptive use in the postpartum period. Am Fam Physician. 2011;84(12):1422–5.
53. Huang CY, Shah SA, Cochrane M, Douglas A, Yang S. Hidradenitis suppurativa disease control associated with type of hormonal contraceptive use. Clin Exp Dermatol. 2024;49(4):375–8. https://doi.org/10.1093/ced/llad385.
54. Chi CC, Wang SH, Wojnarowska F, Kirtschig G, Davies E, Bennett C. Safety of topical corticosteroids in pregnancy. Cochrane Database Syst Rev. 2015;2015(10):CD007346. https://doi.org/10.1002/14651858.CD007346.pub3.
55. Sakhiya J, Sakhiya D, Kaklotar J, et al. Intralesional agents in dermatology: pros and cons. J Cutan Aesthet Surg. 2021;14(3):285–95. https://doi.org/10.4103/JCAS.JCAS_109_20.
56. Park SE, Hsiao JL, Aleshin MA. Management of hidradenitis suppurativa during pregnancy and lactation. Curr Derm Rep. 2024;13(4):293–304. https://doi.org/10.1007/s13671-024-00443-x.
57. Ibarra Barrueta O, García Martín E, López Sánchez P, Ramírez Herráiz E, Merino Bohórquez V, Ais LA. Medicamentos inmunosupresores y biológicos en el embarazo, la lactancia y la fertilidad en enfermedades inmunomediadas. Farm Hosp. 2023;47(1):39–49. https://doi.org/10.1016/j.farma.2022.12.005.
58. Ince-Askan H, Van Den Akker ELT, De Rijke YB, Van Rossum EFC, Hazes JMW, Dolhain RJEM. Associations between antenatal prednisone exposure and long-term cortisol and cortisone concentrations in children born to women with rheumatoid arthritis: results from a nationwide prospective cohort study. RMD Open. 2019;5(1):e000852. https://doi.org/10.1136/rmdopen-2018-000852.
59. Prednisolone. In: Drugs and lactation database (LactMed®). National Institute of Child Health and Human Development; 2006. Accessed 10 Nov 2024. http://www.ncbi.nlm.nih.gov/books/NBK501076/.
60. NHS. Using oral or parenteral corticosteroids during breastfeeding. NHS.
61. Wang H, Hu Y, Chen F, Shen M. Comparative safety of infliximab and adalimumab on pregnancy outcomes of women with inflammatory bowel diseases: a systematic review & meta-analysis. BMC Pregnancy Childbirth. 2022;22(1):854. https://doi.org/10.1186/s12884-022-05191-z.
62. Elmets CA, Korman NJ, Prater EF, et al. Joint AAD–NPF guidelines of care for the management and treatment of psoriasis with topical therapy and alternative medicine modalities for psoriasis severity measures. J Am Acad Dermatol. 2021;84(2):432–70. https://doi.org/10.1016/j.jaad.2020.07.087.
63. Warren RB, Reich K, Langley RG, et al. Secukinumab in pregnancy: outcomes in psoriasis, psoriatic arthritis and ankylosing spondylitis from the global safety database. Br J Dermatol. 2018;179(5):1205–7. https://doi.org/10.1111/bjd.16901.
64. Chugh R, Long MD, Jiang Y, et al. Maternal and neonatal outcomes in Vedolizumab- and Ustekinumab-exposed pregnancies: results from the PIANO registry. Am J Gastroenterol. 2024;119(3):468–76. https://doi.org/10.14309/ajg.0000000000002553.
65. Meyer A, Miranda S, Drouin J, Weill A, Carbonnel F, Dray-Spira R. Safety of vedolizumab and ustekinumab compared with anti-TNF in pregnant women with inflammatory bowel disease. Clin Gastroenterol Hepatol. 2025;23(1):144–53. Published online January 2024:S1542356524000107. https://doi.org/10.1016/j.cgh.2023.12.029.

66. Fritzsche J, Pilch A, Mury D, Schaefer C, Weber-Schoendorfer C. Infliximab and Adalimumab use during breastfeeding. J Clin Gastroenterol. 2012;46(8):718–9. https://doi.org/10.1097/MCG.0b013e31825f2807.
67. Ustekinumab. In: Drugs and lactation database (LactMed®). National Institute of Child Health and Human Development; 2006. Accessed 2 Nov 2024. http://www.ncbi.nlm.nih.gov/books/NBK500594/.
68. Secukinumab. In: Drugs and lactation database (LactMed®). National Institute of Child Health and Human Development; 2006. Accessed 2 Nov 2024. http://www.ncbi.nlm.nih.gov/books/NBK500738/.
69. Yang J, Kang Y, Chang Q, et al. Maternal zinc, copper, and selenium intakes during pregnancy and congenital heart defects. Nutrients. 2022;14(5):1055. https://doi.org/10.3390/nu14051055.
70. Ladipo OA. Nutrition in pregnancy: mineral and vitamin supplements. Am J Clin Nutr. 2000;72(1):280S–90S. https://doi.org/10.1093/ajcn/72.1.280S.
71. Hale T, Kristensen J, Hackett L, Kohan R, Ilett K. Transfer of metformin into human milk. Diabetologia. 2002;45(11):1509–14. https://doi.org/10.1007/s00125-002-0939-x.
72. Sznajder KK, Teti DM, Kjerulff KH. Maternal use of acetaminophen during pregnancy and neurobehavioral problems in offspring at 3 years: a prospective cohort study. PLoS One. 2022;17(9):e0272593. https://doi.org/10.1371/journal.pone.0272593.
73. Koren G, Florescu A, Costei AM, Boskovic R, Moretti ME. Nonsteroidal antiinflammatory drugs during third trimester and the risk of premature closure of the ductus arteriosus: a meta-analysis. Ann Pharmacother. 2006;40(5):824–9. https://doi.org/10.1345/aph.1G428.
74. Lidocaine. In: Mother to baby | fact sheets. Organization of Teratology Information Specialists (OTIS); 1994. Accessed 2 Nov 2024. http://www.ncbi.nlm.nih.gov/books/NBK582791/.
75. Esposito DB, Huybrechts KF, Werler MM, et al. Characteristics of prescription opioid analgesics in pregnancy and risk of neonatal opioid withdrawal syndrome in newborns. JAMA Netw Open. 2022;5(8):e2228588. https://doi.org/10.1001/jamanetworkopen.2022.28588.
76. Bosworth OM, Padilla-Azain MC, Adgent MA, et al. Prescription opioid exposure during pregnancy and risk of spontaneous preterm delivery. JAMA Netw Open. 2024;7(2):e2355990. https://doi.org/10.1001/jamanetworkopen.2023.55990.
77. Ibuprofen. In: Drugs and lactation database (LactMed®). National Institute of Child Health and Human Development; 2006. Accessed 2 Nov 2024. http://www.ncbi.nlm.nih.gov/books/NBK500986/.
78. Acetaminophen. In: Drugs and lactation database (LactMed®). National Institute of Child Health and Human Development; 2006. Accessed 2 Nov 2024. http://www.ncbi.nlm.nih.gov/books/NBK501194/.
79. Lidocaine. In: Drugs and lactation database (LactMed®). National Institute of Child Health and Human Development; 2006. Accessed 2 Nov 2024. http://www.ncbi.nlm.nih.gov/books/NBK501230/.
80. American College of Obstetricians and Gynecologists' Committee on Obstetric Practice. Opioid Use and Opioid Use Disorder in Pregnancy. Published online August 2017. Accessed November 10, 2024. https://www.acog.org/clinical/clinical-guidance/committee-opinion/articles/2017/08/opioid-use-and-opioid-usedisorder-in-pregnancy.
81. Phan K, Charlton O, Smith SD. Hidradenitis suppurativa and polycystic ovarian syndrome: systematic review and meta-analysis. Aust J Dermatol. 2020;61(1). https://doi.org/10.1111/ajd.13110.
82. Özkur E, Erdem Y, Altunay İK, et al. Serum irisin level, insulin resistance, and lipid profiles in patients with hidradenitis suppurativa: a case-control study. An Bras Dermatol. 2020;95(6):708–13. https://doi.org/10.1016/j.abd.2020.04.009.
83. Malara A, Hughes R, Jennings L, et al. Adipokines are dysregulated in patients with hidradenitis suppurativa. Br J Dermatol. 2018;178(3):792–3. https://doi.org/10.1111/bjd.15904.
84. Garg A, Neuren E, Strunk A. Hidradenitis suppurativa is associated with polycystic ovary syndrome: a population-based analysis in the United States. J Invest Dermatol. 2018;138(6):1288–92. https://doi.org/10.1016/j.jid.2018.01.009.

85. Mintoff D, Benhadou F, Pace NP, Frew JW. Metabolic syndrome and hidradenitis suppurativa: epidemiological, molecular, and therapeutic aspects. Int J Dermatol. 2022;61(10):1175–86. https://doi.org/10.1111/ijd.15910.
86. Mathur R. Use of ethinylestradiol/drospirenone combination in patients with the polycystic ovary syndrome. Ther Clin Risk Manag. 2008;4:487–92. https://doi.org/10.2147/TCRM.S6864.
87. Alikhan A, Sayed C, Alavi A, et al. North American clinical management guidelines for hidradenitis suppurativa: a publication from the United States and Canadian Hidradenitis Suppurativa Foundations. J Am Acad Dermatol. 2019;81(1):91–101. https://doi.org/10.1016/j.jaad.2019.02.068.
88. Hambly R, Kearney N, Hughes R, Fletcher JM, Kirby B. Metformin treatment of hidradenitis suppurativa: effect on metabolic parameters, inflammation, cardiovascular risk biomarkers, and immune mediators. Int J Mol Sci. 2023;24(8):6969. https://doi.org/10.3390/ijms24086969.
89. Phan K, Huo YR, Smith SD. Hidradenitis suppurativa and psychiatric comorbidities, suicides and substance abuse: systematic review and meta-analysis. Ann Transl Med. 2020;8(13):821. https://doi.org/10.21037/atm-20-1028.
90. Andersen P, Nielsen R, Sigsgaard V, Jemec G, Riis P. Body image quality of life in patients with hidradenitis suppurativa compared with other dermatological disorders. Acta Derm Venereol. 2020;100(8):adv00107-6. https://doi.org/10.2340/00015555-3464.
91. Yee D, Collier EK, Atluri S, Jaros J, Shi VY, Hsiao JL. Gender differences in sexual health impairment in hidradenitis suppurativa: a systematic review. Int J Women's Dermatol. 2021;7(3):259–64. https://doi.org/10.1016/j.ijwd.2020.10.010.
92. Quinto RM, Mastroeni S, Sampogna F, et al. Sexuality in persons with hidradenitis suppurativa: factors associated with sexual desire and functioning impairment. Front Psych. 2021;12:729104. https://doi.org/10.3389/fpsyt.2021.729104.
93. Esmann S, Jemec G. Psychosocial impact of hidradenitis suppurativa: a qualitative study. Acta Derm Venerol. 2011;91(3):328–32. https://doi.org/10.2340/00015555-1082.
94. Bovill J, Haffner ZK, Towfighi P, et al. A multidisciplinary model to managing patients with hidradenitis suppurativa at a single-center wound-care clinic. Plast Reconstr Surg Glob Open. 2022;10(10S):7–8. https://doi.org/10.1097/01.GOX.0000898340.73697.bc.
95. Timila Touhouche A, Chaput B, Marie Rouquet R, et al. Integrated multidisciplinary approach to hidradenitis suppurativa in clinical practice. Int J Women's Dermatol. 2020;6(3):164–8. https://doi.org/10.1016/j.ijwd.2020.02.006.
96. Caccavale S, Tancredi V, Boccellino MP, Babino G, Fulgione E, Argenziano G. Hidradenitis suppurativa burdens on mental health: a literature review of associated psychiatric disorders and their pathogenesis. Life. 2023;13(1):189. https://doi.org/10.3390/life13010189.
97. Bouwman K, Van Der Weijden DAY, Jiawan VCR, Alizadeh BZ, Horváth B. Mental health in hidradenitis suppurativa: a complex matter. Acad Dermatol Venereol. Published online September 21. 2024:jdv.20358. https://doi.org/10.1111/jdv.20358.
98. Triamcinolone. In: Drugs and lactation database (LactMed®). National Institute of Child Health and Human Development; 2006. Accessed 2 Nov 2024. http://www.ncbi.nlm.nih.gov/books/NBK501124/.
99. Spironolactone. In: Drugs and lactation database (LactMed®). National Institute of Child Health and Human Development; 2006. Accessed 2 Nov 2024. http://www.ncbi.nlm.nih.gov/books/NBK501101/.
100. Cominos DC, van der Walt A, van Rooyen AJ. Suppression of postpartum lactation with furosemide. S Afr Med J. 1976;50(8):251–2.

Chapter 19
HS and Down Syndrome

Allison Kranyak, Wilson Liao, and Jillian Rork

Case Title An 18-year-old female with Down syndrome presents with painful bumps in her axillae

Case

It's Tuesday morning in the office and your first patient of the day is a woman with Down syndrome accompanied by her mother. A few weeks ago, her mother noticed yellow stains on the armpit area of a T-shirt her daughter was wearing, and when she asked her daughter about this, she replied she has "bumps in her armpits." The mother looked and saw red, tender, draining "boils" under each arm and made an appointment. Her mother feels awful about how long this could have been going on; the patient has been independently bathing for many years now. You ask how these have been affecting the patient's life. She says it has been more painful playing basketball, and she avoids swimming because she is afraid her friends will think her arms are gross.

You then ask if it would be okay to examine her skin and private area. The patient agrees and changes into a gown. On your exam, you noticed 3–4 erythematous nodules, some draining clear-yellow fluid, under each armpit with atrophic scarring. You also note two similar lesions in the patient's left inguinal fold and numerous inflammatory papules and pustules on the buttocks and thighs.

A. Kranyak (✉) · W. Liao
University of California, San Francisco, Department of Dermatology, San Francisco, CA, USA
e-mail: akranyak@arizona.edu

J. Rork
Dartmouth Heath, Department of Dermatology, Department of Pediatrics, Lebanon, NH, USA

N. Brownstone (ed.), *Clinical Cases in Hidradenitis Suppurativa*, Clinical Cases in Dermatology, https://doi.org/10.1007/978-3-032-15200-8_19

Board Review Question
What are the US and Canadian Hidradenitis Suppurativa Foundations guidelines for screening for hidradenitis suppurativa in patients with Down syndrome?

A. Once when a patient turns 18. Then, as needed if they report symptoms
B. Annually with no specific age requirement provided
C. Twice: Once at the beginning of puberty and again in early adulthood
D. You should only screen for HS if the patient reports symptoms
E. There are no guidelines

Prevalence, and Pathophysiology of HS in Patients with Down Syndrome

There are approximately 200,000 individuals with Down syndrome (DS) living in the United States(US), and all dermatologists are likely to care for patients with DS, particularly since the average life expectancy has increased from 25 years to 60 years in the last four decades [1]. Individuals with DS have been found to develop HS at a higher rate than the general population in several studies. The largest study to date was a cross-sectional analysis of 11,936 patients with DS and 16,813,290 patients without DS. This study found that individuals with DS had over five times the odds of developing HS compared to other individuals [2]. For 81.8% of individuals with DS and HS, they were diagnosed by age 29 compared to 34% of patients without DS [2]. This suggests that HS is not only more prevalent in the DS population, but also occurs at a younger age. Consistent with this data, a meta-analysis of HS in individuals with DS found the mean age of onset was age 14 [3]. This evidence led to the US and Canadian Hidradenitis Suppurativa Foundations recommending annual screening for HS in individuals with DS. These guidelines did not provide an age to begin screening, but we encourage starting around age 10 years given the potential for pre-pubescent HS [4].

Overall, patients with DS are more likely to develop disorders of follicular occlusion; there may be several pathophysiologic mechanisms for this predisposition. Trisomy 21 causes both immune deficiency and immune dysregulation. Immunodeficiency in individuals with DS includes defective T-helper cell response and reduced lymphocyte numbers, impaired neutrophil chemotaxis and phagocytic activity, and decreased IgM antibody levels [5, 6]. This immunodeficiency may facilitate uncontrolled bacterial proliferation and growth in the skin and hair follicles. Concurrent immune dysregulation includes increased circulating cytokines such as TNF-α, IL-1β, and IFN-γ, downregulation of inhibitors of the complement pathway via micro-RNAs coded by chromosome 21, and aberrant toll-like receptor activation [5, 6]. Furthermore, chromosome 21 has four of the six interferon (IFN) receptor genes: IFNAR2, IL10RB, IFNAR1, and IFNGR2, resulting in increased receptor expression and IFN response [6]. Thus, individuals with DS are prone to autoimmunity and chronic inflammation, such as the inflammation in HS. Amyloid

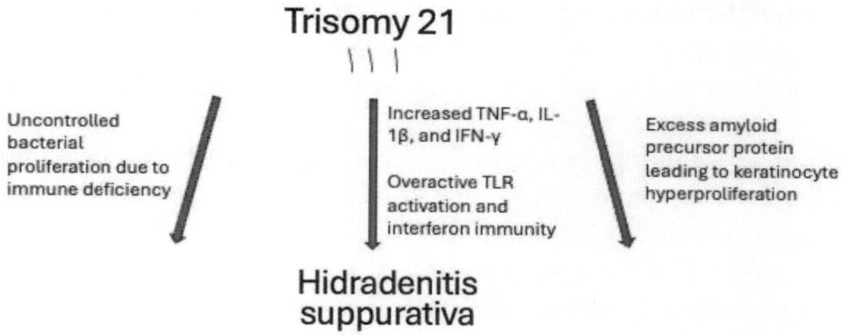

Fig. 19.1 Possible components of the increased predisposition to HS in patients with DS

precursor protein is also located on chromosome 21 and has been associated with Alzheimer's disease [6]. However, excessive amyloid precursor protein can potentially induce keratinocyte hyperproliferation and follicular plugging, which could also contribute to HS developing in those with DS (Fig. 19.1) [3]. Patients with DS may develop folliculitis first and then HS later in life, but patients without folliculitis can also develop HS. Folliculitis should prompt providers to be suspicious of future HS development.

Management and Treatment Considerations Unique to Patients with Down Syndrome

DS is associated with several other co-morbidities, including obesity [7]. However, DS is considered an independent risk factor for HS, regardless of a patient's body mass index (BMI). Obesity itself exacerbates pro-inflammatory states. Furthermore, skin-to-skin friction can worsen follicular occlusion. Thus, weight is an important consideration in all patients with HS, including the DS patient population.

Despite a higher prevalence of elevated BMI in individuals with DS, the DS population is thought to be "cardio-protected" with reduced risks of atherosclerotic disease and hypertension [7]. However, it is not known if this is true for individuals with DS and HS. HS is known to increase the risk of cardiometabolic comorbidities in the general population. Current US and Canadian Hidradenitis Suppurativa Foundations guidelines recommend screening for hypertension, dyslipidemia, diabetes mellitus, metabolic syndrome, and cardiovascular disease for all HS patients, although appropriate intervals are to be determined by medical providers [8]. Until further research indicates otherwise, we recommend individuals with DS be similarly screened for these HS-related cardiometabolic comorbidities.

To best care for patients with DS, providers should strive for inclusive communication. Individuals with DS have a range of speech capabilities; however, speech difficulties do not correlate with difficulties in interpreting language. Efforts should be made to first address patients directly rather than an accompanying guardian or support person. As much as possible, the chief complaint and history should be obtained from the patient directly. Furthermore, providers should make note of any hearing difficulties or loss prior to visits so that proper communication aids are available.

A 2021 review article by Ryan et al. on dermatologic conditions in DS provides in depth guidance on the patient visit, with some suggestions on how to best inquire about a patient's personal hygiene routine [9]. It is important to inquire about bathing, particularly when caring for a patient with HS, since successful therapy may include frequent use of washes. Some possible questions suggested by Ryan et al. include:

> Do you like the way water feels? How often do you take a shower or bath?
>
> Does anyone help you with your bathing routine? If so, who?

It can also be helpful to give the patient autonomy to facilitate a more comfortable environment, as patients with DS may find transitions, like the transition required changing into a gown for a skin exam, difficult. This can include interviewing the patient in their clothes prior to them changing into a gown and asking them where they would like to be examined first. The authors recommend a thorough skin examination of all 'hidden spots' including axilla, under the breasts, and groin area even if a patient does not directly complain of symptoms of HS in these areas.

If a patient with DS is diagnosed with HS, there are certain treatment considerations to review. Sensory differences in patients with DS are relevant when prescribing topical treatments, as some patients may not be able to tolerate the feeling of certain washes, lotions, or creams. Communicating with caregivers about adherence to topical therapy is also important in ensuring that these therapies have the best chance of being effective.

There is more to consider when thinking about systemic options given the comorbidities in a person with DS. There should be careful discussion regarding potential gastrointestinal (GI) effects of commonly prescribed antibiotics such as doxycycline, as patients with DS have a higher rate of both structural and functional GI abnormalities, such as Celiac Disease. Individuals with DS may experience more cheilitis and lip irritation at baseline, making systemic retinoids potentially difficult to tolerate. Oral contraceptive pills are also a potential treatment option for female patients. These can have the added benefit of period regulation in patients with heavy periods. Spironolactone can also be effective in female patients, but screening for a history of syncope, renal disease, and careful blood pressure monitoring is needed given individuals with DS are known to have lower blood pressures than the general population.

Biologics are emerging as effective treatments for moderate-to-severe HS, and the tumor-necrosis factor alpha inhibitor (TNF-i) adalimumab, IL-17A inhibitor secukinumab, and IL17A/F inhibitor bimekizumab are currently approved by the US Food and Drug Administration. However, a thorough risk-benefit discussion should be had with patients with DS and their caretakers before starting biologic therapy. Individuals with DS have a dysregulated immune system and respiratory infection remains a leading cause of death in the DS population [6]. Thus, the risk of serious infection with adalimumab may be further heightened in individuals with DS. Secukinumab and bimekizumab are more targeted with less concern about immunosuppression, but there is still a risk of upper respiratory infection. Furthermore, adalimumab, secukinumab, and bimekizumab all increase the risk of fungal infections, with secukinumab and bimekizumab increasing the risk of candida infections in particular, which individuals with DS are at risk for at baseline.

Another concerning adverse effect for patients with DS when considering adalimumab is the increased risk of lymphoma caused by the medication, which was threefold in clinical trials, necessitating a box warning. Children with DS have a 20-fold increased risk of Acute Lymphoblastic Leukemia (ALL), making the increased risk of a malignancy particularly relevant for adolescents with HS [7]. Whether or not an increased risk of hematologic malignancies carries into adulthood is more uncertain, although individuals with DS appear to have a lower risk of some solid organ malignancies compared to the general population [10]. It is unclear how biologic treatments would impact these malignancy risks.

A recent small retrospective clinical case series of seven patients with DS and psoriasis treated with biologic therapy found the medications to be well-tolerated with no adverse effects over a 52-week period [11]. Three of these patients were under 18 years of age and treated with adalimumab, while one of the four adult patients were treated with secukinumab. This report is limited, however, both in number of patients and follow-up period. Caution should be exercised when prescribing patients with DS biologic therapies, and multidisciplinary approach with patient's primary-care physician and other specialists, including infectious disease, pulmonology, hematology/oncology, and otolaryngology is warranted. Patients and caregivers should also be educated about possible adverse effects and appropriate prevention and monitoring.

In summary, individuals with DS develop HS at a higher rate and younger age than the general population. Several reasons may underlie this, including a propensity for disorders of follicular occlusion and immune dysregulation. Providers should prepare for clinical visits with patients with DS to make patients feel included and empowered. Providers should review treatment options with consideration for comorbidities and side effects seen in individuals with DS.

Board Review Question Explanation

What are the US and Canadian Hidradenitis Suppurativa Foundations guidelines for screening for hidradenitis suppurativa in patients with Down syndrome?

A. Once when a patient turns 18. Then, as needed if they report symptoms
B. Annually with no specific age requirement provided (Correct)
C. Twice: once at the beginning of puberty and again in early adulthood
D. You should only screen for HS if the patient reported symptoms
E. There are no guidelines

Answer Explanation

A is incorrect, as screening should occur before age 18 and annually regardless if a patient endorses symptoms.

B is correct. The authors recommend starting annual screening around age 10.

C is incorrect. More frequent (annual) screening is necessary.

D is incorrect. It is important for providers to build rapport with patients with DS and look at all parts of the body, including groin and under the breasts, to evaluate for HS.

E is incorrect as there are specific guidelines, however no explicit lower age is given in these guidelines.

Key Takeaway Points

- Annual HS screening is needed in patients with DS, regardless of endorsed symptoms.
- The predisposition for individuals with DS to develop HS is multi-factorial.
- Special efforts should be made to prepare for and conduct clinical visits with patients with DS.
- Increased risk of infection and lymphoma are important considerations when deciding if biologic treatment is appropriate for patients with DS and moderate-to-severe HS.

References

1. Tsou AY, Bulova P, Capone G, Chicoine B, Gelaro B, Harville TO, Martin BA, McGuire DE, McKelvey KD, Peterson M, Tyler C, Wells M, Whitten MS, Global Down Syndrome Foundation. Medical care guidelines for adults with Down syndrome workgroup. Medical care of adults with Down syndrome: a clinical guideline. JAMA. 2020;324(15):1543–56. https://doi.org/10.1001/jama.2020.17024. PMID: 33079159.
2. Garg A, Strunk A, Midura M, Papagermanos V, Pomerantz H. Prevalence of hidradenitis suppurativa among patients with Down syndrome: a population-based cross-sectional analysis. Br J Dermatol. 2018;178(3):697–703. https://doi.org/10.1111/bjd.15770. Epub 2018 Jan 17. PMID: 28662304.
3. Lam M, Lai C, Almuhanna N, Alhusayen R. Hidradenitis suppurativa and Down syndrome: a systematic review and meta-analysis. Pediatr Dermatol. 2020;37(6):1044–50. https://doi.org/10.1111/pde.14326. Epub 2020 Sep 6. PMID: 32892406.
4. Garg A, Malviya N, Strunk A, Wright S, Alavi A, Alhusayen R, Alikhan A, Daveluy SD, Delorme I, Goldfarb N, Gulliver W, Hamzavi I, Jaleel T, Kimball AB, Kirby JS, Kirchhof MG, Lester J, Lev-Tov H, Lowes MA, Micheletti R, Orenstein LA, Piguet V, Sayed C, Tan J, Naik HB. Comorbidity screening in hidradenitis suppurativa: evidence-based recommendations from the US and Canadian Hidradenitis Suppurativa Foundations. J Am Acad Dermatol. 2022;86(5):1092–101. https://doi.org/10.1016/j.jaad.2021.01.059. Epub 2021 Jan 23. PMID: 33493574; PMCID: PMC8298595.
5. Huggard D, Doherty DG, Molloy EJ. Immune dysregulation in children with Down syndrome. Front Pediatr. 2020;8:73. https://doi.org/10.3389/fped.2020.00073. PMID: 32175298; PMCID: PMC7056667.
6. Ramba M, Bogunovic D. The immune system in Down syndrome: autoimmunity and severe infections. Immunol Rev. 2024;322(1):300–10. https://doi.org/10.1111/imr.13296. Epub 2023 Dec 5. PMID: 38050836; PMCID: PMC10950520.
7. Lagan N, Huggard D, Mc Grane F, Leahy TR, Franklin O, Roche E, Webb D, O' Marcaigh A, Cox D, El-Khuffash A, Greally P, Balfe J, Molloy EJ. Multiorgan involvement and management in children with Down syndrome. Acta Paediatr. 2020;109(6):1096–111. https://doi.org/10.1111/apa.15153. Epub 2020 Jan 24. PMID: 31899550.

8. Alikhan A, Sayed C, Alavi A, et al. North American clinical management guidelines for hidradenitis suppurativa: a publication from the United States and Canadian Hidradenitis Suppurativa Foundations: part II: topical, intralesional, and systemic medical management. J Am Acad Dermatol. 2019;81(1):91–101. https://doi.org/10.1016/j.jaad.2019.02.068.
9. Ryan C, Vellody K, Belazarian L, Rork JF. Dermatologic conditions in Down syndrome. Pediatr Dermatol. 2021;38(Suppl 2):49–57. https://doi.org/10.1111/pde.14731.
10. Rethoré MO, Rouëssé J, Satgé D. Cancer screening in adults with down syndrome, a proposal. Eur J Med Genet. 2020;63(4):103783. https://doi.org/10.1016/j.ejmg.2019.103783.
11. Tancredi V, Licata G, Calabrese G, et al. Down syndrome and biological treatments in dermatology: efficacy and safety in our real-life experience and review of literature. Australas J Dermatol. 2023;64(2):285–8. https://doi.org/10.1111/ajd.14006.

Chapter 20
Comorbidities of HS

Meha Aggarwal and Cindy Wassef

Case Title A 29-year-old female presents with intermittently recurring boils in abdominal folds and axilla

Case
A 29-year-old female with PCOS presents for concerns of intermittently recurring boils in her axillae. These boils have been occurring for several years, and the time between recurrences is becoming shorter. The boils have been painful and have drained pus, causing significant discomfort. Social history is significant for a 15 pack-year smoking history. Physical exam shows tender, erythematous draining nodules in both axillae.

You determine that her symptoms are likely caused by hidradenitis suppurativa. The patient asks you if she is at higher risk for other conditions due to this diagnosis.

Board Review Question
Which of the following comorbidities is most commonly associated with hidradenitis suppurativa?

A. Generalized anxiety disorder
B. Pyoderma gangrenosum
C. Rheumatoid arthritis
D. Obesity
E. Septic arthritis

M. Aggarwal (✉) · C. Wassef
Robert Wood Johnson University Hospital, Department of Dermatology, New Brunswick, NJ, USA
e-mail: ma1493@rwjms.rutgers.edu; wassefci@rutgers.edu

N. Brownstone (ed.), *Clinical Cases in Hidradenitis Suppurativa*, Clinical Cases in Dermatology, https://doi.org/10.1007/978-3-032-15200-8_20

Cardiovascular Disease

The association between HS and cardiovascular disease has been demonstrated at the cellular and clinical level. Although the precise pathogenesis of HS remains unclear, increased expression of pro-inflammatory cytokines IL-1β, IL-10, IL-17, and TNF-α is seen, suggesting that a chronic inflammatory state may be responsible [1]. HS patients additionally have greater inflammatory load than the general population, with increased CRP and lymphocyte counts [2]. Upregulation of IL-1β is particularly inflammatory; IL-1β levels are 130-fold greater in HS lesions compared to skin from a healthy patient, and together with the augmenting effect of TNF-α, lead to significantly upregulated IL-6 levels systemically [3]. Higher baseline IL-6 levels are independently associated with worse cardiovascular disease outcomes and higher risk of all-cause mortality [4, 5]. Similarly, in patients with established cardiovascular disease, elevated CRP levels are an independent risk marker for heart failure [6]. Pro-inflammatory cytokines seen in HS are associated with worse cardiovascular outcomes; this may be explained by their roles in endothelial dysregulation, atherosclerosis, and thrombosis [3, 7, 8]. This association persists after TNF-α inhibitor therapy, which improves HS outcomes in moderate-to-severe disease, but does not prevent progression of atherosclerosis as measured by carotid intima-media thickness [9, 10].

The cellular-level findings are supported clinically, with HS patients experiencing cardiovascular disease at higher rates and with greater severity. Patients with HS are four times more likely to develop dyslipidemia and are three times more likely to develop carotid plaques with subclinical impact [11–13]. This population also faces higher risk of developing hypertension, diabetes mellitus, and coronary artery disease [11]. Overall, HS is independently associated with significantly increased risk for myocardial infarctions, ischemic strokes, cardiovascular-associated death, and all-cause mortality [14]. Its association with cardiovascular-associated death risk persists when compared with severe psoriasis controls, suggesting that HS possesses a uniquely destructive inflammatory profile towards cardiovascular health [14]. Taken together, these findings suggest that HS patients should be screened for cardiovascular comorbidities and treated accordingly, even when HS disease burden is low.

Endocrine Comorbidities

Patients with HS are twice as likely to develop metabolic syndrome [15]. HS patients are also significantly more likely to develop obesity, with one meta-analysis suggesting a 3.5 times greater risk [16]. The risk of developing HS increases with increasing BMI, and obesity can cause poor treatment response and is associated with more severe HS symptoms [17, 18]. Causality has not yet been established; it remains unclear whether metabolic syndrome increases mechanical friction and systemic inflammation through obesity, leading to HS, or if the chronic inflammatory state characteristic of HS development also leads to metabolic syndrome. The present understanding of HS pathogenesis involves impaired Notch signaling in HS, which leads to dysregulation of TNF-α [19]. TNF-α is thought to impair insulin signaling through multiple pathways, potentially leading to insulin resistance and metabolic syndrome [19, 20]. In addition, mTORC1 is upregulated in patients with HS [21]. Overproduction of mTORC1 is associated with impaired pancreatic B-cell functioning and contributes to insulin resistance [22, 23]. Conversely, hyperinsulinemia may lead to overactivation of the mTOR pathway. mTORC1 mediates keratinocyte and sebaceous gland proliferation and lipogenesis, possible contributing to follicular occlusion and thus, HS [19, 24]. The risk of diabetes mellitus (DM), one component of metabolic syndrome, is significantly higher in patients with HS [25]. Notably, metformin, which is commonly used to treat type 2 DM, has also demonstrated improvement in HS symptoms [26, 27]. While the mechanism through which metformin attenuates HS severity is unclear, it is hypothesized to improve insulin sensitivity, lower glucose levels, and modulate androgen levels through its antiandrogen effects [25, 26].

Polycystic ovary syndrome (PCOS) is also overrepresented in the HS patient population. PCOS and HS share an association with metabolic syndrome, obesity, and hyperinsulinemia, and both respond to antiandrogen therapy [12]. When adjusted for complicating factors such as obesity and T2DM, patients with HS are twice as likely to have PCOS, suggesting that obesity is not the only modulator of the association between PCOS and HS [28]. While both HS and PCOS respond to metformin, one key difference is that PCOS is marked by high androgen levels whereas HS presents with normal androgen levels [28, 29].

Psychiatric Comorbidities

Patients with HS are more likely than the general population to have depression, anxiety, anxiolytic use, and antidepressant use, along with being twice as likely to die by suicide [30, 31]. Patients may develop depression and anxiety as a result of psychological stress due to painful lesions, frequent clothing changes due to draining lesions, shame or embarrassment, or social isolation. IL-17 has been speculated to play a role in the association between HS and depression. Mouse models have shown that administration of IL-17 prompts susceptibility to depression-like behaviors, and elevated levels of IL-17 have been found in patients with psoriasis and depression. IL-17 is notably upregulated in HS. Moreover, targeting IL-17 in psoriasis patients using ixekizumab led to depression remission and improvement of systemic inflammation, whereas etanercept, a TNF-α inhibitor, improved systemic inflammation but did not improve depressive symptoms [32–34].

Patients with HS are more likely to have bipolar disorder, personality disorders, substance use disorders, and alcohol use disorder. Substances most commonly abused include alcohol, opioids, and cannabis; all three can be abused to treat pain and highlight the importance of treating pain appropriately in patients with HS [35, 36].

Schizophrenia is also more prevalent in HS patients, although the pathophysiologic mechanism relating the two remains unclear [35]. Notably, depression and anxiety occur around 3 years after HS onset, whereas schizophrenia occurs approximately 3 years prior to HS onset [37]. While depression and anxiety can be partially explained by disease burden, schizophrenia appears to be associated with HS through a different mechanism. One possible relation is that schizophrenia treatment with second-generation antipsychotics, which have been known to increase the risk of developing metabolic syndrome and obesity, may contribute to a subclinical inflammatory state that then pre-disposes patients to HS. The risk of schizophrenia, obesity, and metabolic syndrome increase with higher Hurley stages, whereas no such association exists for depression and anxiety [37]. Psychiatric comorbidities contribute to poorer quality of life in patients with HS through biological and psychological mechanisms. Dermatologists should screen patients for psychiatric disorders at HS symptom onset and over the course of treatment.

Gastrointestinal Comorbidities

Inflammatory bowel disease (IBD) consists of Crohn's disease (CD) and ulcerative colitis (UC). Multiple studies have concluded that IBD is overrepresented in the HS patient population, with CD being more prevalent than UC [38, 39]. Their association is likely multifactorial and may be driven in part by the disorders' similar inflammatory profiles and their relationships with smoking. The IL-23/Th17 pathway is dysregulated in both intestinal inflammation and lesional skin [40, 41]. TNF-α is also overexpressed in IBD and HS and both diseases show response to anti-TNF-α therapy [1, 40–43]. Smoking increases the risk of CD and HS, although it is protective for UC, with UC risk rising after smoking cessation [44]. Immune dysregulation thus seems to drive both IBD and HS with CD and HS sharing several risk factors and pathogenetic factors. CD and HS also share similar presentations such as tunneling, deep-seated fistulas, and abscesses.

Patients with HS are three times more likely to have CD, and the association between both disorders is strongest for men, non-obese patients, non-smokers, and patients ages 45–64 [45]. Conversely, patients with CD and UC are nine and seven times more likely to develop HS, respectively [46]. IBD is associated with later HS onset; IBD onset usually precedes HS diagnosis by 10 years [37, 46]. Dermatologists should thus have a lower threshold of suspicion for HS in patients with diagnosed IBD or gastrointestinal symptoms.

Musculoskeletal Comorbidities

HS is associated with inflammatory arthritis, with studies reporting a three to eleven-fold increase in risk [47, 48]. The prevalence of spondyloarthritis is thus significantly higher in the HS population [49, 50]. The risk of spondyloarthritis (SpA) is significantly increased, as well as that of rheumatoid arthritis (RA) and ankylosing spondylitis (AS); however, subgroup analyses in a Korea-based study found that the association between AS and HS is only significant for men, whereas the association between RA and HS is significant for both men and women [35, 48]. Notably, HS symptoms generally precede inflammatory arthritis symptoms by about 3.6 years, reaffirming the need for early detection in recently-diagnosed HS patients [49].

The mechanism underlying these associations is likely complex and remains unclear, although the IL-23/IL-17 axis may play a role in the pathogenesis of both SpA and HS [41, 51]. IL-1 and TNF dysregulation could also fuel both disorders, and TNF-blockade ameliorates symptoms in both SpA and HS to some degree [1, 51]. Further, smoking is a known trigger for both HS and SpA and is associated with more severe disease [52, 53].

PASH/PAPASH

Co-occurrence of pyoderma gangrenosum, acne, and HS comprises PASH syndrome and is a rare constellation of diseases with similar cytokine profiles. Pyoderma gangrenosum (PG) consists of painful cutaneous ulcers with violaceous and undermined borders, often in response to trauma. Given the combined burden of these painful and often disfiguring diseases, patients with PASH often experience higher morbidity and poorer quality of life than patients with HS alone. Pro-inflammatory cytokines IL-1β, TNF-α, and IL-17 are overexpressed in PASH lesions, although the blood levels of these cytokines are normal, suggesting that the inflammatory process of PASH is restricted to skin [54]. The syndrome is newly established and limited case studies have shown early onset with acne, and later development of HS and PG. [55] PASH appears to disproportionately affect young men and presents with more severe lesions of PG, acne, and HS than each disease alone [55]. Anti-TNF therapy has shown promising results, with infliximab and adalimumab being most commonly used [55–57]. Remission of PG lesions is seen earlier than HS lesions, which appear to be more resistant to most therapies [56, 57].

PAPASH syndrome includes PG, acne, HS, with the addition of pyogenic arthritis (PA). Previously, PAPA syndrome (pyogenic arthritis, acne, and pyoderma gangrenosum) was found to be marked by mutations in the proline-serine-threonine-phosphatase protein 1 (PSTPIP1) gene. While this mutation is not found in PASH syndrome, it is reported to be found in PAPASH syndrome in the few patients that have been diagnosed since its establishment in 2013 [58, 59]. Unlike PASH, it has been treated most effectively by IL-1 receptor antagonist anakinra [58].

Psoriasis

HS patients are 2–3 times more likely to have psoriasis [60]. Conversely, patients with psoriasis are significantly more likely to develop HS. Both diseases share key features such as upregulation of Th1/Th17-related cytokines and IL-23/IL-17 axis dysregulation, but only HS displays markedly overexpressed TNF [61]. Psoriasis onset generally occurs before HS diagnosis, although patients who experience HS symptoms first tend to follow a more severe disease course [62]. Patients who have both diseases are typically younger than 65 years old, a trend also seen for HS alone [63–65]. This finding could be explained by possible hormonal influence on HS, as HS symptoms are often reported to be exacerbated during menses and attenuated following menopause [66]. Patients with HS and psoriasis are predominantly women and have higher rates of smoking, obesity, hypertension, diabetes, and inflammatory bowel disease than psoriasis-only patients or healthy controls [65, 67]. HS/psoriasis patients additionally tend to have higher BMIs than HS-only patients [67]. Having both diseases also places a greater mental and emotional burden on patients: HS/psoriasis patients are more likely to be depressed than psoriasis-only or HS-only patients [64, 67]. Whereas several biologic agents have shown excellent results in psoriasis treatment, there are fewer such therapies for HS and are often unsatisfactory [68]. Overall, HS displays a significantly greater inflammatory burden, which may explain its relative resistance to therapies that are very effective against psoriasis such as adalimumab [61]. IL-17 receptor antagonist brodalumab and IL-23 receptor antagonist risankizumab have also shown efficacy in patients with concurrent and refractory HS and psoriasis [69, 70]. Table 20.1 reviews the comorbidities of HS.

Board Review Question Explanation
Which of the following comorbidities is most commonly associated with hidradenitis suppurativa?

A. Generalized anxiety disorder
B. Pyoderma gangrenosum
C. Rheumatoid arthritis
D. Obesity (Correct)
E. Pyogenic arthritis

Answer Explanation
Patients with HS are several times more likely to be obese, and obesity is associated with poorer treatment response and disease severity. Obesity is part of the metabolic syndrome, which is one of the most prevalent comorbidities associated with HS. While HS patients do have increased risk for depression and anxiety,

Table 20.1 Comorbidities of HS

Patients with HS are at higher risk for:	
Cardiovascular	Dyslipidemia Coronary artery disease Hypertension Myocardial infarction Ischemic stroke Cardiovascular-caused death
Endocrine	Metabolic syndrome Obesity Type 2 diabetes mellitus Polycystic ovary syndrome
Psychiatric	Depression Anxiety Death by suicide Substance use disorder Alcohol use disorder Schizophrenia Bipolar disorder Personality disorders
Gastrointestinal	Crohn's disease Ulcerative colitis
Musculoskeletal	Spondyloarthritis (including ankylosing spondylitis and psoriatic arthritis) Rheumatoid arthritis
Dermatological	PASH (pyogenic gangrenosum, acne, hidradenitis suppurativa) PAPASH (pyogenic arthritis, pyogenic gangrenosum, acne, hidradenitis suppurativa) Psoriasis

generalized anxiety disorder is not as common as obesity. Pyoderma gangrenosum and pyogenic arthritis rarely co-occur with HS as part of PAPASH syndrome and are far less prevalent in the HS population than obesity. Rheumatoid arthritis is an inflammatory arthritis that can co-occur with HS, but this is not common.

Key Takeaway Points

- Cardiovascular and endocrine comorbidities such as metabolic syndrome, obesity, and type 2 diabetes mellitus are among the most common comorbidities with HS and can occur even with controlled HS.
- HS, Crohn's disease, and spondyloarthritis share smoking as a risk factor, which may explain HS patients' increased risk for developing these comorbidities.
- Multiple biologic agents have shown some efficacy in treating HS as well as its comorbidities such as psoriasis, pyogenic gangrenosum, and inflammatory bowel disease.
- HS places a significant emotional and physical burden on patients and can cause social isolation, embarrassment, and mental stress. Patients with HS should be screened for psychiatric comorbidities and substance use disorders.

References

1. van der Zee HH, de Ruiter L, van den Broecke DG, Dik WA, Laman JD, Prens EP. Elevated levels of tumour necrosis factor (TNF)-α, interleukin (IL)-1β and IL-10 in hidradenitis suppurativa skin: a rationale for targeting TNF-α and IL-1β. Br J Dermatol. 2011;164(6):1292–8.
2. Riis PT, Søeby K, Saunte DM, Jemec GBE. Patients with hidradenitis suppurativa carry a higher systemic inflammatory load than other dermatological patients. Arch Dermatol Res. 2015;307(10):885–9.
3. Witte-Händel E, Wolk K, Tsaousi A, Irmer ML, Mößner R, Shomroni O, et al. The IL-1 pathway is hyperactive in hidradenitis suppurativa and contributes to skin infiltration and destruction. J Invest Dermatol. 2019;139(6):1294–305.
4. Khan MS, Talha KM, Maqsood MH, Rymer JA, Borlaug BA, Docherty KF, et al. Interleukin-6 and cardiovascular events in healthy adults: MESA. JACC Adv. 2024;3(8):101063.
5. Kaptoge S, Seshasai SRK, Gao P, Freitag DF, Butterworth AS, Borglykke A, et al. Inflammatory cytokines and risk of coronary heart disease: new prospective study and updated meta-analysis. Eur Heart J. 2014;35(9):578–89.
6. Burger P, Koudstaal S, Mosterd A, et al. C-reactive protein and risk of incident heart failure in patients with cardiovascular disease. J Am Coll Cardiol. 2023;82(5):414–26.
7. Amezcua-Castillo E, González-Pacheco H, Sáenz-San Martín A, Méndez-Ocampo P, Gutierrez-Moctezuma I, Massó F, et al. C-reactive protein: the quintessential marker of systemic inflammation in coronary artery disease-advancing toward precision medicine. Biomedicine. 2023;11(9). https://doi.org/10.3390/biomedicines11092444.
8. Golia E, Limongelli G, Natale F, Fimiani F, Maddaloni V, Pariggiano I, et al. Inflammation and cardiovascular disease: from pathogenesis to therapeutic target. Curr Atheroscler Rep. 2014;16(9):435.
9. Oba MC, Askin O, Gunver MG, Kocaarslan G, Alis DC, Engin B. Subclinical atherosclerosis in patients with hidradenitis suppurativa treated with TNF inhibitors. Skin Res Technol. 2023;29(3):e13302.
10. Kimball AB, Kerdel F, Adams D, Mrowietz U, Gelfand JM, Gniadecki R, et al. Adalimumab for the treatment of moderate to severe Hidradenitis suppurativa: a parallel randomized trial. Ann Intern Med. 2012;157(12):846–55.
11. Hung CT, Chiang CP, Chung CH, Tsao CH, Chien WC, Wang WM. Increased risk of cardiovascular comorbidities in hidradenitis suppurativa: a nationwide, population-based, cohort study in Taiwan. J Dermatol. 2019;46(10):867–73.
12. Garg A, Malviya N, Strunk A, Wright S, Alavi A, Alhusayen R, et al. Comorbidity screening in hidradenitis suppurativa: evidence-based recommendations from the US and Canadian Hidradenitis Suppurativa Foundations. J Am Acad Dermatol. 2022;86(5):1092–101.
13. González-López MA, Hernández JL, Lacalle M, Mata C, López-Escobar M, López-Mejías R, et al. Increased prevalence of subclinical atherosclerosis in patients with hidradenitis suppurativa (HS). J Am Acad Dermatol. 2016;75(2):329–35.
14. Egeberg A, Gislason GH, Hansen PR. Risk of major adverse cardiovascular events and all-cause mortality in patients with hidradenitis suppurativa. JAMA Dermatol. 2016;152(4):429–34.
15. Phan K, Charlton O, Smith SD. Hidradenitis suppurativa and metabolic syndrome – systematic review and adjusted meta-analysis. Int J Dermatol. 2019;58(10):1112–7.
16. Tzellos T, Zouboulis CC, Gulliver W, Cohen AD, Wolkenstein P, Jemec GBE. Cardiovascular disease risk factors in patients with hidradenitis suppurativa: a systematic review and meta-analysis of observational studies. Br J Dermatol. 2015;173(5):1142–55.
17. Mintoff D, Agius R, Benhadou F, Das A, Frew JW, Pace NP. Obesity and hidradenitis suppurativa: targeting meta-inflammation for therapeutic gain. Clin Exp Dermatol. 2023;48(9):984–90.
18. Jørgensen AHR, Aarestrup J, Baker JL, Thomsen SF. Association of birth weight, childhood body mass index, and height with risk of hidradenitis suppurativa. JAMA Dermatol. 2020;156(7):746–53.

19. Garg A, Birabaharan M, Strunk A. Prevalence of type 2 diabetes mellitus among patients with hidradenitis suppurativa in the United States. J Am Acad Dermatol. 2018;79(1):71–6.
20. Hotamisligil GS, Budavari A, Murray D, Spiegelman BM. Reduced tyrosine kinase activity of the insulin receptor in obesity-diabetes. Central role of tumor necrosis factor-alpha. J Clin Invest. 1994;94(4):1543–9.
21. Monfrecola G, Balato A, Caiazzo G, De Vita V, Di Caprio R, Donnarumma M, et al. Mammalian target of rapamycin, insulin resistance and hidradenitis suppurativa: a possible metabolic loop. J Eur Acad Dermatol Venereol. 2016;30(9):1631–3.
22. Blagosklonny MV. TOR-centric view on insulin resistance and diabetic complications: perspective for endocrinologists and gerontologists. Cell Death Dis. 2013;4(12):e964.
23. De Vita V, Melnik BC. Activated mTORC1 signaling: the common driving force of type 2 diabetes and hidradenitis suppurativa. J Am Acad Dermatol. 2018;78(5):e121.
24. Ueno M, Carvalheira JBC, Tambascia RC, Bezerra RMN, Amaral ME, Carneiro EM, et al. Regulation of insulin signalling by hyperinsulinaemia: role of IRS-1/2 serine phosphorylation and the mTOR/p70 S6K pathway. Diabetologia. 2005;48(3):506–18.
25. Bui TL, Silva-Hirschberg C, Torres J, Armstrong AW. Hidradenitis suppurativa and diabetes mellitus: a systematic review and meta-analysis. J Am Acad Dermatol. 2018;78(2):395–402.
26. Verdolini R, Clayton N, Smith A, Alwash N, Mannello B. Metformin for the treatment of hidradenitis suppurativa: a little help along the way. J Eur Acad Dermatol Venereol. 2013;27(9):1101–8.
27. Kraft JN, Searles GE. Hidradenitis suppurativa in 64 female patients: retrospective study comparing oral antibiotics and antiandrogen therapy. J Cutan Med Surg. 2007;11(4):125–31.
28. Garg A, Neuren E, Strunk A. Hidradenitis suppurativa is associated with polycystic ovary syndrome: a population-based analysis in the United States. J Invest Dermatol. 2018;138(6):1288–92.
29. Wang K, Li Y, Chen Y. Androgen excess: a hallmark of polycystic ovary syndrome. Front Endocrinol (Lausanne). 2023;14:1273542.
30. Patel KR, Lee HH, Rastogi S, Vakharia PP, Hua T, Chhiba K, et al. Association between hidradenitis suppurativa, depression, anxiety, and suicidality: a systematic review and meta-analysis. J Am Acad Dermatol. 2020;83(3):737–44.
31. Ragi SD, Lin Z, Moseley I, Ahmed F, Ouellette S, Rao B. Psychiatric comorbidities of Hidradenitis suppurativa in underrepresented groups: a case-control study utilizing the all of us research program. Arch Dermatol Res. 2023;315(5):1457–9.
32. Griffiths CEM, Fava M, Miller AH, Russell J, Ball SG, Xu W, et al. Impact of Ixekizumab treatment on depressive symptoms and systemic inflammation in patients with moderate-to-severe psoriasis: an integrated analysis of three phase 3 clinical studies. Psychother Psychosom. 2017;86(5):260–7.
33. Beurel E, Harrington LE, Jope RS. Inflammatory T helper 17 cells promote depression-like behavior in mice. Biol Psychiatry. 2013;73(7):622–30.
34. Krueger JG, Brunner PM. Interleukin-17 alters the biology of many cell types involved in the genesis of psoriasis, systemic inflammation and associated comorbidities. Exp Dermatol. 2018;27(2):115–23.
35. Lee JW, Heo YW, Lee JH, Lee S. Epidemiology and comorbidity of hidradenitis suppurativa in Korea for 17 years: a nationwide population-based cohort study. J Dermatol. 2023;50(6):778–86.
36. Phan K, Huo YR, Smith SD. Hidradenitis suppurativa and psychiatric comorbidities, suicides and substance abuse: systematic review and meta-analysis. Ann Transl Med. 2020;8(13):821.
37. Jørgensen AHR, Yao Y, Ghazanfar MN, Ring HC, Thomsen SF. Burden, predictors and temporal relationships of comorbidities in patients with hidradenitis suppurativa: a hospital-based cohort study. J Eur Acad Dermatol Venereol. 2020;34(3):565–73.
38. Shalom G, Freud T, Ben Yakov G, Khoury R, Dreiher J, Vardy DA, et al. Hidradenitis suppurativa and inflammatory bowel disease: a cross-sectional study of 3,207 patients. J Invest Dermatol. 2016;136(8):1716–8.

39. Egeberg A, Jemec GBE, Kimball AB, Bachelez H, Gislason GH, Thyssen JP, et al. Prevalence and risk of inflammatory bowel disease in patients with hidradenitis suppurativa. J Invest Dermatol. 2017;137(5):1060–4.
40. Abraham C, Cho JH. Inflammatory bowel disease. N Engl J Med. 2009;361(21):2066–78.
41. Schlapbach C, Hänni T, Yawalkar N, Hunger RE. Expression of the IL-23/Th17 pathway in lesions of hidradenitis suppurativa. J Am Acad Dermatol. 2011;65(4):790–8.
42. Cholapranee A, Hazlewood GS, Kaplan GG, Peyrin-Biroulet L, Ananthakrishnan AN. Systematic review with meta-analysis: comparative efficacy of biologics for induction and maintenance of mucosal healing in Crohn's disease and ulcerative colitis controlled trials. Aliment Pharmacol Ther. 2017;45(10):1291–302.
43. Nazary M, van der Zee HH, Prens EP, Folkerts G, Boer J. Pathogenesis and pharmacotherapy of Hidradenitis suppurativa. Eur J Pharmacol. 2011;672(1–3):1–8.
44. Rosenfeld G, Bressler B. The truth about cigarette smoking and the risk of inflammatory bowel disease. Am J Gastroenterol. 2012;107(9):1407–8.
45. Garg A, Hundal J, Strunk A. Overall and subgroup prevalence of Crohn disease among patients with hidradenitis suppurativa: a population-based analysis in the United States. JAMA Dermatol. 2018;154(7):814–8.
46. Yadav S, Singh S, Edakkanambeth Varayil J, Harmsen WS, Zinsmeister AR, Tremaine WJ, et al. Hidradenitis suppurativa in patients with inflammatory bowel disease: a population-based cohort study in Olmsted County, Minnesota. Clin Gastroenterol Hepatol. 2016;14(1):65–70.
47. Fauconier M, Reguiai Z, Barbe C, Colosio A, Eschard JP, Salmon JH, et al. Association between hidradenitis suppurativa and spondyloarthritis. Joint Bone Spine. 2018;85(5):593–7.
48. Almuhanna N, Finstad A, Alhusayen R. Association between hidradenitis suppurativa and inflammatory arthritis: a systematic review and meta-analysis. Dermatology. 2021;237(5):740–7.
49. Richette P, Molto A, Viguier M, Dawidowicz K, Hayem G, Nassif A, et al. Hidradenitis suppurativa associated with spondyloarthritis—results from a multicenter national prospective study. J Rheumatol. 2014;41(3):490–4.
50. Shlyankevich J, Chen AJ, Kim GE, Kimball AB. Hidradenitis suppurativa is a systemic disease with substantial comorbidity burden: a chart-verified case-control analysis. J Am Acad Dermatol. 2014;71(6):1144–50.
51. Hreggvidsdottir HS, Noordenbos T, Baeten DL. Inflammatory pathways in spondyloarthritis. Mol Immunol. 2014;57(1):28–37.
52. Chung HY, Machado P, van der Heijde D, D'Agostino MA, Dougados M. Smokers in early axial spondyloarthritis have earlier disease onset, more disease activity, inflammation and damage, and poorer function and health-related quality of life: results from the DESIR cohort. Ann Rheum Dis. 2012;71(6):809–16.
53. Acharya P, Mathur M. Hidradenitis suppurativa and smoking: a systematic review and meta-analysis. J Am Acad Dermatol. 2020;82(4):1006–11.
54. Marzano AV, Ceccherini I, Gattorno M, Fanoni D, Caroli F, Rusmini M, et al. Association of pyoderma gangrenosum, acne, and suppurative hidradenitis (PASH) shares genetic and cytokine profiles with other autoinflammatory diseases. Medicine (Baltimore). 2014;93(27):e187.
55. Gasparic J, Theut Riis P, Jemec GB. Recognizing syndromic hidradenitis suppurativa: a review of the literature. J Eur Acad Dermatol Venereol. 2017;31(11):1809–16.
56. Saint-Georges V, Peternel S, Kaštelan M, Brajac I. Tumor necrosis factor antagonists in the treatment of pyoderma gangrenosum, acne, and suppurative hidradenitis (PASH) syndrome. Acta Dermatovenerol Croat. 2018;26(2):173–8.
57. Yan A, Gallardo M, Savu A, Kaffenberger B. Pyoderma gangrenosum, acne, and suppurative hidradenitis (PASH) syndrome: a single-institution case series with a focus on management. Arch Dermatol Res. 2024;316(7):397.
58. Marzano AV, Trevisan V, Gattorno M, Ceccherini I, De Simone C, Crosti C. Pyogenic arthritis, pyoderma gangrenosum, acne, and hidradenitis suppurativa (PAPASH): a new autoinflammatory syndrome associated with a novel mutation of the PSTPIP1 gene. JAMA Dermatol. 2013;149(6):762–4.

59. Cugno M, Borghi A, Marzano AV. PAPA, PASH and PAPASH syndromes: pathophysiology, presentation and treatment. Am J Clin Dermatol. 2017;18(4):555–62.
60. Gau SY, Preclaro IAC, Wei JCC, Lee CY, Kuan YH, Hsiao YP, et al. Risk of psoriasis in people with hidradenitis suppurativa: a systematic review and meta-analysis. Front Immunol. 2022;13:1033844.
61. Navrazhina K, Renert-Yuval Y, Frew JW, Grand D, Gonzalez J, Williams SC, et al. Large-scale serum analysis identifies unique systemic biomarkers in psoriasis and hidradenitis suppurativa. Br J Dermatol. 2022;186(4):684–93.
62. Pinter A, Sarlak M, Zeiner KN, Malisiewicz B, Kaufmann R, Romanelli M, et al. Coprevalence of hidradenitis suppurativa and psoriasis: detailed demographic, disease severity and comorbidity pattern. Dermatology. 2021;237(5):759–68.
63. Li CP, Lo SW, Tsai RY, Chang HC, Gau SY. New-onset hidradenitis suppurativa in psoriasis patients: a multi-center, retrospective cohort study. Life (Basel). 2024;14(6). https://doi.org/10.3390/life14060730.
64. Pinter A, Kokolakis G, Rech J, Biermann MHC, Häberle BM, Multmeier J, et al. Hidradenitis suppurativa and concurrent psoriasis: comparison of epidemiology, comorbidity profiles, and risk factors. Dermatol Ther (Heidelb). 2020;10(4):721–34.
65. Kridin K, Shani M, Schonmann Y, Fisher S, Shalom G, Comaneshter D, et al. Psoriasis and hidradenitis suppurativa: a large-scale population-based study. J Am Acad Dermatol. 2023;88(5):e231–6.
66. von der Werth JM, Williams HC. The natural history of hidradenitis suppurativa. J Eur Acad Dermatol Venereol. 2000;14(5):389–92.
67. Patel M, Cohen JM, Wright NA, Merola JF, Qureshi AA, Vleugels RA. Epidemiology of concomitant psoriasis and hidradenitis suppurativa (HS): experience of a tertiary medical center. J Am Acad Dermatol. 2015;73(4):701–2.
68. Macca L, Li Pomi F, Ingrasciotta Y, Morrone P, Trifirò G, Guarneri C. Hidradenitis suppurativa and psoriasis: the odd couple. Front Med (Lausanne). 2023;10:1208817.
69. Yoshida Y, Oyama N, Iino S, Shimizu C, Hasegawa M. Long-standing refractory hidradenitis suppurativa responded to a brodalumab monotherapy in a patient with psoriasis: a possible involvement of Th17 across the spectrum of both diseases. J Dermatol. 2021;48(6):916–20.
70. Licata G, Gambardella A, Buononato D, De Rosa A, Calabrese G, Pellerone S, et al. A case of moderate hidradenitis suppurativa and psoriasis successfully treated with risankizumab. Int J Dermatol. 2022;61(4):e126–9.

Chapter 21
Complications of HS

Madeline Tchack and Cindy Wassef

Case Title A 33-year-old male with recurrent, painful draining nodules and abscesses in the axillary, inguinal, and perineal regions

Case

A 33-year-old male with a 10-year history of hidradenitis suppurativa presents with recurrent, painful draining nodules and abscesses in the axillary, inguinal, and perineal regions. The patient has a 20-pack-year smoking history and is obese with a body mass index (BMI) of 32.86 kg/m^2. The patient is febrile (100.9 °F) but otherwise hemodynamically stable. On physical examination, the patient has multiple erythematous nodules, abscesses, and draining sinus tracts in the axilla, groin, and perianal regions. The overlying skin is hyperpigmented with evidence of significant scarring and surface verrucous changes. The patient also exhibits marked lymphedema in both lower extremities, contributing to impaired mobility. Laboratory studies identify a leukocytosis; microcytic anemia (hemoglobin 8.4 g/dL); low iron saturation (15%); a normal ferritin, iron, and total iron binding capacity; and an elevated C-reactive protein (6.7 mg/dL), serum creatinine (1.5 mg/dL), blood urea nitrogen (37 mg/dL), and estimated glomerular filtration rate ($\geq$120 mL/min/1.73 m^2). Urinalysis demonstrates proteinuria without hematuria.

M. Tchack
Rutgers Robert Wood Johnson Medical School, Piscataway, NJ, USA

Rutgers Robert Wood Johnson Department of Dermatology, Somerset, NJ, USA
e-mail: mst122@rwjms.rutgers.edu

C. Wassef (✉)
Premier Health Associates, Randolph, NJ, USA
e-mail: cindy.wassef@atlantichealth.org

N. Brownstone (ed.), *Clinical Cases in Hidradenitis Suppurativa*, Clinical Cases in Dermatology, https://doi.org/10.1007/978-3-032-15200-8_21

Board Review Question

A 45-year-old woman presents with painful, draining nodules and abscesses in her axilla and groin that have progressively worsened over the past 10 years. She reports fatigue, intermittent fever, and weight loss over the last few months. On physical examination, there are multiple inflamed nodules, sinus tracts, and scarring in the axillary and inguinal areas. Laboratory studies reveal:

- Hemoglobin: 9.5 g/dL (Normal: 12.1–15.1 g/dL)
- C-reactive protein: 48 mg/L (Normal: <0.3 mg/dL)
- Serum creatinine: 1.6 mg/dL (Normal: 0.6–1.1 mg/dL)
- Estimated glomerular filtration rate: 45 mL/min/1.73 m^2 (Normal: ≥90 mL/min/1.73 m^2)

A urinalysis shows proteinuria without hematuria. Blood cultures are negative. Imaging reveals hepatosplenomegaly and no evidence of abscesses outside the skin. Which of the following is the most likely explanation for her systemic findings?

A. AA amyloidosis
B. Sarcoidosis
C. Iron-deficiency anemia secondary to chronic blood loss
D. Diabetic nephropathy
E. Lupus nephritis with anemia of chronic disease

Hidradenitis suppurativa (HS) is a chronic, recurrent, inflammatory skin disorder that is characterized by painful nodules, pustules, and abscesses primarily in the axillae, inguinal, perineal, buttocks, and inframammary regions [1]. Acute HS often presents with a single or few deep nodules that may develop into cord-like structures [2–4]. As the disease progresses, new lesions in adjacent skin may develop and spontaneously rupture or coalesce to form deep, dermal, exquisitely painful abscesses [5] that can lead to complex networks of cutaneous complications. If uncontrolled, inflammation can promote sinus tract and fistula formation, contractures and scarring, ulceration, increased risk of infection, or systemic complications. Potential lab abnormalities that may be seen in cutaneous and systemic complications secondary to HS can be found in Table 21.1.

Table 21.1 Potential lab abnormalities that may be seen with systemic or cutaneous complications of HS and their associated complication

Order	Notable labs	Potential abnormalities seen with HS	Associated complication
Erythrocyte Sedimentation Rate (ESR)		Elevated	General inflammation
C-reactive protein (CRP)		Elevated	
Wound cultures		Positive	Cutaneous infection Systemic infection
Blood cultures		Positive	
Complete blood count (CBC)	White blood cells (WBC)	Elevated	
	Hemoglobin (Hb)	Low	Anemia Renal disease AA amyloidosis
	Mean corpuscular volume (MCV)	Low	Anemia
Iron panel	Serum iron	Low	Anemia
	Serum ferritin	Low[a]	
	Total iron binding capacity (TIBC)	Elevated	
	Transferrin saturation	Low	
Comprehensive metabolic panel (CMP)	Blood urea nitrogen (BUN)	Elevated	Renal disease AA amyloidosis
	Creatinine	Elevated	
	Albumin	Low	
	Total protein	Low	Renal disease
		Elevated	AA amyloidosis
	Alkaline phosphatase	Elevated	
Coagulation studies	Prothrombin time-international normalized ratio (PT-INR)	Prolonged	
	Partial thromboplastin time (PTT)		
N-terminal pro-B-type natriuretic peptide (NT-proBNP)		Elevated	
Estimated glomerular filtration rate (eGFR)	Glomerular Filtration Rate (GFR)	Low	
		Elevated (early in disease) [53] or Low (later in disease)	Renal disease
Urinalysis		Hematuria	
		Proteinuria	AA amyloidosis

[a]Inflammation can cause elevations in ferritin

Cutaneous Complications

Sinus Tracts, Fistulas, and Scarring/Contractures

HS has a complex and poorly understood pathophysiology and etiology that have been linked to several genetic loci, upregulation of proinflammatory cytokines, and the activation of immune cells [6–9]. These processes are believed to initially promote occlusion of hair follicles which ruptures and re-epithelializes. This eventually leads to sinus tract formation that becomes a nidus for foreign material and bacteria [4, 10]. Furthermore, recent studies suggest that biofilm formation may play an important role in the chronic and recurring nature of the disease [11, 12]. Biofilms, which adhere to sinus tracts and hair follicles, complicate bacterial eradication and contribute to persistent infection and inflammation [12]. As HS advances, these biofilm-laden tracts can coalesce into large regions of fibrous, scarred networks. The Hurley staging system, commonly used to classify the severity of HS, distinguishes between three stages: Stage I is characterized by recurrent abscesses without sinus tracts, stage II involves at least one sinus tract, and stage III features multiple interconnected sinus tracts with extensive fibrosis and little to no intervening healthy skin [11, 13]. In severe HS cases, sinus tracts can invade deeper tissues, including muscle, fascia, and even internal organs, creating a labyrinth of tracts that may lead to anal, rectal, or urethral fistulas [5].

Perianal HS, in particular, can resemble conditions like Crohn's disease, perianal abscesses, or pilonidal disease, presenting with swelling, pain, pruritus, bleeding, and/or purulent discharge [5, 14]. Risk of anal fistula formation [4, 15] and infection may also be increased in severe or long-standing cases of perianal HS as lumbosacral epidural abscesses and sacral bacterial osteomyelitis have both been reported as perianal complications [4, 16, 17]. Regardless of the location of HS lesions, later-stage disease is often accompanied by classic signs of infection (e.g., pain, swelling, warmth, erythema) [12].

With time, inflammatory abscesses heal, producing dermal contractures, induration of the skin, and excessive scarring that impair mobility, especially in the axilla. Additionally, chronic inflammation may lead to ulceration in later-stage disease, characteristically presenting with rolled, boggy, ragged edges and a clean granulating base [4, 16]. These abscesses and inflamed areas often leave behind fibrous, indurated scars that contribute to both cosmetic and functional impairment. In the genitofemoral region, this scarring may result in strictures or anal sphincter fixation that may potentially result in fecal incontinence [4, 18].

Lymphedema

Though relatively rare, lymphedema is a debilitating complication of HS that most commonly affects anogenital regions, including the scrotum, penis, labia majora, perineum, groin, buttocks, and abdomen [19]. While HS disproportionately affects females and most frequently involves the axillae, HS-associated lymphedema is more common in male patients and is seldom reported in the axilla [2, 4, 19]. Most HS patients who develop lymphedema have long-standing disease, with an HS duration ranging from 4 to 30 years, and an average of 18 years [19].

Lymphedema exacerbates the already diminished quality of life in HS patients, contributing to significant psychosocial morbidity due to impaired functionality, pain, and disfiguring swelling [19–21]. In severe cases, the swelling can be extreme, presenting as scrotal elephantiasis that can completely bury the penis [19, 22]. Swelling is often accompanied by induration or a "woody" appearance, but may occasionally present with lymphangiectasis, persistent clusters of clear vesicles on thickened plaques commonly seen on the scrotal skin or labia majora. Verrucous papules and polypoid masses that mimic verrucous carcinoma have also been reported, indicating a low threshold for biopsy when these changes are present [19]. HS-associated lymphedema may lead to ulceration and recurrent infections, like cellulitis and erysipelas, and has also been found to increase the risk of developing malignancies, such as angiosarcoma [19, 23] and squamous cell carcinoma [19, 24, 25].

Cutaneous Squamous Cell Carcinoma (SCC)

Cutaneous SCC is one of the most severe cutaneous complications associated with chronic HS, with a prevalence of 4.6% and more commonly seen in male patients [26, 27]. Like HS-associated lymphedema, SCC development in HS typically occurs after a long disease duration, with the mean duration prior to SCC diagnosis being 26 years [26, 27], and most commonly occurs in the buttocks and perineal regions [26–28]. Although SCC associated with HS is often well-differentiated, the prognosis can be poor due to a tendency for early metastasis and high mortality rates, despite the theoretically good prognosis of well-differentiated SCC [26, 29].

The malignant transformation of chronic HS into SCC is thought to be driven primarily by chronic inflammation that fosters an environment conducive to oncogenesis. Studies suggest that dysregulation of Notch, a known tumor suppressor in nonmelanoma skin cancer, may potentially play a significant role [26, 30, 31]. Additionally, chronic infection, inflammation, and oxidative damage from free radicals may lead to genetic mutations, which are missed by DNA damage checkpoints and tumor suppressor mechanisms, further increasing the risk for malignancy [26, 32]. One study also demonstrated that changes in cytokeratin (CK) expression, particularly the downregulation of CK1 and CK10, may signal the early stages of SCC in HS [26, 33].

Environmental factors, like smoking and obesity, may also increase the risk for SCC development in HS. Jourabchi et al. found that 80% of individuals who developed SCC in the context of chronic HS were tobacco users and noted strong associations between HPV infection and cutaneous SCC, with 72.7% of HS patients with SCC testing positive for alpha-HPV and 87.5% positive for beta-HPV. In general, a low threshold for biopsy is recommended in chronic HS lesions, as distinguishing malignant transformation from the usual painful and inflammatory lesions of HS can be challenging [26, 27]. Furthermore, clinicians should consider sending any specimens from HS deroofing procedures to histopathology for evaluation of potential SCC, particularly in atypical or nonhealing lesions [27], though more research is needed to investigate the percent transformation into SCC of deroofing lesions.

Systemic Complications

Anemia

Though cutaneous complications are more commonly observed, systemic complications associated with HS may arise. Studies have shown that hemoglobin (Hb) levels inversely correlate with C-reactive protein (CRP) levels and HS severity, suggesting that anemia may be secondary to systemic inflammation and that individuals with more advanced HS may be at higher risk of developing anemia [34, 35]. Notably, Hurley stage III HS patients are nearly six times more likely to be anemic than Hurley stage I HS patients [36]. In general, anemia secondary to HS is more prevalent among non-Caucasians, females, and older individuals who may also have additional comorbidities, but is disproportionately experienced by African American women [34, 37, 38].

Mechanistically, high inflammatory states may lead to serum iron sequestration in macrophages and the release of inflammatory cytokines that restrict erythropoiesis, contributing to the development of anemia of chronic disease (ACD) [34, 39, 40]. Others have postulated that bacteria may also contribute to anemia as infections are thought to reduce serum transferrin, but the exact mechanism is unknown [41]. In addition to causing ACD, some studies have also found HS to be associated with iron deficiency anemia (IDA) [42], likely resulting from an increased release of hepcidin in response to inflammatory cytokines that reduce intestinal iron absorption [43]. Still, Hb levels in HS patients typically fail to respond to iron supplementation alone unless the underlying inflammatory process is also medically addressed [35].

Surgical procedures are sometimes indicated in severe HS cases, but studies suggest that surgical treatment may also increase the risk of IDA. Hospitalized patients with severe HS have been found to have significantly higher rates of acute hemorrhagic anemia from both significant surgical blood loss and the use of NSAIDs for postoperative pain management [42, 44].

Amyloidosis

Amyloid A amyloidosis (AA amyloidosis) is a rare but serious complication of HS with limited cases reported in the literature. AA amyloidosis is a progressive, multiorgan disease that most commonly affects the kidneys but may also involve the cardiovascular, gastrointestinal, musculoskeletal, and integumentary systems [1]. Patients with HS-associated AA amyloidosis typically have had chronic HS for 9–25 years and are aged between 39 and 62 [45–47], and most frequently present with hypoalbuminemia and proteinuria [1], though it's been reported that some patients have also experienced diarrhea, edema, and bilateral pleural effusions [47]. Biopsies of the kidneys and colon often confirm the presence of amyloid deposits in affected patients [1, 47, 48].

With renal involvement, HS-associated AA amyloidosis can present with asymptomatic proteinuria or progress to nephrotic syndrome that can potentially lead to fatal renal failure if left untreated [1, 49]. One study noted that 45% of HS patients with renal AA amyloidosis secondary to HS developed renal failure [49]. While cardiac involvement is rarer and usually asymptomatic, echocardiographic findings appear to present identically to other forms cardiac amyloidosis and even presented as a dynamic left ventricular outflow tract obstruction in one case [50]. Observed musculoskeletal manifestations included arthropathy, likely from amyloid deposits in joints or pseudohypertrophy from muscle infiltration. Skin changes in AA amyloidosis may involve waxy thickening, easy bruising, and the formation of subcutaneous nodules or plaques. Gastrointestinal involvement of HS-associated AA amyloidosis can lead to hepatosplenomegaly, bowel perforation, or gastrointestinal hemorrhage, resulting from the fragility of blood vessels from protein deposition. Additionally, HS-associated AA amyloidosis has resulted in mixed sensory and motor peripheral neuropathy or autonomic neuropathy and has been associated with impaired coagulation and anemia [1].

Renal Disease

Several mechanisms have been proposed to explain chronic kidney disease (CKD) as a complication of HS. Though HS is primarily a skin condition, its systemic inflammatory nature and common comorbidities, such as diabetes, hypertension, and obesity, may contribute significantly to renal risks [51–53]. Additionally, HS-associated immune dysregulation, particularly the involvement of Th1 and Th17 cells, may directly impact renal tissue, potentially leading to tubular and mesangial cell damage [54, 55]. Chronic inflammation in HS can disrupt the structural integrity of the cutaneous basement membrane zone, and it's possible that this defect that may also extend to renal basement membrane, potentially causing proteinuria and changes in glomerular filtration rate (GFR) [53, 56]. Evidence also suggests that chronic inflammation and the influence of cytokines (e.g., TNF-alpha) may affect vascular formation and renal cell apoptosis [53, 57].

In general, CKD appears to be more prevalent in HS patients (6.3%) than in non-HS individuals (4.3%) [56], with the highest prevalence presenting in HS patients with severe disease (3.1%) [58]. Further, estimated GFR (eGFR) was notably higher for hospital and population-based HS groups compared to non-HS controls, potentially suggesting a causal relationship between HS and eGFR that causes initial eGFR elevations in early renal dysfunction [53]. This association is particularly pronounced among HS patients who are older (≥60 years), male, obese, diabetic, hyperlipidemic, and/or have cardiovascular disease [56]. Routine renal screening has been recommended for all HS patients, but especially those with additional risk factors and comorbidities, and should include serum creatinine, GFR, and blood urea nitrogen as well as a urinalysis to evaluate for proteinuria and hematuria [56]. Any abnormal investigations should be assessed by a nephrologist.

Infections

Factors inherent to the disease, such as bacterial colonization of lesions, epidermal barrier disruption, and immune dysregulation, increase one's susceptibility to developing acute, chronic, cutaneous, extracutaneous, and systemic infections in HS patients [9, 59]. Multiple studies have observed high rates of soft-tissue and skin infections, such as cellulitis and erysipelas, colonized by *S. aureus*, coagulase-negative *Staphylococci*, and/or mixed anaerobic bacteria in HS lesions [6–8, 60–62]. Systemically, HS has been found to be associated with acute infections (herpes simplex virus, herpes zoster, necrotizing fasciitis, septicemia, bone infection, *C. difficile*, methicillin-sensitive and -resistant *S. aureus*, *Streptococcus*, *Pseudomonas*, mycobacterial, fungal, viral), chronic infections (HIV and hepatitis B), and antibiotic-resistant infections [9, 63]. Studies that have demonstrated associations of HS with *C. difficile* and antibiotic-resistant infections suggest that risk of infection may increase with over-use of topical and/or oral antibiotic treatments (e.g., clindamycin and tetracyclines) [64–66].

While HS patients, including those without other comorbidities, have higher rates of infection compared to healthy controls [9], several risk factors appear to make HS patients more prone to developing infection. Compared to HS alone, serious infection occurred more commonly in patients with coexisting psoriasis, autoimmune disease, acne, mental illness, HIV, cancer, and cardiometabolic disease (e.g., diabetes) [9, 67], as well as those being treated with immunosuppressants, topical agents, and/or oral antibiotics [61]. Hospitalization in HS patients may also be associated with increased risk of infection, as one study noted an infection prevalence of 34% in this population [9, 68]. Interestingly, one study found that patients with coexisting atopic dermatitis were less likely to develop serious infection compared to patients with HS alone [9]. Long-term systemic corticosteroid use was also not found to be associated with increased risk of infection [9].

HS patients treated with biologic or systemic therapies may also be at risk for developing infection with an overall pooled incidence of nearly 25%, though the development of severe or opportunistic infections is rare, occurring in <1% of cases [68]. Research suggests that infection risk varies depending on the medications mechanism of action, as anti-IL1 agents demonstrated the lowest infection rates (7.77%) followed by apremilast (14.24%), anti-TNF therapies (21.96%), and anti-IL17 agents (33.63%) as demonstrated in one systematic review [68]. Notably, studies suggest that patients receiving anti-TNF therapy are not at higher risk of infection compared to those receiving a placebo, an important clinical finding as adalimumab, an anti-TNF, is an FDA-approved biologic treatment for moderate-to-severe HS [68]. Nevertheless, long-term anti-TNF use has been associated with a slight increase in opportunistic infections [68, 69], underscoring the need for preventive measures, including baseline and ongoing screenings for hepatitis, HIV, tuberculosis, and recommended vaccinations to mitigate infection risk [68].

Public health research also suggests that socioeconomic factors influence infection outcomes, with higher infection rates noted in patients with government/public insurance or no insurance, suggesting that limited access to comprehensive dermatologic care may positively correlate with risk of serious infection [9]. A higher number of untreated, chronic comorbidities is also more common in lower socioeconomic populations and was associated with rates of serious infections in hospitalized HS patients [9], particularly in the summer months when heat, sweat, and stress may be more likely to trigger [9, 70].

Board Review Question Explanation

A 45-year-old woman presents with painful, draining nodules and abscesses in her axilla and groin that have progressively worsened over the past 10 years. She reports fatigue, intermittent fever, and weight loss over the last few months. On physical examination, there are multiple inflamed nodules, sinus tracts, and scarring in the axillary and inguinal areas. Laboratory studies reveal:

- Hemoglobin: 9.5 g/dL (Normal: 12.1–15.1 g/dL)
- C-reactive protein: 48 mg/L (Normal: <0.3 mg/dL)
- Serum creatinine: 1.6 mg/dL (Normal: 0.6–1.1 mg/dL)
- Estimated glomerular filtration rate: 45 mL/min/1.73 m^2 (Normal: ≥ 90 mL/min/1.73 m^2)

A urinalysis shows proteinuria without hematuria. Blood cultures are negative. Imaging reveals hepatosplenomegaly and no evidence of abscesses outside the skin. Which of the following is the most likely explanation for her systemic findings?

A. AA amyloidosis (Correct)
B. Sarcoidosis
C. Iron-deficiency anemia secondary to chronic blood loss
D. Diabetic nephropathy
E. Lupus nephritis with anemia of chronic disease

Answer Explanation

This patient's cutaneous findings suggest long-standing, severe HS. Her systemic findings, including proteinuria, hepatosplenomegaly, anemia, and reduced eGFR, are most consistent with AA amyloidosis. Chronic inflammation in HS leads to excessive production of serum amyloid A protein, which can deposit in tissues, causing multiorgan dysfunction, including renal impairment (e.g., proteinuria, CKD) and hepatosplenomegaly.

Key Takeaways

- HS causes painful nodules, abscesses, and sinus tracts that can lead to scarring, contractures, and deep fistulas in advanced stages.
- Lymphedema is a rare, debilitating complication of HS that can significantly impair quality of life and increase the risk of developing malignancy.
- Cutaneous SCC is the most serious cutaneous complication of HS that's associated with high rates of metastasis and mortality compared to the general population.
- HS can lead to systemic complications, including anemia, AA amyloidosis, and renal disease that may lead to increased morbidity and mortality.
- HS patients are prone to cutaneous and systemic infections due to immune dysregulation and barrier disruption, with biologic therapies varying in associated infection risks.

References

1. Girouard SD, Falk RH, Rennke HG, Merola JF. Hidradenitis suppurativa resulting in systemic amyloid A amyloidosis: a case report and review of the literature. Dermatol Online J. 2012;18(1):2.
2. Anderson MJ Jr, Dockerty MB. Perianal hidradenitis suppurativa; a clinical and pathologic study. Dis Colon Rectum. 1958;1(1):23–31.
3. Ching CC, Stahlgren LH. Clinical review of hidradenitis suppurativa. Dis Colon Rectum. 1965;8:349–52. https://doi.org/10.1007/BF02627258.
4. Alikhan A, Lynch PJ, Eisen DB. Hidradenitis suppurativa: a comprehensive review. J Am Acad Dermatol. 2009;60(4):539–61. https://doi.org/10.1016/j.jaad.2008.11.911; quiz 562–3.
5. Slade DE, Powell BW, Mortimer PS. Hidradenitis suppurativa: pathogenesis and management. Br J Plast Surg. 2003;56(5):451–61. https://doi.org/10.1016/s0007-1226(03)00177-2.
6. Kurayev A, Ashkar H, Saraiya A, Gottlieb AB. Hidradenitis suppurativa: review of the pathogenesis and treatment. J Drugs Dermatol. 2016;15(8):1017–22.
7. Balato A, Caiazzo G, Annunziata MC, Marasca C, Scala E, Cacciapuoti S, Fabbrocini G. Anti-TNF-α therapy modulates mTORC1 signalling in hidradenitis suppurativa. J Eur Acad Dermatol Venereol. 2019;33(1):e43–5. https://doi.org/10.1111/jdv.15160.
8. Monfrecola G, Balato A, Caiazzo G, De Vita V, Di Caprio R, Donnarumma M, Lembo S, Fabbrocini G. Mammalian target of rapamycin, insulin resistance and hidradenitis suppurativa: a possible metabolic loop. J Eur Acad Dermatol Venereol. 2016;30(9):1631–3. https://doi.org/10.1111/jdv.13233.
9. Lee HH, Patel KR, Singam V, Rastogi S, Silverberg JI. Associations of cutaneous and extracutaneous infections with hidradenitis suppurativa in U.S. children and adults. Br J Dermatol. 2020;182(2):327–34. https://doi.org/10.1111/bjd.18093.
10. Habif TP. Clinical dermatology: a color guide to diagnosis and therapy. New York: Mosby; 2004.
11. Gill L, Williams M, Hamzavi I. Update on hidradenitis suppurativa: connecting the tracts. F1000Prime Rep. 2014;6:112. https://doi.org/10.12703/P6-112.
12. Kathju S, Lasko LA, Stoodley P. Considering hidradenitis suppurativa as a bacterial biofilm disease. FEMS Immunol Med Microbiol. 2012;65(2):385–9. https://doi.org/10.1111/j.1574-695X.2012.00946.x.
13. Hurley HJ. Axillary hyperhidrosis, apocrine bromhidrosis, hidradenitis suppurativa and familial benign pemphigus: surgical approach. In: Roenigk RK, Roenigk HH, editors. Dermatologic surgery. New York: Marcel Dekker; 1989. p. 729–39.

14. Church JM, Fazio VW, Lavery IC, Oakley JR, Milsom JW. The differential diagnosis and comorbidity of hidradenitis suppurativa and perianal Crohn's disease. Int J Color Dis. 1993;8(3):117–9. https://doi.org/10.1007/BF00341181.
15. Wiltz O, Schoetz DJ Jr, Murray JJ, Roberts PL, Coller JA, Veidenheimer MC. Perianal hidradenitis suppurativa. The Lahey Clinic experience. Dis Colon Rectum. 1990;33(9):731–4. https://doi.org/10.1007/BF02052316.
16. Anderson BB, Cadogan CA, Gangadharam D. Hidradenitis suppurativa of the perineum, scrotum, and gluteal area: presentation, complications, and treatment. J Natl Med Assoc. 1982;74(10):999–1003.
17. Russ E, Castillo M. Lumbosacral epidural abscess due to hidradenitis suppurativa. AJR Am J Roentgenol. 2002;178(3):770–1. https://doi.org/10.2214/ajr.178.3.1780770.
18. Williams ST, Busby RC, DeMuth RJ, Nelson H. Perineal hidradenitis suppurativa: presentation of two unusual complications and a review. Ann Plast Surg. 1991;26(5):456–62.
19. Micieli R, Alavi A. Lymphedema in patients with hidradenitis suppurativa: a systematic review of published literature. Int J Dermatol. 2018;57(12):1471–80. https://doi.org/10.1111/ijd.14173.
20. Passik SD, McDonald MV. Psychosocial aspects of upper extremity lymphedema in women treated for breast carcinoma. Cancer. 1998;83(12 Suppl American):2817–20. https://doi.org/10.1002/(sici)1097-0142(19981215)83:12b+<2817::aid-cncr32>3.0.co;2-2.
21. Fu MR, Ridner SH, Hu SH, Stewart BR, Cormier JN, Armer JM. Psychosocial impact of lymphedema: a systematic review of literature from 2004 to 2011. Psychooncology. 2013;22(7):1466–84. https://doi.org/10.1002/pon.3201.
22. Konety BR, Cooper T, Flood HD, Futrell JW. Scrotal elephantiasis associated with hidradenitis suppurativa. Plast Reconstr Surg. 1996;97(6):1243–5. https://doi.org/10.1097/00006534-199605000-00023.
23. Grada AA, Phillips TJ. Lymphedema: pathophysiology and clinical manifestations. J Am Acad Dermatol. 2017;77(6):1009–20. https://doi.org/10.1016/j.jaad.2017.03.022.
24. Lapins J, Ye W, Nyrén O, Emtestam L. Incidence of cancer among patients with hidradenitis suppurativa. Arch Dermatol. 2001;137(6):730–4.
25. Maclean GM, Coleman DJ. Three fatal cases of squamous cell carcinoma arising in chronic perineal hidradenitis suppurativa. Ann R Coll Surg Engl. 2007;89(7):709–12. https://doi.org/10.1308/003588407X209392.
26. Chapman S, Delgadillo D III, Barber C, Khachemoune A. Cutaneous squamous cell carcinoma complicating hidradenitis suppurativa: a review of the prevalence, pathogenesis, and treatment of this dreaded complication. Acta Dermatovenerol Alp Pannonica Adriat. 2018;27(1):25–8.
27. Jourabchi N, Fischer AH, Cimino-Mathews A, Waters KM, Okoye GA. Squamous cell carcinoma complicating a chronic lesion of hidradenitis suppurativa: a case report and review of the literature. Int Wound J. 2017;14(2):435–8. https://doi.org/10.1111/iwj.12671.
28. Pena ZG, Sivamani RK, Konia TH, Eisen DB. Squamous cell carcinoma in the setting of chronic hidradenitis suppurativa; report of a patient and update of the literature. Dermatol Online J. 2015;21(4):13030/qt9q9707dp.
29. Lavogiez C, Delaporte E, Darras-Vercambre S, Martin De Lassalle E, Castillo C, Mirabel X, Laurent F, Patenotre P, Gheit T, Talmant JC, Beylot-Barry M, Martinot V, Piette F, Aubin F, Mortier L. Clinicopathological study of 13 cases of squamous cell carcinoma complicating hidradenitis suppurativa. Dermatology. 2010;220(2):147–53. https://doi.org/10.1159/000269836.
30. Prens E, Deckers I. Pathophysiology of hidradenitis suppurativa: an update. J Am Acad Dermatol. 2015;73(5 Suppl 1):S8–11. https://doi.org/10.1016/j.jaad.2015.07.045.
31. Panelos J, Massi D. Emerging role of Notch signaling in epidermal differentiation and skin cancer. Cancer Biol Ther. 2009;8(21):1986–93. https://doi.org/10.4161/cbt.8.21.9921.
32. Rakoff-Nahoum S. Why cancer and inflammation? Yale J Biol Med. 2006;79(3–4):123–30.

33. Kurokawa I, Nishimura K, Yamanaka K, Mizutani H, Tsubura A, Revuz J. Cytokeratin expression in squamous cell carcinoma arising from hidradenitis suppurativa (acne inversa). J Cutan Pathol. 2007;34(9):675–8. https://doi.org/10.1111/j.1600-0560.2006.00680.x.
34. Farrugia F, Mintoff D, Pace NP. Anaemia in the hidradenitis suppurativa population. Arch Dermatol Res. 2024;316(5):193. https://doi.org/10.1007/s00403-024-02943-z.
35. Huang CM, Lowes MA, Cserti C, Alavi A. Hemoglobin levels and serum C-reactive protein in patients with moderate to severe hidradenitis suppurativa. J Cutan Med Surg. 2019;23(5):501–6. https://doi.org/10.1177/1203475419858963.
36. Soliman YS, Chaitowitz M, Hoffman LK, Lin J, Lowes MA, Cohen SR. Identifying anaemia in a cohort of patients with hidradenitis suppurativa. J Eur Acad Dermatol Venereol. 2020;34(1):e5–8. https://doi.org/10.1111/jdv.15837.
37. Kassebaum NJ, Jasrasaria R, Naghavi M, Wulf SK, Johns N, Lozano R, Regan M, Weatherall D, Chou DP, Eisele TP, Flaxman SR, Pullan RL, Brooker SJ, Murray CJ. A systematic analysis of global anemia burden from 1990 to 2010. Blood. 2014;123(5):615–24. https://doi.org/10.1182/blood-2013-06-508325.
38. Chaparro CM, Suchdev PS. Anemia epidemiology, pathophysiology, and etiology in low- and middle-income countries. Ann N Y Acad Sci. 2019;1450(1):15–31. https://doi.org/10.1111/nyas.14092.
39. Ghias MH, Johnston AD, Babbush KM, Kutner AJ, Hosgood HD, Lowes MA, Gil MR, Cohen SR. Hepcidin levels can distinguish anemia of chronic disease from iron deficiency anemia in a cross-sectional study of patients with hidradenitis suppurativa. J Am Acad Dermatol. 2022;86(4):954–6. https://doi.org/10.1016/j.jaad.2021.03.090.
40. Jørgensen AR, Nielsen VW, Yao Y, Ring HC, Thomsen SF. Anemia in patients with hidradenitis suppurativa: prevalence and risk factors in a hospital-based cohort. Skinmed. 2021;19(6):432–7.
41. Weiss G, Goodnough LT. Anemia of chronic disease. N Engl J Med. 2005;352(10):1011–23. https://doi.org/10.1056/NEJMra041809.
42. Patel S, Patel S, Shah S, Lio PA. Identifying prevalence and inpatient outcomes of anemia and hidradenitis suppurativa. Arch Dermatol Res. 2023;315(5):1287–91. https://doi.org/10.1007/s00403-022-02515-z.
43. Hurrell RF. Influence of inflammatory disorders and infection on iron absorption and efficacy of iron-fortified foods. Nestle Nutr Inst Workshop Ser. 2012;70:107–16. https://doi.org/10.1159/000337673.
44. Sheth KR, Bernthal NM, Ho HS, Bergese SD, Apfel CC, Stoicea N, Jahr JS. Perioperative bleeding and non-steroidal anti-inflammatory drugs: an evidence-based literature review, and current clinical appraisal. Medicine (Baltimore). 2020;99(31):e20042. https://doi.org/10.1097/MD.0000000000020042.
45. Özer İ, Karaçin C, Adışen E, Güz G, Ali Gürer M. Two diseases one remedy? Systemic amyloidosis secondary to hidradenitis suppurativa: treatment with infliximab. Dermatol Ther. 2017;30(2). https://doi.org/10.1111/dth.12445.
46. Montes-Romero JA, Callejas-Rubio JL, Sánchez-Cano D, González-Martínez FJ, Navas-Parejo A, Ortego-Centeno N. Amyloidosis secondary to hidradenitis suppurativa. Exceptional response to infliximab. Eur J Intern Med. 2008;19(6):e32–3. https://doi.org/10.1016/j.ejim.2007.11.014.
47. Titze J, Schneider M, Krause H, Jacobi J, Stolte M, Linke RP, Rupprecht HD. Diarrhea, nephrotic syndrome and hidradenitis suppurativa: an unusual case. Nephrol Dial Transplant. 2003;18(1):192–4. https://doi.org/10.1093/ndt/18.1.192.
48. Rubaian NFB, Al Zamami HF, Almuhaidib SR, Al Breiki SH. Hidradenitis supparativa complicated by penoscrotal lymphedema and renal amyloidosis. Saudi Med J. 2022;43(7):751–4. https://doi.org/10.15537/smj.2022.43.7.20220352.
49. Real de Asúa D, Costa R, Galván JM, Filigheddu MT, Trujillo D, Cadiñanos J. Systemic AA amyloidosis: epidemiology, diagnosis, and management. Clin Epidemiol. 2014;6:369–77. https://doi.org/10.2147/CLEP.S39981.

50. Dinwoodey DL, Skinner M, Maron MS, Davidoff R, Ruberg FL. Light-chain amyloidosis with echocardiographic features of hypertrophic cardiomyopathy. Am J Cardiol. 2008;101(5):674–6. https://doi.org/10.1016/j.amjcard.2007.10.031.
51. Kazancioğlu R. Risk factors for chronic kidney disease: an update. Kidney Int Suppl (2011). 2013;3(4):368–71. https://doi.org/10.1038/kisup.2013.79.
52. Maarouf M, Clark AK, Lee DE, Shi VY. Targeted treatments for hidradenitis suppurativa: a review of the current literature and ongoing clinical trials. J Dermatolog Treat. 2018;29(5):441–9. https://doi.org/10.1080/09546634.2017.1395806.
53. Miller IM, Carlson N, Mogensen UB, Ellervik C, Jemec GB. A population- and hospital-based cross-sectional study of renal function in hidradenitis suppurativa. Acta Derm Venereol. 2016;96(1):68–71. https://doi.org/10.2340/00015555-2072.
54. Alikhan A, Sayed C, Alavi A, Alhusayen R, Brassard A, Burkhart C, Crowell K, Eisen DB, Gottlieb AB, Hamzavi I, Hazen PG, Jaleel T, Kimball AB, Kirby J, Lowes MA, Micheletti R, Miller A, Naik HB, Orgill D, Poulin Y. North American clinical management guidelines for hidradenitis suppurativa: a publication from the United States and Canadian Hidradenitis Suppurativa Foundations: part I: diagnosis, evaluation, and the use of complementary and procedural management. J Am Acad Dermatol. 2019;81(1):76–90. https://doi.org/10.1016/j.jaad.2019.02.067.
55. Turner JE, Paust HJ, Steinmetz OM, Panzer U. The Th17 immune response in renal inflammation. Kidney Int. 2010;77(12):1070–5. https://doi.org/10.1038/ki.2010.102.
56. Almuhanna N, Tobe SW, Alhusayen R. Risk of chronic kidney disease in hospitalized patients with hidradenitis suppurativa. Dermatology. 2023;239(6):912–8. https://doi.org/10.1159/000531960.
57. Schonmann Y, Mansfield KE, Mulick A, Roberts A, Smeeth L, Langan SM, Nitsch D. Inflammatory skin diseases and the risk of chronic kidney disease: population-based case-control and cohort analyses. Br J Dermatol. 2021;185(4):772–80. https://doi.org/10.1111/bjd.20067.
58. Mahé E, Morelon E, Lechaton S, Sang KH, Mansouri R, Ducasse MF, Mamzer-Bruneel MF, de Prost Y, Kreis H, Bodemer C. Cutaneous adverse events in renal transplant recipients receiving sirolimus-based therapy. Transplantation. 2005;79(4):476–82. https://doi.org/10.1097/01.tp.0000151630.25127.3a.
59. Lowe MM, Naik HB, Clancy S, Pauli M, Smith KM, Bi Y, Dunstan R, Gudjonsson JE, Paul M, Harris H, Kim E, Shin US, Ahn R, Liao W, Hansen SL, Rosenblum MD. Immunopathogenesis of hidradenitis suppurativa and response to anti-TNF-α therapy. JCI Insight. 2020;5(19):e139932. https://doi.org/10.1172/jci.insight.139932. Erratum in: JCI Insight. 2022 Oct 24;7(20):e165502. doi: 10.1172/jci.insight.165502.
60. Guet-Revillet H, Coignard-Biehler H, Jais JP, Quesne G, Frapy E, Poirée S, Le Guern AS, Le Flèche-Matéos A, Hovnanian A, Consigny PH, Lortholary O, Nassif X, Nassif A, Join-Lambert O. Bacterial pathogens associated with hidradenitis suppurativa, France. Emerg Infect Dis. 2014;20(12):1990–8. https://doi.org/10.3201/eid2012.140064.
61. Shanmugam VK, Zaman NM, McNish S, Hant FN. Review of current immunologic therapies for hidradenitis suppurativa. Int J Rheumatol. 2017;2017:8018192. https://doi.org/10.1155/2017/8018192.
62. Katoulis AC, Koumaki D, Liakou AI, Vrioni G, Koumaki V, Kontogiorgi D, Tzima K, Tsakris A, Rigopoulos D. Aerobic and anaerobic bacteriology of hidradenitis suppurativa: a study of 22 cases. Skin Appendage Disord. 2015;1(2):55–9. https://doi.org/10.1159/000381959.
63. Kimball AB, Sundaram M, Gauthier G, Guérin A, Pivneva I, Singh R, Ganguli A. The comorbidity burden of hidradenitis suppurativa in the United States: a claims data analysis. Dermatol Ther (Heidelb). 2018;8(4):557–69. https://doi.org/10.1007/s13555-018-0264-z.
64. Cohen SH, Gerding DN, Johnson S, Kelly CP, Loo VG, McDonald LC, Pepin J, Wilcox MH, Society for Healthcare Epidemiology of America, Infectious Diseases Society of America. Clinical practice guidelines for Clostridium difficile infection in adults: 2010 update by the society for healthcare epidemiology of America (SHEA) and the infectious diseases society of America (IDSA). Infect Control Hosp Epidemiol. 2010;31(5):431–55. https://doi.org/10.1086/651706.

65. Giet G, Lebas E, Libon F, Dezfoulian B, Nikkels AF. Quoi de neuf dans le traitement de l'hidradénite suppurative en 2018 ? [What's new in the treatment of suppurative hidradenitis in 2018 ?]. Rev Med Liege. 2018;73(9):468–73. French.
66. Ochi H, Tan LC, Oon HH. The effect of oral clindamycin and rifampicin combination therapy in patients with hidradenitis suppurativa in Singapore. Clin Cosmet Investig Dermatol. 2018;11:37–9. https://doi.org/10.2147/CCID.S136730.
67. Abu Rached N, Gambichler T, Ocker L, Dietrich JW, Quast DR, Sieger C, Seifert C, Scheel C, Bechara FG. Screening for diabetes mellitus in patients with hidradenitis suppurativa-a monocentric study in Germany. Int J Mol Sci. 2023;24(7):6596. https://doi.org/10.3390/ijms24076596.
68. Lazaridou I, Vassilopoulos A, Vassilopoulos S, Shehadeh F, Kalligeros M, Mylonakis E, Qureshi A. Risk of infection in patients with hidradenitis suppurativa on biologics or other immunomodulators: a systematic review and meta-analysis. Int J Dermatol. 2024;63(2):139–49. https://doi.org/10.1111/ijd.16885.
69. Gómez-Reino JJ, Carmona L, Valverde VR, Mola EM, Montero MD, BIOBADASER Group. Treatment of rheumatoid arthritis with tumor necrosis factor inhibitors may predispose to significant increase in tuberculosis risk: a multicenter active-surveillance report. Arthritis Rheum. 2003;48(8):2122–7. https://doi.org/10.1002/art.11137.
70. von der Werth JM, Williams HC. The natural history of hidradenitis suppurativa. J Eur Acad Dermatol Venereol. 2000;14(5):389–92. https://doi.org/10.1046/j.1468-3083.2000.00087.x.

Chapter 22
Patient Resources and Support Groups for HS

Zane Sejdiu, Alexis Morgenstern, and Nicholas Brownstone

Case Title The role of social support in managing hidradenitis suppurativa

Case
A 34-year-old female presents to the dermatology clinic with a longstanding history of recurrent painful nodules and abscesses of the axillary and inguinal regions. These lesions have intermittently drained purulent material, often leaving the patient with scars and sinus tracts. Over the years, the patient has tried various treatments including oral antibiotics, dietary modifications, and a short course of biologic therapy, with minimal improvement. During her visit, the patient appears anxious and guarded, frequently avoiding eye contact and fidgeting with the hem of her oversized sweater. Despite expressing that her condition significantly impacts her daily activities, including limiting her physical mobility and work options, she downplays the emotional toll, merely stating, "I manage." The patient lives alone, minimally engages in social activities due to embarrassment of her condition, works remotely, and mentions that her support system is limited to family members who live in a different state. When asking about coping strategies, the patient endorses a sense of hopelessness, embarrassment, and fear of judgement from others. Physical examination reveals active, fluctuant nodules and sinus tracts, along with extensive scarring in the affected areas.

Z. Sejdiu (✉)
Drexel University College of Medicine, Philadelphia, PA, USA
e-mail: zs368@drexel.edu

A. Morgenstern
Temple University Lewis Katz School of Medicine, Philadelphia, PA, USA
e-mail: alexis.morgenstern@temple.edu

N. Brownstone
The Kimberly and Eric J. Waldman Department of Dermatology,
Mount Sinai Icahn School of Medicine, New York, NY, USA

N. Brownstone (ed.), *Clinical Cases in Hidradenitis Suppurativa*, Clinical Cases in Dermatology, https://doi.org/10.1007/978-3-032-15200-8_22

Board Review Question

What would be the most appropriate next step in managing this patient?

A. Initiate surgical intervention for her Hidradenitis Suppurativa immediately
B. Recommend referral to a mental health professional and introduce the idea of support groups as a beneficial resource for emotional support
C. Discontinue all current treatments and begin a course of high-dose corticosteroids
D. Schedule patient for weekly office visits focused on lesion drainage

Introduction

Hidradenitis suppurativa (HS) is a chronic, inflammatory skin disease characterized by painful nodules, abscesses, sinus tracts, and scaring that primarily impacts regions of the body with apocrine glands, namely, the armpits, groin, and genital areas [1–4]. Pathogenesis of HS includes occlusion and subsequent inflammation of the hair follicle, which, when combined with immune dysregulation, cause HS [5]. HS is categorized in severity by three Hurley Stages, with Hurley Stage I being single or multiple abscesses without scarring or sinus tracts, Hurley Stage II being recurrent abscesses with scarring and sinus tracts, and Hurley Stage III being interconnected or diffuse abscesses and sinus tracts with severe scarring and involvement of an entire region [2]. The estimated global prevalence of HS has been found to be between 0.00033 and 4.1% with a higher prevalence of 0.7–1.2% in US and European populations [6, 7]. Black patients are disproportionally impacted by HS in the United States and research in White women has shown an increased prevalence compared to men, with a 3:1 ratio [7, 8]. Numerous studies have identified risk factors for HS which include both environmental and genetic factors. Autosomal dominant genetic influences have been suggested in research that showed, in individuals with HS, 34% of their first-degree relatives had HS [9–11]. HS has been linked to mutations in the γ-secretase complex, affecting the NOTCH signaling pathway [4]. In addition to genetic risk factors, environmental risk factors such as obesity and smoking are established [4, 12, 13]. Typically, patients with HS will experience pain, malodor, itch, and a burning sensation, which are all very uncomfortable for the patient [7, 14].

In addition to the physical discomfort patients with HS experience, HS has also been shown to have psychosocial impacts. Research has shown that quality of life, determined by the Dermatology Life Quality Index (DLQI), is significantly lower in patients with HS, with worsened DLQI in more severe Hurley stages [1]. The same cross-sectional study showed that women with HS experience sexual dysfunction across all stages of HS, noting difficulties with sexual desire and pain during sexual activity [1]. Studies have highlighted the psychosocial impacts of HS and have all consistently shown negative impacts on quality of life, emotional burdens including feelings of shame and embarrassment, higher levels of anxiety and depression, and sexual dysfunction [1–3].

This chapter explores various resources and support groups for patients with HS, highlights patient perspectives, and examines the impact of these groups along with the role of social media in providing support.

The HS Foundation and Other Resources

The HS Foundation is an incredible resource for patients struggling with HS. The foundation was created to positively impact the lives of individuals who are affected by HS through advocacy, education, and research [15]. Their educational efforts are evidenced by the existence of programs and conferences such as the Annual Symposium on Hidradenitis Suppurativa Advances (SHSA), HS Spotlight, and HS Academy [15]. Each program has a specific target audience to ensure both patients and medical professionals are knowledgeable and up to date with advancements occurring within the HS sphere. SHSA plays a particularly critical role in education by presenting the latest advancements in the causes, diagnosis, management, and potential cures for HS during a 3-day conference [15]. The HS foundation website offers valuable resources for both patients and healthcare professionals, including comprehensive information on the definition, symptoms, causes, and treatments of HS, as well as related health issues. For providers, the site features the latest treatment guidelines, research updates, and online courses aimed at addressing the unmet needs of patients [16].

The HS Foundation website provides patients and providers with an easy-to-use interface to explore various facets of the disease. For patients, the website provides resources and information on how to talk to their providers regarding HS [17]. As many individuals who suffer with HS may feel uncomfortable or embarrassed to discuss their symptoms, having information on how to broach the topic so that the patient can effectively discuss their experience and begin treatment is beneficial. Additionally, the site provides patients with information on how they can identify the signs and symptoms of HS [18]. Arguably, one of the most important tools on the HS Foundation website is the resources tab. Here, resources for investigators, clinicians, and, most critically, patients, can be found. Patients can find access to HS specialty clinics, information about biologics, summary of research, educational videos and content, and ongoing clinical trials [19].

The HS Foundation also offers access to available support groups and encourages individuals to seek support from others. Hope for HS is a support group that was founded in 2013, and is the first face-to-face support group in the United States for individuals with HS and their loved ones and caregivers [20]. As a fully volunteer patient and caregiver directed non-profit organization, Hope for HS offers both in-person and virtual support groups across 12 different cities in the United States. The HS Foundation offers another support organization, HS Connect, on their website [21]. HS Connect is an organization whose goal is to eradicate the stigmas associated with HS, change the narrative, and educate as many individuals as possible, including family members, caretakers, surgeons, and non-HS specialized dermatologists. Founded by Brindley Brooks, who has bravely battled HS since she was 11 years old, HS Connect was born from her personal journey of living with the disease. After years of suffering in silence, Brindley shared her struggles publicly, embraced vulnerability, and found strength in her support system. Her resilience and desire to help others led to the creation of HS Connect, an organization dedicated to empowering those with HS to share their experiences, amplify their voices, and ensure that no one has to face this condition alone. HS Connect offers a plethora of resources for individuals with HS, ranging from in person events to online resources. Their site offers links to books and articles that community members have found helpful for mental health, webinars from dermatologists and psychiatrists, podcasts, and HS stories by patients. Additionally, HS Connects offers links to 11 different Facebook support groups, where individuals can find support and community with those struggling with HS.

The Role of Social Media in HS Support Groups

HS is a painful and often stigmatizing chronic skin condition, making social media platforms such as Facebook, Reddit, and Instagram increasingly important as spaces for connection and support [22]. The internet offers patients a lifeline where traditional healthcare models may fall short. Due to the chronic and conspicuous nature of HS (i.e., abscesses, scarring, and malodor), this can often lead to isolation and withdrawal from everyday life. One patient encapsulated this dilemma, remarking, "When a big rupture or explosion happens, there is no dressing or anything you can apply that can contain the mess, and it does lead to social embarrassment." This sense of humiliation, coupled with a lack of control over symptoms, can push patients into feelings of isolation and emotional distress. This often leads to psychological conditions such as depression and anxiety, and there has even been shown to be a heightened risk of suicide among HS patients [23–25].

Social media support groups could help destigmatize these feelings. They create a community where patients can share their stories, obtain practical advice, and most importantly, not feel alone. While medical professionals provide essential guidance, these day-to-day lived experiences can provide additional support. Individuals can supplement the advice they receive from healthcare providers by turning to these groups, using them for practical insights and understanding [26].

However, these platforms are not without challenges. Misinformation is a growing concern in online health communities [27, 28]. Most influencers on social media platforms, such as X (formerly, Twitter) are from a non-medical background [26]. Users should be conscious about where information is coming from and approach the information with caution in any social media platform or forum as medical advice could be sourced from laypersons. Patients often trade tips about home remedies and alternative treatments, which can be helpful but also may be ineffective or cause adverse events. Without reliable oversight, the wrong piece of advice could lead to ineffective or harmful treatment strategies. The lack of effective fact-checking on social media platforms also heightens the risk of misinformation spreading unchecked, which is especially concerning in vulnerable populations seeking medical support [29, 30].

Still, the benefits cannot be understated. Social media platforms serve as an easily accessible, and crucial source of emotional support, offering understanding and validation from others with shared experiences [31, 32]. One member of a social media platform focused on HS remarked, “I am so thankful for this group and the support and help I have gotten.” For many, these groups are more than just a source of information—they are emotional lifelines.

Patient Perspectives

HS patients’ participation in these groups has profound impacts on their coping strategies and mental health [32]. As mentioned, HS can feel isolating, but as one patient and support group member pointed out, “I’m exhausted. I wake up in pain, I go to work in pain, I fall asleep in pain. I can’t tell y’all how many times I wanted to give up, how many times I thought of ending it. Knowing I’m not alone in this suffering helps.” These online spaces foster emotional resilience by offering patients a place where they can vent frustrations, ask questions, and find solidarity. The shared understanding helps combat feelings of loneliness, which are particularly prevalent in patients who struggle with severe and visible symptoms [33].

In addition to emotional support, patients can find advice that helps them identify or manage their condition; as one patient shared, “I had no idea there was a name for these devilish boil things.” Another commented with a similar sentiment, “I’ve learned more here [in the Facebook support group] in 10 min than I’ve learned in 3.5 years seeing the specialist once every 6 months.” In this regard, some patients feel that they cannot find the help they need from doctors, “The sad part is that it’s hard to find a doctor here who really knows cases like this. So it’s really nice to finally found this support group.” When patients connect with others who understand these struggles, it can lessen the stigma and allows for more productive coping strategies [34].

Moreover, the experience of patients with skin of color in support groups has demonstrated how valuable these platforms are for underserved communities. Many have reported gaining more knowledge about managing their HS through group participation, as access to medical care is often uneven across different demographic groups [35]. Online spaces help bridge these gaps, offering a sense of empowerment and knowledge where the healthcare system may be lacking.

Patients in support groups often express relief at finding a community where they can seek help without feeling judged. As one participant shared, “It’s hard to find the line between annoying and wanting support,” a sentiment that likely resonates with individuals managing both the physical and emotional burdens of HS. This highlights how people value the opportunity to connect with others facing similar struggles, offering them a space to be vulnerable while navigating the complexities of asking for help. It allows patients to share their challenges without fear of imposing on those close to them. These patient insights highlight the crucial role of online support groups in fostering both emotional resilience and practical problem-solving for those living with HS. These platforms provide a safe environment where individuals can connect, share their experiences, and receive guidance, helping to ease the burden of managing the condition while reducing feelings of isolation.

The Impact of Support Groups on Quality of Life

Historically, the significance of the role social support plays in mitigating stress was emphasized by John Cassel, an epidemiologist and public health expert, in 1974 [36]. Cassel's research laid the foundation in which numerous studies that followed assessed the influence of social networks on health. Research showed that social support is consistently associated with positive mental health outcomes through ways of reducing anxiety and depression [37]. There are several theories of how social support works, involving behavioral, psychological, and physiological mechanisms. Behavioral theories suggest that social support leads to healthier behaviors, like improved treatment compliance. Psychological theories propose that social support can enhance self-esteem and promote a sense of self-control. Finally, physiological theories suggest that social support can help in reducing the body's stress response, such as lowering elevated blood pressure during stressful situations [37]. The buffering hypothesis, first proposed by Sidney Cobb in 1976 suggested that social support protects individuals from harmful effects of stress on health by reducing the perception of stress or providing resources to help cope with it [38]. This hypothesis was further supported through decades of research, bringing us to today's age, where support groups for individuals with chronic diseases have shown to be impactful.

Social support, through the means of support groups, have historically shown positive impacts on quality of life. As previously mentioned, support groups can offer patients and families educational and emotional support, addressing the psychosocial impacts of disease. They can facilitate adaptive coping skills, improve emotional well-being, and reduce social isolation in patients are caregivers [39]. Song et al. investigated the role of web-based patient communities in health goal attainment for patients in chronic disease, focusing on how social support and self-reflection in these support groups contribute to researching patient goals [40]. Data were collected across 13 online support groups for patients with chronic diseases including hypertension, diabetes, and breast cancer, which showed emotional support from these groups significantly increased the likelihood of goal attainment [40]. Interestingly, informational support did not show a significant improvement in goal attainment, highlighting the importance of emotional bonds in support groups rather than just informational exchanges [40].

Studies in individuals with other chronic diseases such as idiopathic pulmonary fibrosis have shown that support groups increased psychological wellbeing-indexes (PGWBI) across anxiety, depression, positivity, self-control, general health, and vitality [39]. Research on support groups for individuals with HIV have shown that they improve morbidity, care adherence and retention, and quality of life in individuals through means such as reducing stigma of disease and promoting adherence to medication [41]. Although there have not been any studies specifically examining the impact of support groups on quality of life in HS patients, data from other chronic diseases suggest that social support, particularly through support groups, has a positive effect on patients.

Conclusion

In conclusion, HS is a chronic and debilitating skin condition that significantly impacts both physical and mental well-being of patients. Support groups and online communities have emerged as invaluable resources for patients, providing emotional support, advice, and a sense of connection that helps to combat feelings of isolation related to the disease. Support groups underscore the importance in improving psychological health and coping strategies for those living with HS and their support group, as evidenced by positive effects of support groups in other chronic conditions. Future research and efforts should focus on expanding access to and increasing the number of HS support groups, while also exploring the direct impact of these HS support groups on quality of life.

Board Review Question Explanation
What would be the most appropriate next step in managing this patient?

A. Initiate surgical intervention for her Hidradenitis Suppurativa immediately
B. Recommend referral to a mental health professional and introduce the idea of support groups as a beneficial resource for emotional support (Correct)
C. Discontinue all current treatments and begin a course of high-dose corticosteroids
D. Schedule patient for weekly office visits focused on lesion drainage

Answer Explanation
Addressing both the physical and psychological burdens of HS is crucial in providing comprehensive care. Support groups have been shown to improve quality of life in patients, reduce feelings of isolation, anxiety, and depression. Many support groups exist for patients with HS across different platforms, both in-person or virtually, allowing patients flexibility. This approach to the patient complements medical treatment and acknowledges the psychosocial impact of the disease.

Key Takeaway Points

- Hidradenitis suppurativa (HS) is a chronic and debilitating skin condition that significantly impacts both physical and mental well-being of patients.
- Support groups and online communities have emerged as invaluable resources for patients, providing emotional support, advice, and a sense of connection to help combat feelings of isolation related to the disease.
- Support groups underscore the importance of improving psychological health and coping strategies for those living with HS.
- Positive effects of support groups in other chronic conditions highlight their potential benefits for HS patients.
- Future research and efforts should focus on expanding access to, increasing the number of, and exploring the direct impacts on quality of life of HS support groups.

References

1. Alavi A, Farzanfar D, Rogalska T, Lowes MA, Chavoshi S. Quality of life and sexual health in patients with hidradenitis suppurativa. Int J Womens Dermatol. 2018;4(2):74–9. https://doi.org/10.1016/j.ijwd.2017.10.007. Published 2018 Feb 1.
2. Maghfour J, Sivesind TE, Dellavalle RP, Dunnick C. Trends in hidradenitis suppurativa disease severity and quality of life outcome measures: scoping review. JMIR Dermatol. 2021;4(2):e27869. https://doi.org/10.2196/27869. Published 2021 Oct 1.
3. Sampogna F, Fania L, Mastroeni S, et al. Correlation between depression, quality of life and clinical severity in patients with hidradenitis suppurativa. Acta Derm Venereol. 2020;100(18):adv00319. https://doi.org/10.2340/00015555-3647. Published 2020 Nov 12.
4. Scala E, Cacciapuoti S, Garzorz-Stark N, et al. Hidradenitis suppurativa: where we are and where we are going. Cells. 2021;10(8):2094. https://doi.org/10.3390/cells10082094. Published 2021 Aug 15.
5. Napolitano M, Megna M, Timoshchuk EA, Patruno C, Balato N, Fabbrocini G, Monfrecola G. Hidradenitis suppurativa: from pathogenesis to diagnosis and treatment. Clin Cosmet Investig Dermatol. 2017;10:105–15. https://doi.org/10.2147/CCID.S111019.
6. Alotaibi HM. Incidence, risk factors, and prognosis of hidradenitis suppurativa across the globe: insights from the literature. Clin Cosmet Investig Dermatol. 2023;16:545–52. https://doi.org/10.2147/CCID.S402453. Published 2023 Mar 2.
7. Nguyen TV, Damiani G, Orenstein LAV, Hamzavi I, Jemec GB. Hidradenitis suppurativa: an update on epidemiology, phenotypes, diagnosis, pathogenesis, comorbidities and quality of life. J Eur Acad Dermatol Venereol. 2021;35(1):50–61. https://doi.org/10.1111/jdv.16677.
8. Shahi V, Alikhan A, Vazquez BG, Weaver AL, Davis MD. Prevalence of Hidradenitis suppurativa: a population-based study in Olmsted County, Minnesota. Dermatology. 2014;229:154–8.
9. Fitzsimmons JS, Guilbert PR. A family study of hidradenitis suppurativa. J Med Genet. 1985;22(5):367–73. https://doi.org/10.1136/jmg.22.5.367.
10. Vinkel C, Thomsen SF. Hidradenitis suppurativa: causes, features, and current treatments. J Clin Aesthet Dermatol. 2018;11:17–23.
11. Von Der Werth JM, Williams HC, Raeburn JA. The clinical genetics of hidradenitis suppurativa revisited. Br J Dermatol. 2000;142:947–53. https://doi.org/10.1046/j.1365-2133.2000.03476.x.

12. Bettoli V, Naldi L, Cazzaniga S, Zauli S, Atzori L, Borghi A, Capezzera R, Caproni M, Cardinali C, De Vita V, et al. Overweight, diabetes and disease duration influence clinical severity in hidradenitis suppurativa-acne inversa: evidence from the national Italian registry. Br J Dermatol. 2016;174:195–7. https://doi.org/10.1111/bjd.13864.
13. Acharya P, Mathur M. Hidradenitis suppurativa and smoking: a systematic review and meta-analysis. J Am Acad Dermatol. 2020;82:1006–11. https://doi.org/10.1016/j.jaad.2019.10.044.
14. Lipsker D, Severac F, Freysz M, Sauleau E, Boer J, Emtestam L, Matusiak Ł, Prens E, Velter C, Lenormand C, et al. The ABC of hidradenitis suppurativa: a validated glossary on how to name lesions. Dermatology. 2016;232:137–42. https://doi.org/10.1159/000443878.
15. HS Foundation. Mission and vision. HS Foundation. https://www.hs-foundation.org/mission. Accessed 23 Oct 2024.
16. HS Foundation. For clinicians. HS Foundation. https://www.hs-foundation.org/for-clinicians. Accessed 23 Oct 2024.
17. HS Foundation. Talking about HS. HS Foundation. https://www.hs-foundation.org/talking-about-hs. Accessed 23 Oct 2024.
18. HS Foundation. How to identify HS. HS Foundation. https://www.hs-foundation.org/how-to-identify-hs. Accessed 23 Oct 2024.
19. HS Foundation. HS Foundation. https://www.hs-foundation.org/. Accessed 23 Oct 2024.
20. Hope for HS. Online support group. Hope for HS. https://hopeforhs.org/online/. Accessed 23 Oct 2024.
21. HS Connect. HS Connect. https://www.hsconnect.org/. Accessed 23 Oct 2024.
22. Yesantharao LV, Suresh R, Lerman SF, Cox C, Caffrey J. Hidradenitis Suppurativa Reddit Support Group: finding new meaning in social media during the COVID-19 pandemic. J Burn Care Res. 2023;44(2):373–80. https://doi.org/10.1093/jbcr/irac183.
23. Singh R, Kelly KA, Senthilnathan A, Feldman SR, Pichardo RO. Stigmatization, a social perception which may have a debilitating impact on hidradenitis suppurativa patients: an observational study. Arch Dermatol Res. 2023;315(4):1049–52. https://doi.org/10.1007/s00403-022-02412-5.
24. Thorlacius L, Cohen AD, Gislason GH, Jemec GBE, Egeberg A. Increased suicide risk in patients with hidradenitis suppurativa. J Invest Dermatol. 2018;138(1):52–7. https://doi.org/10.1016/j.jid.2017.09.008.
25. Kouris A, Platsidaki E, Christodoulou C, et al. Quality of life and psychosocial implications in patients with hidradenitis suppurativa. Dermatology. 2017;232(6):687–91. https://doi.org/10.1159/000453355.
26. Wortsman X, Ramírez-Cornejo C, Ferreira-Wortsman C, Howes R. Perspectives on the Twitter presence of hidradenitis suppurativa. Int J Dermatol. 2021;60(10):e402–3. https://doi.org/10.1111/ijd.15631.
27. Gill H, Murphy M, O'Connor C. Pits and perils: a qualitative analysis of online misinformation and conspiracy theories in hidradenitis suppurativa. JEADV Clin Pract. 2023;2(4):955–7. https://doi.org/10.1002/jvc2.213.
28. Méndez A, Rao M, Rahnama-Moghadam S, Gomaa B, Walsh-Buhi ER. Describing hidradenitis suppurativa misinformation diffusion among Facebook users: a content analysis. J Clin Aesthet Dermatol. 2023;16(6):50.
29. Wasike B. You've been fact-checked! Examining the effectiveness of social media fact-checking against the spread of misinformation. Telemat Inform Rep. 2023;11:100090. https://doi.org/10.1016/j.teler.2023.100090.
30. Bozarth L, Im J, Quarles C, Budak C. Wisdom of two crowds: misinformation moderation on Reddit and how to improve this process—a case study of COVID-19. Proc ACM Hum Comput Interact. 2023;7(CSCW1):1–33. https://doi.org/10.1145/3579631.
31. Butt M, Cotton C, Kirby JS. Support group utilization and impact for patients with hidradenitis suppurativa. J Am Acad Dermatol. 2020;83(1):216–9. https://doi.org/10.1016/j.jaad.2019.09.023.

32. Longest K, Kang JA. Social media, social support, and mental health of young adults during COVID-19. Front Commun. 2022;7. https://doi.org/10.3389/fcomm.2022.828135.
33. Perche PO, Singh R, Senthilnathan A, Feldman SR, Pichardo RO. Hidradenitis suppurativa's impact on social activities: an observational study. Cureus. 2022;14(5):e25292. https://doi.org/10.7759/cureus.25292.
34. Sun X, Li BJ, Zhang H, Zhang G. Social media use for coping with stress and psychological adjustment: a transactional model of stress and coping perspective. Front Psychol. 2023;14:1140312. https://doi.org/10.3389/fpsyg.2023.1140312.
35. De D, Shih T, Atluri S, et al. Support group utilization and perspectives among hidradenitis suppurativa patients. SKIN J Cutan Med. 2022;6:507–10. https://doi.org/10.25251/skin.6.6.8.
36. Cassel J. An epidemiological perspective of psychosocial factors in disease etiology. Am J Public Health. 1974;64(11):1040–3. https://doi.org/10.2105/ajph.64.11.1040.
37. Ganster DC, Victor B. The impact of social support on mental and physical health. Br J Med Psychol. 1988;61(Pt 1):17–36. https://doi.org/10.1111/j.2044-8341.1988.tb02763.x.
38. Cobb S. Presidential Address-1976. Social support as a moderator of life stress. Psychosom Med. 1976;38(5):300–14. https://doi.org/10.1097/00006842-197609000-00003.
39. Magnani D, Lenoci G, Balduzzi S, Artioli G, Ferri P. Effectiveness of support groups to improve the quality of life of people with idiopathic pulmonary fibrosis a pre-post test pilot study. Acta Biomed. 2017;88(5S):5–12. https://doi.org/10.23750/abm.v88i5-S.6870. Published 2017 Nov 30.
40. Song J, Xu P, Paradice DB. Health goal attainment of patients with chronic diseases in web-based patient communities: content and survival analysis. J Med Internet Res. 2020;22(9):e19895. https://doi.org/10.2196/19895. Published 2020 Sep 11.
41. Bateganya MH, Amanyeiwe U, Roxo U, Dong M. Impact of support groups for people living with HIV on clinical outcomes: a systematic review of the literature. J Acquir Immune Defic Syndr. 2015;68 Suppl 3(03):S368–74. https://doi.org/10.1097/QAI.0000000000000519.

Chapter 23
Artificial Intelligence in the Management of HS

Andrea Leung, Georgia Marquez-Grap, Allison Kranyak, and Wilson Liao

Case Title Role of artificial intelligence in the management of HS

Case
The year is 2030, and you are the director of a busy HS clinic. You have a long of list of patients who have been referred to your clinic for evaluation of possible HS, but your new patient availability is limited. Your existing HS patients have asked you for information about the role of lifestyle factors and weight loss medications in HS, but you have not had a chance to develop a patient handout on these topics. You also notice that you have many unread patient messages in your in-basket. Feeling overwhelmed with the tasks needed to be done, you consider utilizing artificial intelligence (AI) tools to help you manage HS care.

Board Review Question
All of the following are ways in which artificial intelligence could be integrated into clinical workflow except:

A. Provide educational information regarding HS pathogenesis and management
B. Provide a definitive diagnosis of HS in a new symptomatic patient
C. Triage patient messages to identify and prioritize a flare
D. Grade Hurley stage based on photographs
E. All of the above

Andrea Leung and Georgia Marquez-Grap contributed equally with all other contributors.

A. Leung (✉) · G. Marquez-Grap · A. Kranyak · W. Liao
University of California, San Francisco, Department of Dermatology,
San Francisco, CA, USA
e-mail: Andrea.Leung@ucsf.edu; Georgia.Marquez@ucsf.edu; allison.kranyak@ucsf.edu; wilson.liao@ucsf.edu

N. Brownstone (ed.), *Clinical Cases in Hidradenitis Suppurativa*, Clinical Cases in Dermatology, https://doi.org/10.1007/978-3-032-15200-8_23

Introduction

Artificial intelligence (AI) is increasingly utilized in medicine, from research applications to real clinical scenarios. The utilization of AI in dermatology is especially relevant given the specialty's reliance on visualization for disease diagnosis and management. Artificial neural networks can be created to connect inputs, such as clinical records or images, to outputs, such as specific disease diagnoses or outcomes. This type of AI technology is referred to as deep learning (DL), and it has the potential to learn from inputs, generate models of connection, and predict outcomes [1]. In a meta-analysis investigating the use of AI to diagnose melanoma, DL models performed just as well as humans [2]. Apart from image learning and diagnosis, however, AI may also be harnessed for research, patient management, education, and clinical administrative needs. OpenAI's ChatGPT has the ability to draft patient facing handouts for disease education, and write after-visit summaries for the provider [3, 4].

The applications of AI in hidradenitis suppurativa (HS) diagnosis and disease management are explored in the following sections. AI has the potential to address some of the most pressing problems in HS care, including aiding in earlier diagnosis, triaging patient messages, contributing to patient education, and assisting providers with clinical management of HS patients. The limitations of AI in HS care are also explained below, and include data privacy concerns, ethical considerations, and feasibility of implementation.

Prioritizing HS Referrals and Enhancing HS Diagnosis

HS is an underrecognized medical condition, often with a delay in diagnosis of 7–10 years [5]. This is due to several factors, including a lack of awareness and education surrounding HS among patients and providers. Additionally, available information is often difficult to interpret and can lead to missed or underdiagnosed cases. With the rise of AI, there has been an increase in patients who look to platforms like Google AI and ChatGPT for information about their symptoms. Chat GPT has the ability to generate readable education and resources for HS patients, but a study investigating the readability of generated responses revealed an average readability grade of 15, which was higher than resources found from the HS foundation, HSpatient guide, and HS-related websites [6]. This complexity in available information further contributes to the difficulty in HS diagnosis and management.

While not explicitly created to help diagnose HS, the HS bot made by Walss et al., 2021 has potential to aid in disease diagnosis. This particular HS chatbot was publicly available online for a period of 15 months and had pre-defined "jumps," meaning specific phrases or questions would lead the user down specific paths [7]. Several of these jump categories included diagnostics, pathogenesis, therapy, and other [7]. 254 cases using the chatbot were analyzed, and 211 or 83% of cases were from users that were not yet diagnosed with HS. 164 users completed the entire diagnostics jump, and 138 or 84% received a tentative positive diagnosis [7]. Given the well-characterized delays that many patients experience in receiving an official HS diagnosis, the outcome of this study is not surprising. With a limited number of dermatologists and month-long delays for referrals and appointments, patients may seek out AI tools to help them better understand their disease and receive a diagnosis, even if that diagnosis was not made by a human provider. HS Chatbot and similar AI models could be used as tools to identify possible undiagnosed patients and quickly connect them to expert care. However, these tools cannot replace a dermatologist's assessment, and providers and patients should remain skeptical of AI diagnosis in the absence of a holistic review that takes into account visual changes, medical history, and clinical signs indicative of HS.

HS Severity Assessment

The time between referral to first dermatology appointment can often be extensive. A Canadian retrospective study found a median time of 9.1 weeks from referral to appointment for HS patients [8]. This contributes to issues with accessibility and timely assessment and treatment of HS. Additionally, there are a number of HS scoring systems and severity rating tools, however in a review of 12 randomized control trials utilizing 30 HS coring tools, Ingram et al. found that only 10% of these tools had been validated [9]. AI and DL have been employed to aid disease diagnosis via visual assessment in dermatology, and expansion of this into HS severity scoring can potentially address these two issues.

The International Hidradenitis Suppurativa Severity Score System (IHS4) was developed to standardize HS severity scoring among providers in both clinical and research settings [10]. The scoring system subdivides lesions into three categories (inflammatory nodules, abscesses, and draining tunnels) and assigns a score to each category [10]. However, using IHS4 may be time-consuming for providers and thus not always practical for to utilize in clinic. There is also high variability of scores between users due to differences in users' experience in HS management [11]. To reduce user variability and increase feasibility of utilizing the scoring system, Hernandez et al., 2023 developed Automatic International Hidradenitis Suppurativa Severity Score System (AIHS4), which is a DL version of ISH4 based on a machine learning architecture called YOLOv5. Legit.Health-HS-IHS4, an image collection comprised of 221 HS cases manually scored by six providers, was used to train a DL model and create AIHS4 [11]. The tool was close in performance to senior dermatologists when assessing moderate and severe HS cases, but behind most other dermatologists when assessing mild cases [11]. While AIHS4 did not outperform the six dermatologists when averaged, AIHS4 did perform better than some dermatologists on specific cases [6]. Areas of improvement for AIHS4 include training the model on a larger data set with a greater number of mild cases, and having the data set rated by a larger group of experts [11].

Another study created a convolutional neural network (CNN) to automatically assess severity of HS using the IHS4 [12]. The CNN was fed 777 photos taken on smartphones from patients with HS, as well as physician severity scoring of those same reference photos [12]. The model was able to categorize cases as no disease, mild, moderate, and severe, with a high level of sensitivity and specificity [12]. Limitations of this CNN induced difficulty assessing severity on hairy skin, as well as relatively few mild cases included in the data set [12]. Nonetheless, CNN's are promising tools for quickly and automatically assessing HS severity, with the potential to reduce human variability and error.

Treatment Selection and Efficacy

HS is a highly complex condition that requires treatment stacking and combination therapy, and it is common for providers who are unfamiliar with HS to pursue unrecommended treatments, such as serial incision and drainages. The question of what the most effective treatment is for a patient is also pervasive across all providers, as patients will have variable responses to different treatments. Current clinical trials investigating biologic and non-biologic therapeutics for HS have advanced the way in which we understand and treat HS, but there still remain many gaps in our understanding of HS treatment by factors like severity.

Clinical trials are the gold standard for evaluating treatment efficacy. However, these studies are often expensive, long, and inadequately capture patient-reported experiences and outcomes. Investigators have evaluated the potential role for AI to assist in HS research to fill these gaps in knowledge. A recent study by Barak-Levitt et al. aimed to create a reproducible AI-based platform for patient-reported outcomes. Through a retrospective patient-reported outcome study based on online questionnaires, clinical characteristics, comorbidities, treatment, and patient satisfaction were evaluated and recoded using machine learning, manual coding, and validation to generate a model of treatment effectiveness. With a cohort of 1050 patients, this AI-based platform found that depression, anxiety, and polycystic ovary syndrome were the most frequent comorbidities. This study also assessed which treatments, such as topical agents, dietary changes, pain relief measures, and biologics, were rated by patients as the most effective for each Hurley stage. The model of treatment effectiveness contributed to a more comprehensive picture of evaluating treatment effectiveness, comorbidities, and patient satisfaction [13].

Patient Communication, Flare Monitoring, and Education

Another major challenge that providers and clinics face is the volume of patient messages and ability to triage patient questions and symptoms. HS flares are characterized by extreme pain and symptomatology that require timely communication with their provider to first assess their condition and subsequently what the proper management should be. However, when providers receive hundreds of messages a day, it may be difficult to find and respond to these messages efficiently. AI is emerging as a tool to assist providers and patients in the triage process, which can potentially improve patient outcomes and quality of life.

The effective management of HS requires timely patient-provider communication and evidence-based education and information on treatment guidelines. AI has been tested and integrated into resources that can address both.

The use of digital technology like language learning models (LLM) may help to manage patient messages and improve patient-centered care [14]. Through the recognition of topics and patterns within patient messages, LLM tools can identify, categorize, and prioritize messages related to concerns like flares, scheduling, and medication refills [14]. This can be utilized to effectively triage patient messages and evaluate the need for in-office evaluations versus questions that can be addressed remotely. Additionally, evaluation of patterns in patient messages may have the potential to predict an individual's risk of HS comorbidities [14]. For patients, this can also positively increase perceived access to care [14].

Current limitations of utilizing this technology include errors, such as the misclassification of message topics and sentiments, more limited use when messages are unrelated to HS, lack ICD-9 codes, Hurley staging, and other information pertinent to classification [14].

AI has promising potential to serve as an accessible and timely resource for patients to learn more about their symptoms and health. Platforms like ChatGPT can generate readable education for HS patients, though additional work must be done to ensure these generated responses are at an accessible reading level and linguistic complexity. Additionally, the chatbot interface for information accessibility has emerged as a widely used tool. A medical chatbot, the *HS Chatbot*, was studied to assess its ability to enable individual-level communication with a virtual database [7]. Many individuals with HS or HS-similar symptoms turn to the internet for information, and tools like this have the potential to connect patients to answers in a way that can supplement their clinical care. However, a limitation of utilizing generative platforms for assessment of patient symptoms is the potential risk of misclassification, which can contribute to increased patient anxiety. It is important to ensure these tools are trained on data that has a high level of evidence.

Conclusion

The applications of AI have the potential to improve many aspects of HS diagnosis and management. Patient-facing medical chatbots like HS Chatbot have shown potential for assisting with preemptive diagnosis, which can shorten time to clinical evaluation and diagnosis. AIHS4 and convolutional neural networks are examples of tools trained on HS images that may be able to assist clinicians in making more timely assessments of HS severity in the future with reliable accuracy. AI interfaces can provide instant patient and provider-facing resources and education, while

AI-based studies are helping to build a more comprehensive understanding of treatment effectiveness and the patient experience with HS. With continuous advancements in technology, AI has potential to supplement, but not replace, current strategies and tools in HS care. Figure 23.1 reviews the applications of AI in HS care.

Board Review Question Explanation
All of the following are ways in which artificial intelligence could be integrated into clinical workflow except:

A. Provide educational information regarding HS pathogenesis and management
B. Provide a definitive diagnosis of HS in a new symptomatic patient (Correct)
C. Triage patient messages to identify and prioritize a flare
D. Grade Hurley stage based on photographs
E. All of the above

Answer Explanation
B is correct answer. The role of AI is not to provide a definitive diagnosis of HS. Rather, it has the potential to give a presumptive diagnosis that can prompt patients to connect with clinicians sooner, such that they can be evaluated for a clinical, definitive diagnosis. AI can be integrated into many areas of HS care. AI chatbots like ChatGPT and HS Chatbot are patient-facing tools that can be utilized to answer questions regarding HS (A). Current technology is being developed to help sort through patient messages to identify themes, topics, and clues for flares that can help triage these patients (C). Research is investigating the role of AI and tools like convolutional neural networks in creating technology to assess HS Hurley stage and severity based on photographs (D).

Key Takeaway Points
- AI may help address some of the challenges in HS care.
- AI cannot yet be used to diagnose or manage HS by itself.
- Deep learning AI tools can assess HS severity.
- Patient communication and education may be enhanced with AI tools such as LLMs.

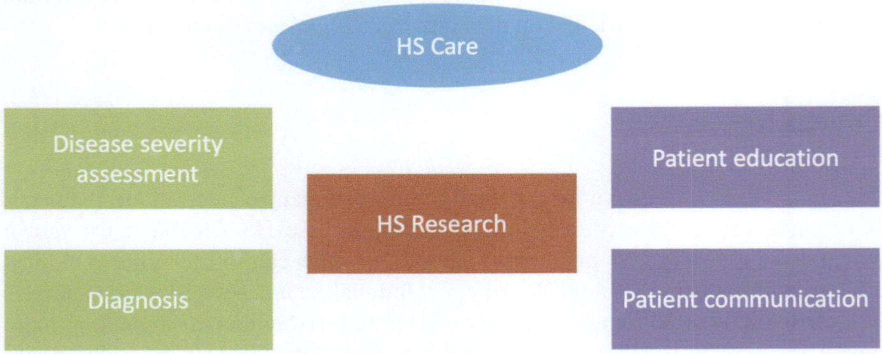

Fig. 23.1 Applications of AI in HS care

References

1. Young AT, Xiong M, Pfau J, Keiser MJ, Wei ML. Artificial intelligence in dermatology: a primer. J Invest Dermatol. 2020;140(8):1504–12. https://doi.org/10.1016/j.jid.2020.02.026.
2. Dick V, Sinz C, Mittlböck M, Kittler H, Tschandl P. Accuracy of computer-aided diagnosis of melanoma: a meta-analysis. JAMA Dermatol. 2019;155(11):1291. https://doi.org/10.1001/jamadermatol.2019.1375.
3. Baker MN, Burruss CP, Wilson CL. ChatGPT: a supplemental tool for efficiency and improved communication in rural dermatology. Cureus. 2023;15(8):e43812. https://doi.org/10.7759/cureus.43812.
4. Young AT, Lane BN, Ozog D, Matthews NH. Patients and dermatologists are largely satisfied with ChatGPT-generated after-visit summaries: a pilot study. JAAD Int. 2024;15:33–5. https://doi.org/10.1016/j.jdin.2023.12.004.
5. Saunte DM, Boer J, Stratigos A, et al. Diagnostic delay in hidradenitis suppurativa is a global problem. Br J Dermatol. 2015;173(6):1546–9. https://doi.org/10.1111/bjd.14038.
6. Gawey L, Dagenet CB, Tran KA, Park S, Hsiao JL, Shi V. Readability of information generated by ChatGPT for hidradenitis suppurativa. JMIR Dermatol. 2024;7:e55204. https://doi.org/10.2196/55204.
7. Walss M, Anzengruber F, Arafa A, Djamei V, Navarini AA. Implementing medical chatbots: an application on hidradenitis suppurativa. Dermatology. 2021;237(5):712–8. https://doi.org/10.1159/000511706.
8. Johnston LA, Poelman SM. Hidradenitis suppurativa patient referrals to a Canadian community dermatology practice: a retrospective chart review. J Cutan Med Surg. 2024;28(2):136–40. https://doi.org/10.1177/12034754231223451.
9. Ingram JR, Hadjieconomou S, Piguet V. Development of core outcome sets in hidradenitis suppurativa: systematic review of outcome measure instruments to inform the process. Br J Dermatol. 2016;175(2):263–72. https://doi.org/10.1111/bjd.14475.
10. Zouboulis CC, Tzellos T, Kyrgidis A, et al. Development and validation of the International Hidradenitis Suppurativa Severity Score System (IHS 4), a novel dynamic scoring system to assess HS severity. Br J Dermatol. 2017;177(5):1401–9. https://doi.org/10.1111/bjd.15748.
11. Hernández Montilla I, Medela A, Mac Carthy T, et al. Automatic International Hidradenitis Suppurativa Severity Score System (AIHS4): a novel tool to assess the severity of hidradenitis suppurativa using artificial intelligence. Skin Res Technol. 2023;29(6):e13357. https://doi.org/10.1111/srt.13357.
12. Wiala A, Ranjan R, Schnidar H, Rappersberger K, Posch C. Automated classification of hidradenitis suppurativa disease severity by convolutional neural network analyses using calibrated clinical images. Acad Dermatol Venereol. 2024;38(3):576–82. https://doi.org/10.1111/jdv.19639.
13. Barak-Levitt J, Held R, Synett Y, Kremer N, Hodak E, Sherman S. Hidradenitis suppurativa international online community: patient characteristics and a novel model of treatment effectiveness. Acta Derm Venereol. 2022;102:adv00686. https://doi.org/10.2340/actadv.v102.1056.
14. Chen ML, Kim J, Naik HB, et al. Analysing common topics of secure patient messages in hidradenitis suppurativa: a text-embedding and natural language-processing approach. Br J Dermatol. 2024;191(4):633–5. https://doi.org/10.1093/bjd/ljae222.

Chapter 24
Biologic, Off-label, and Pipeline Therapies for HS

Milaan Shah, Graham H. Litchman, and James Q. Del Rosso

Case Title A young female patient inquires if there is a new and/or better alternative she can try for her HS disease

Case

A 29-year-old female presents with Hurley stage III hidradenitis suppurativa (HS) primarily involving the bilateral axillae, inframammary folds, and buttocks. She notes that her HS initially presented at the age of 13 with an outbreak of painful nodules in her axillae. As she got older, she subsequently started to experience new lesions in the anogenital region. The pain and location of her HS lesions limit her from being active when she is flaring, which she finds particularly distressing as the mother of two young children. Additionally, she is very self-conscious about the malodorous discharge from her underarms and is worried about how it will impact her coworkers' assessment of her, as she works in a professional setting. She has a strong family history of HS with her mother and maternal aunt both also being afflicted by the condition. She was diagnosed with HS almost 8 years after her initial flare and repeated visits to the Emergency Department for "boils" and "infections." She has tried numerous topical and oral medications including metformin, spironolactone, numerous different antibiotics, and prednisone, with limited benefit.

M. Shah
Department of Dermatology, Medical University of South Carolina, Charleston, SC, USA

G. H. Litchman (✉)
Vivida Dermatology, Las Vegas, NV, USA

JDR Dermatology Research, Las Vegas, NV, USA

J. Q. Del Rosso
JDR Dermatology Research, Las Vegas, NV, USA

Touro University Nevada, Henderson, NV, USA

N. Brownstone (ed.), *Clinical Cases in Hidradenitis Suppurativa*, Clinical Cases in Dermatology, https://doi.org/10.1007/978-3-032-15200-8_24

Intralesional corticosteroids have previously been effective in alleviating associated pain, but she notes that the resolution is only temporary and within 1–2 weeks her pain returns. Her dermatologist eventually started her on adalimumab 80 mg injections every 2 weeks. She initially noticed substantial improvement, although she didn't have complete clearance, but after 3 years of therapy, she began having more frequent and severe flares. Given her persistent symptoms despite being on the maximum dose of her current biologic, she would like to know more about potential alternative treatment options and if there are any medications in development for HS.

Board Review Question
Which of the following is NOT a key cytokine involved in the pathogenesis of hidradenitis suppurativa?

A. TNF-alpha
B. IL-1
C. IL-13
D. IL-17
E. IL-23
F. IL-36

This case depicts an all-too-common course for many patients affected by hidradenitis suppurativa (HS). This disorder, which commonly starts after puberty, is characterized by exacerbations and relative remissions, with many patients experiencing low-grade inflammation for several days of the year between more severe flares. While not fully understood, the pathogenesis of HS is complex and multifactorial and is precipitated by a combination of genetic, hormonal, behavioral, and environmental factors that cause immune overactivation [1]. Dysregulation of inflammatory pathways in the hair follicle subunit, mediated by cytokine activity, leads to the development of inflammation around the hair follicle, causing follicular rupture and abscess formation which are the hallmark cutaneous manifestations of HS [2]. Key cytokines involved in the pathophysiology of HS include tumor necrosis factor-alpha (TNF-α), interleukin-1 (IL-1), interleukin-6 (IL-6), interleukin-10 (IL-10), interleukin-12 (IL-12), interleukin-17 (IL-17), interleukin-23 (IL-23), and interleukin-36 (IL-36) [3]. Additionally, the complement system, nucleotide-binding oligomerization domain 2 (NOD2) protein, and granulocyte colony-stimulating factor (G-CSF) are thought to play crucial roles in the pathophysiology of HS [2, 3]. A robust analysis of the molecular mechanisms of HS allows clinicians to better understand how the disease functions and progresses and provides potential targets for novel clinical interventions. Several medications approved for the treatment of HS, and numerous other pipeline agents, are being developed with this concept in mind. Table 24.1 provides a summary of medications evaluated in clinical studies for the treatment of hidradenitis suppurativa.

Table 24.1 Summary of medications evaluated in clinical studies for the treatment of hidradenitis suppurativa[a]

Mechanism of action	Medication	Route	Initiation dosing	Maintenance dosing
TNF-α inhibitors	Adalimumab[b]	SC	160 mg at week 0 and 80 mg at week 2	40 or 80 mg weekly or q2weeks
	Infliximab	IV	7.5 mg/kg at weeks 0, 2, and 6	5–10 mg/kg q4–8weeks
IL-17 inhibitors	Secukinumab[b]	SC	300 mg at weeks 0, 1, 2, 3, and 4	300 mg q4weeks
	Bimekizumab[b]	SC	320 mg q2weeks for 16 weeks	320 mg q4weeks
	Izokibep	SC	80 or 160 mg q2weeks for 12 weeks	80 or 160 mg q4weeks
	Sonelokimab	SC	120 mg q2weeks from Weeks 0 to 6	120 mg q4weeks
	CJM112	SC	300 mg at weeks 0, 1, 2, 3, and 4	300 mg q2weeks
IL-1 inhibitors	Anakinra	SC	n/a	100 mg daily
	Bermekimab	SC	n/a	400 mg weekly
	Lutikizumab	SC	n/a	300 mg weekly or q2weeks
IL-12/23 inhibitor	Ustekinumab	SC	45 mg (<100 kg) or 90 mg (>100 kg) at weeks 0 and 4	45 or 90 mg q12weeks; can be increased to q8weeks
IL-36 inhibitor	Spesolimab	IV	1200 mg for weeks 0, 1, and 2	1200 mg q2weeks
JAK inhibitors	Upadacitinib	Oral	n/a	15 or 30 mg daily
	Povorcitinib	Oral	n/a	45 or 75 mg daily
	Deucravacitinib	Oral	n/a	6 mg daily
PDE-4 inhibitors	Apremilast	Oral	Increase from 10 mg to 50 mg by 10 mg per day for days 1 to 5	30 mg BID
	Roflumilast	Oral	n/a	500 mcg daily
	Orismilast	Oral	n/a	40 mg BID
CXC chemokine receptor inhibitor	Eltrekibart	IV	n/a	600 mg q2weeks
IRAK4 degrader	KT-474	Oral	1600 mg on day 1	200 mg daily
C5a inhibitors	Vilobelimab	IV	n/a	1200 mg q2weeks
	Avacopan	Oral	n/a	30 mg BID
Tyrosine kinase inhibitors	Remibrutinib	Oral	n/a	25 mg BID
	Fostamatinib	Oral	100 mg BID for 4 weeks	150 mg BID
OX-40 inhibitors	Amlitelimab	SC	500 mg	250 mg q4weeks
	SAR-442970	SC	n/a	150 mg q2weeks

(continued)

Table 24.1 (continued)

Mechanism of action	Medication	Route	Initiation dosing	Maintenance dosing
GLP-1 agonists	Semaglutide	SC	0.25 mg at weeks 0, 1, 2, 3, and 4	0.5 mg weekly
	Liraglutide	SC	0.6 mg daily for 1 week; increase dose by 0.6 mg each week	3 mg daily

Abbreviations: Subcutaneous (SC); Intravenous (IV); Twice daily (BID); every 2 weeks (q2 weeks); every 4 weeks (q4 weeks); every 8 weeks (q8 weeks); every 12 weeks (q12 weeks)
[a]Not all agents are currently commercially available
[b]Approved by the United States Food and Drug Administration (FDA) for treatment of HS

Approved Therapies

As discussed in earlier chapters, several treatment options, including topical and oral antibiotics, oral antiandrogen agents, oral retinoids, and metformin, may be started in isolation or combination for the initial treatment of HS [1]. However, many patients will have extensive and/or recalcitrant disease that requires further intervention beyond the scope of traditional medications. More efficacious treatments should be trialed for these patients, and biologic agents provide a more efficacious therapeutic option. Adalimumab, secukinumab, and bimekizumab are the three biologic agents currently US Food and Drug Administration (FDA) approved for the treatment of moderate-to-severe HS following the success of their pivotal phase III trials.

Clinical trials for agents that treat HS generally examine several endpoint parameters including Hidradenitis Suppurativa Physician Global Assessment (HS-PGA), International Hidradenitis Suppurativa Severity Scoring System (IHS4), Hidradenitis Suppurativa Clinical Response (HiSCR), and abscess and inflammatory nodule (AN) count [4]. HS-PGA is a severity scale ranging from clear (0) to very severe (5) based on the number of abscesses and draining fistulas, inflammatory nodules, and non-inflammatory nodules. Similarly, IHS4 is a scoring system based on the number of fistulae/sinuses (x4 points), abscesses (x2 points), and nodules (x1 point) the patient has and is stratified by severity into mild (0–3), moderate (4–10), or severe (11+). HiSCR represents the degree of reduction from baseline in abscess and inflammatory nodule count from baseline, with the associated number indicating the percentage of improvement: HiSCR50, HiSCR75, and HiSCR90 are the percentage of patients who have a 50%, 75%, and 90% or greater reduction in abscess and inflammatory nodule counts, respectively. AN count is defined as the patient's total abscess and inflammatory nodule count, which is compared from baseline to the end time point.

Adalimumab represented a major breakthrough in the treatment armamentarium of HS. It was the first FDA-approved biologic for moderate-to-severe HS, which gained approval in 2015. Adalimumab, a TNF- α inhibitor also approved for the treatment of Crohn's disease, rheumatoid arthritis, ankylosing spondylitis, psoriatic arthritis, and plaque psoriasis, showed success in its phase II trial where 13.7% of patients receiving 40 mg of adalimumab weekly achieved clinical response, defined as at least a 2-grade improvement in HS-PGA, compared to 3.9% of placebo patients at week 16 [5]. In the two pivotal phase III trials that followed significantly more patients on weekly adalimumab had an improvement in HiSCR50 compared to those on placebo [6, 7]. The rates of adverse events (AEs), serious AEs (sAEs), infectious events, and discontinuations were generally similar between those on adalimumab and placebo [7]. Long-term extension trial data after 3 years demonstrated that rates of HiSCR50 scores were maintained (52.3% at week 168 and 50.6% at week 12), and the safety profile largely mirrored that seen in the phase III trials [8]. Contraindications and relative contraindications to adalimumab include malignancy, demyelinating conditions, cytopenias, heart failure, and active infections, particularly hepatitis B and tuberculosis [6].

Secukinumab is an IL-17A inhibitor that was the next biologic approved for the treatment of HS in 2023 [9]. An initial phase II trial with 20 patients had 70% of patients achieve HiSCR50 by week 24 [10]. In the subsequent SUNSHINE and SUNRISE phase III trials of secukinumab for moderate-to-severe HS demonstrated efficacy at both week 16 and week 52 endpoints when the medication was administered every 2 and 4 weeks [9]. Additionally, a 52-week real-life study on the use of secukinumab in 21 HS patients who had previously failed treatment with adalimumab showed that 57.1% of them achieved the primary endpoint and had significant reductions in disease severity, impact on quality of life, and pain scores [11]. In the 2-year follow-up of the SUNSHINE and SUNRISE trials analyzing how long clinical response was maintained, some patients were switched to placebo while others continued on secukinumab [12]. Loss of response, the primary endpoint, was defined as a 50% increase in AN count at any visit or an increase of 3 or greater in absolute AN count versus the average of the previous three visits or the week 52 visit, depending on which was lower. The median time to loss of response for patients on secukinumab every 2 and 4 weeks was 283 and 365 days compared to 239 and 171 days for patients that were switched to placebo, respectively. These results showed that response to secukinumab was sustained following 1 year of treatment, and the medication was also well tolerated during this time period. The most commonly reported adverse events (AEs) include headache, nasopharyngitis, and worsening of HS, and it is relatively contraindicated in patients with inflammatory bowel disease, although hypersensitivity reaction to secukinumab is the only contraindication listed in the label [9].

Bimekizumab, an IL-17A and IL-17F inhibitor, became the newest biologic therapy FDA-approved for the treatment of HS in 2024 [13]. In a phase II trial with 167 participants, patients receiving bimekizumab every 2 weeks had higher rates of HiSCR50 compared to placebo (57.3% vs. 26.1%) and greater improvements in mean IHS4 compared to placebo (16.0 vs. 40.2) [14]. In the following BE HEARD I and BE HEARD II phase III trials, participants treated with bimekizumab every 4 weeks also showed a significant improvement in HiSCR50 scores compared to placebo at 16 weeks, with response maintained or increased to week 48 [13]. Bimekizumab was the first agent to have Phase III trials that reported HiSCR75 and

HiSCR90 scores for which responses were improved and maintained to week 48 [13]. HiSCR90 and HiSCR100 responses from week 16 improved to week 48 with treatment in both trials [13]. Additionally, investigators incorporated a new and validated assessment scale, called the hidradenitis suppurativa symptom daily diary (HSSDD), to determine the absolute change in skin pain and pain response. At week 16, participants on both bimekizumab every 2 weeks and every 4 weeks had numerically greater improvements in HSSDD worst skin pain and clinically meaningful improvements in pain response. The most common AEs in the pivotal trials were worsening of hidradenitis, oral candidiasis, headache, and diarrhea, and bimekizumab has no formal contraindications but should be prescribed with caution in patients with inflammatory bowel disease, suicidal ideation and behavior, and/or liver enzyme abnormalities [13, 15].

Given the recent FDA approval of these agents, familiarity with their efficacy and availability grows among clinicians. All three currently approved biologic agents can and should be considered in patients with moderate-to-severe HS and, of note, no head-to-head trials exist comparing the efficacy of these medications. When selecting the appropriate therapy, the authors recommend that agent selection be guided by a consideration of the absolute and relative contraindications, ability to obtain access, and patient preference.

Off-Label/Pipeline Therapies

While the treatment armamentarium for hidradenitis has expanded, a notable subsection of patients with HS are still unable to achieve adequate clinical response with currently approved medications. For these patients, off-label use with agents that have demonstrated efficacy in studies and clinical practice for treating HS but do not carry formal FDA approval may warrant consideration. In addition, several pipeline biologics and oral systemic medications are undergoing rigorous analysis in various phase II and III clinical trials for HS with the hope of providing further treatment options for this chronic and difficult to treat disease. These treatment options and the evidence surrounding them are explored in the rest of this chapter.

TNF-α Inhibitors

Infliximab is a chimeric monoclonal antibody targeting TNF-α that may be used for the treatment of Crohn's disease, ulcerative colitis, rheumatoid arthritis, plaque psoriasis, and psoriatic arthritis [16]. While not FDA-approved for the treatment of HS, substantial evidence supports its efficacy; a systematic review and meta-analysis including 19 studies with 299 patients with moderate-to-severe HS treated with infliximab by Shih et al. found that participants had a pooled response rate of 83% (largely based on clinician reported outcomes) [17]. Infliximab is generally administered intravenously at 5 mg/kg every 6–8 weeks, but a prospective study of 42 patients with HS receiving 7.5 mg/kg of infliximab every 4 weeks showed 47.6%

and 70.8% of participants experienced clinical response [defined as achieving a Physician Global Assessment score of clear, minimal, or mild (0–2) HS with at least a 2-grade improvement from baseline] at week 4 and week 12, respectively [18]. These results support that infliximab can be considered in doses as high as 10 mg/kg administered every 4 weeks for rapid clinical response [18]. AEs for infliximab include non-serious infections and infusion reactions [12].

Etanercept, a soluble TNF-α receptor that competitively binds to TNF receptors 1 and 2, is FDA approved for ankylosing spondylitis, juvenile idiopathic arthritis, plaque psoriasis, psoriatic arthritis, and rheumatoid arthritis with several additional off-label uses as well [19]. However, the current evidence does not support the use of etanercept for HS, with a Phase II trial including 20 patients with HS showing no statistical difference in clinical response between 50 mg of subcutaneous etanercept twice a week and placebo at 12 or 24 weeks, and another Phase II trial with 15 patients on etanercept (50 mg weekly) showing a clinical response rate of only 20% [20, 21].

IL-17 Inhibitors

Two IL-17 inhibitors, discussed above, are currently approved for the treatment of HS, but several other agents within this class are actively being investigated, with the preliminary results showing great promise.

Izokibep is a selective inhibitor of IL-17A being investigated for the treatment of HS as well as plaque psoriasis [22]. The current trial data on izokibep is mixed. In an initial Phase IIb/III trial, izokibep failed to meet the primary endpoint of at least a 75% reduction from baseline in abscess and inflammatory-nodule count (HiSCR75) response in a statistically significant proportion of patients at week 16 [23]. However, another randomized, double-blind, placebo-controlled Phase III trial showed promising results with 33% of patients receiving 160 mg of izokibep weekly achieving HiSCR75 at week 12 compared to 21% of patients on placebo [24]. Injection-site reactions were the most common AE noted, occurring in 65.1% of participants on izokibep compared to 7.8% on placebo [24]. However, only one patient had an injection-site reaction greater than Grade 1 or 2, and this contributed to discontinuation in 4.7% of patients [24]. Further release and analysis of trial data will be needed to better characterize the impact of izokibep in HS.

Sonelokimab is a trivalent nanobody derived from camel-like mammals that selectively targets IL-17A and IL-17F and is being studied in the treatment of both adolescent and adult HS as well as numerous other inflammatory conditions [25]. In a phase II trial, 43.3% and 34.8% of patients with moderate-to-severe HS treated with 120 mg or 240 mg of sonelokimab every 4 weeks achieved HiSCR75 compared to 14.7% on placebo at week 12 [26]. Additionally, similar trends in efficacy results were demonstrated in data presented on outcomes at week 24 [27, 28]. The medication was overall well tolerated. The safety profile of sonelokimab was similar to that of other IL-17 inhibitors, with oral candidiasis being seen more frequently in the treatment arms [26]. Phase 3 trials of sonelokimab are ongoing.

CJM112, an anti-IL17A monoclonal antibody, was effective in treating HS based on initial data from a Phase II trial completed in 2016, but further Phase III trials were not subsequently commenced [28, 29]. Of note, the primary endpoint for the Phase II trial was at least a 2-point reduction in HS-Physician Global Assessment (HS-PGA), which varies from HiSCR scores employed in other trials [29].

Of the IL-17 inhibitors already approved for plaque psoriasis, there is some preliminary evidence that supports that brodalumab and ixekizumab may be effective in HS [30, 31].

IL-1 Inhibitors

A number of agents that inhibit IL-1 through different subunits, including anakinra, AVTX-009, bermekimab, canakinumab, gevokizumab, lutikizumab, MEDI8968, and rilonacept, have been studied for HS treatment [32]. While further investigation is either needed and/or is ongoing for all of the above agents, we review the available data to date that exists for anakinra, bermekimab, and lutikizumab.

Anakinra is a recombinant human IL-1 receptor antagonist with established efficacy in the treatment of rheumatoid arthritis and early evidence supporting its role in the treatment of HS [33]. In an open-label trial of six patients treated with anakinra for 8 weeks, the five patients who completed treatment showed significant improvements in physician and patient global assessment and Dermatology Life Quality Index (DLQI) [34]. In a subsequent double-blinded, randomized, placebo-controlled trial where 20 patients received either anakinra subcutaneously daily or placebo for 12 weeks, HS clinical response was achieved in 78% of participants in the treatment arm (30% in placebo) [35]. One patient discontinued treatment at week 4 due to diarrhea, but no major safety signals were identified [35]. Limitations of both studies include the small number of patients included.

Bermekimab, an IL-1α inhibitor, demonstrated safety and efficacy in the treatment of moderate-to-severe HS in an initial Phase II trial [36]. 42 patients who had either failed prior anti-TNF-α use (group A, $n = 24$) or were treatment naive (group B, $n = 18$) received 400 mg of bermekimab weekly for 12 weeks. At week 12, 63% and 61% of patients in groups A and B, respectively, achieved HiSCR50. Injection site reactions were the only AEs seen. These promising results may warrant further investigation in a larger, placebo-controlled trial.

Lutikizumab is a dual IL-1α and IL-1β neutralizing antibody that has shown promise in the treatment of moderate-to-severe HS from the early reported results of its Phase II trial [37]. A cohort of 153 patients were equally randomized to receive either 300 mg of lutikizumab weekly, 300 mg of lutikizumab every other week, 100 mg of lutikizumab every other week, or placebo for 16 weeks, with the primary endpoint being HiSCR50. Patients in the 300 mg of lutikizumab weekly arm achieved HiSCR50 significantly more than those in placebo (59.5% vs. 35%, no statistical significance with other two treatment arms). However, HiSCR75 was achieved significantly more in both the 300 mg of lutikizumab weekly and 300 mg of lutikizumab every other week groups compared to placebo, demonstrating greater efficacy at a higher clinical endpoint. Rates of AEs were similar between treatment arms and placebo, with the most common being diarrhea, headache, pruritus, contact dermatitis, and nasopharyngitis.

IL-23 Inhibitors

IL-23 inhibitors that have been investigated for use in HS include risankizumab and guselkumab. While both treatments showed early evidence of efficacy, risankizumab was found to not be effective for HS in its Phase II trial, and guselkumab showed higher rates of HiSCR50 in patients on treatment than placebo, but these results were not statistically significant [38, 39].

Ustekinumab is a dual IL-12 and IL-23 inhibitor that is not FDA-approved for the treatment of HS but has supporting evidence for its efficacy. A systematic review and meta-analysis of patients with HS treated with ustekinumab conducted in 2024, including 10 studies with 88 patients, of which the majority had failed a prior biologic (80.7%), showed a pooled response rate of 67% [40]. Additionally, the treatment was well tolerated, but these results are limited by the small sample size.

IL-36 Receptor Inhibitors

The evidence for IL-36 receptor inhibitors in the treatment of HS is continuing to be developed, but the initial results have been promising. Spesolimab is an IL-36 receptor inhibitor FDA approved for the treatment of generalized pustular psoriasis which showed positive results in its proof-of-concept study [41]. In this randomized, double-blinded, placebo-controlled trial with 52 HS patients (2:1 on spesolimab vs. placebo), there were greater improvements in the IHS4 and HiSCR50 in the treatment arm compared to placebo, but there was no statistical difference seen in total abscess and inflammatory nodule (AN) count, which was the primary endpoint. Spesolimab was also well tolerated, and these results may warrant further study with a larger scale trial.

Imsidolimab is another IL-36 receptor inhibitor investigated for use in HS but development was discontinued due to a lack of demonstrated efficacy [42].

JAK Inhibitors

As the therapeutic indications of JAK inhibitors continue to expand, so has the investigation of their use in HS. While isolated cases suggesting efficacy have been documented for numerous JAK inhibitors, tofacitinib, upadacitinib, povorcitnib, and deucravacitinib have the most available data for this potential indication.

Tofacitinib is an inhibitor of JAK1 and JAK3 and is FDA approved for use in numerous inflammatory conditions including rheumatoid arthritis, psoriatic arthritis, and ulcerative colitis [43]. There are no particular trials investigating this indication, but four case reports in the literature demonstrate efficacy with good clinical response of patients with severe HS being treated with 5 mg of tofacitinib BID [44]. However, in one case, the patient had to discontinue therapy due to COVID-19 infection and subsequent drug resistance [44]. Additionally, another patient experienced elevations in liver function tests which necessitated reduction in dose to 5 mg every other day; the patient continued to have sustained clinical clearance at this dose, and his liver enzymes normalized [44]. The evidence is clouded by a suspected case of paradoxical HS in a juvenile patient with rheumatoid arthritis after 6 months of tofacitinib treatment [45]. Overall, the efficacy of tofacitinib in HS appears inconclusive and further case reports and larger scale randomized controlled trials are needed for clarity.

Upadacitinib is a JAK1 inhibitor that has shown efficacy in treating HS in its early Phase II trial [46, 47]. In a randomized, placebo-controlled cohort of 68 patients with moderate-to-severe HS receiving either once-daily upadacitinib 30 mg or placebo for 12 weeks, higher proportions of patients treated with upadacitinib achieved HiSCR50 compared to historical placebos of adalimumab studies on HS (statistical significance not achieved with in-trial placebo group). At week 12, placebo patients were switched to upadacitinib 15 mg daily until week 48, and HiSCR50 achievement was maintained in the original treatment arm through week 40. One discontinuation was seen due to worsening HS. A subsequent Phase III trial may present further support for this treatment.

Povorcitinib (INCB054707) is a promising JAK1 inhibitor being studied for use in HS. In a Phase II trial, 209 patients were randomized 1:1:1:1 to receive povorcitinib 15, 45, or 75 mg or placebo for 16 weeks, with the endpoints being AN, HiSCR75, HiSCR90, and HiSCR100 [48]. At week 16, all treatment arms had significantly larger decrease in AN count compared to placebo. Additionally, a higher dosage of medication appeared to be more effective with higher rates of HiSCR, but all treatment groups achieved higher HiSCRs (75/90/100) compared to placebo, although the differences were not statistically different. More patients on placebo reported AEs compared to those on povorcitinib (65.4% vs. 60%), with the most common including fatigue, headache, and diarrhea. Preliminary results from the two Phase III trials show that povorcitinib 45 mg and 75 mg achieve significantly greater rates of HiSCR50 and further reduction in AN count compared to placebo with no new safety signals [49]. Completed Phase III trials will improve clarity regarding the duration of this positive response.

Lastly, deucravacitinib, a selective inhibitor of tyrosine kinase 2 (TYK2), is being investigated in a Phase II trial for use in hidradenitis suppurativa, but the results of this trial have not yet been reported [50].

Phosphodiesterase 4 Inhibitors

Phosphodiesterase 4 (PDE4) inhibitors are a class of medications that primarily function to cause bronchial muscle relaxation in the lungs but also blunt inflammatory cascade responses, allowing for treatment of certain dermatoses [51]. The two primary agents in this class investigated for the treatment of HS are apremilast and roflumilast.

An early, small randomized control trial on apremilast in HS showed promising initial results, with 53.3% of 15 patients on therapy achieving HiSCR50 compared to 0% (0/5) in the placebo group [52]. A long-term follow-up to this study followed the eight patients who appropriately responded to therapy for 2 years and revealed that four patients maintained HiSCR50 until 2 years after drug initiation (the other 4 participants discontinued medication use before the end of year 1) [53]. GI side effects were seen, and one patient discontinued therapy due to associated nausea [53]. In an additional phase II trial with 20 patients with mild-to-moderate HS on apremilast, 65% of patients achieved HiSCR30 at week 16 and 24, and significant improvements were seen in pain scores and quality of life assessments [54]. Impressions are limited given smaller sample sizes, but apremilast is generally well tolerated and has been efficacious in preliminary studies.

Oral roflumilast demonstrated similar results to apremilast in a recently studied paper that included 16 patients with moderate-to-severe HS [55]. At week 16, patients on treatment had significant improvements in IHS4, DLQI scores, and weight loss compared to baseline, and 44% of patients achieved HiSCR, for which the threshold for percentage of improvement is unclear based on the limited information available in the published abstract. The associated AEs were largely GI-related and consistent with those expected for this class of medication. Of note, five patients discontinued medication use due to GI symptoms or lack of benefit. Medication associated weight loss in combination with HS treatment may make roflumilast an attractive treatment option for certain patients once efficacy is further established.

Orismilast is a novel PDE4 inhibitor with favorable results seen in its Phase II trial [56]. 20 patients with moderate-to-severe HS were to gradually titrate their dosage of orismilast up to 40 mg BID and continue treatment for 16 weeks. However, due to associated GI symptoms, 11 patients discontinued treatment early, and six of the nine patients who completed therapy were not on the full dosage. Those patients that completed treatment saw a mean AN count reduction of 33% compared to 12% in the early discontinuation group. Additionally, HiSCR50 was achieved in 67% in the complete treatment group versus 27% in the early discontinuation group. The most common side effects were diarrhea, abdominal pain, and nausea. Despite concerns with tolerability in the Phase II trial, orismilast presents a viable oral treatment option for HS.

Chemokine Receptor Antibody

CXC chemokine receptors 1 (CXCR1) and 2 (CXCR2), part of the CXC chemokine family, are G-protein coupled receptors found on numerous cell types, such as granulocytes, monocytes, and mast cells, and are involved in signaling needed for neutrophil migration in sites of inflammation and angiogenesis [57]. Targeting this mechanism may help in HS treatment, and thus, LY3041658 (also known as eltrekibart), which is a monoclonal antibody targeting CXCR1 and CXCR2, has an ongoing Phase 2 trial for use in moderate-to-severe HS [58]. Results show that 65.6% of patients receiving 600 mg of eltrekibart intravenously every 2 weeks for 16 weeks achieved HiSCR50 compared to 41.4% for patients receiving placebo. Additionally, average AN count reduction was 52.1% in the treatment arm and 14.5% in placebo, but this result was not statistically significant ($p = 0.14$) likely due to small sample size ($n = 67$). Most AEs were mild to moderate, and infections were the most common AE. Both the treatment arm and placebo group are to be continued on 20 additional weeks of eltrekibart, but the preliminary results for this novel mechanism of action in HS are reassuring.

IRAK4 Degrader

Interleukin-1 receptor associated kinase 4 (IRAK4) is a protein kinase that plays a role in the activation of the IL-1 pathway, which is known to be amplified in HS [59]. Additionally, IRAK4 is overexpressed in HS skin and correlates with other associated inflammatory biomarkers [59]. KT-474 (SAR444656) is a novel IRAK4 degrader being investigated as a treatment for HS. A Phase I trial including 105 healthy volunteers (13 with HS, although 1 patient discontinued the study early) tolerated a loading dose of 1600 mg followed by 14 days of 200 mg of KT-474 taken orally with no serious safety signals found [60]. Patients with HS in the cohort showed substantial reductions in the proinflammatory cytokines analyzed [54]. A Phase 2 trial examining the therapeutic effects of KT-474 in HS is ongoing (NCT06028230) [61].

Complement C5a Inhibitors

Dysregulation of complement activation may contribute to the pathogenesis of HS by promoting neutrophil migration and stimulating the overproduction of TNF-α [62]. Additionally, increased levels of C5a are present in the blood of HS patients, making it an inflammatory marker of HS [62].

Vilobelimab (IFX-1) is a monoclonal antibody targeting C5a that has demonstrated efficacy for HS in a single-arm open label trial where 9 out 12 patients, all with Hurley stage III disease, reached HiSCR50 at day 50 [63]. However, five patients had sAEs, four of which were flares of HS and the other being a soft tissue infection requiring IV antibiotics. The initial Phase 2 study data further supports the efficacy of vilobelimab, with 63.2% of patients on treatment showing reduction in tunnels compared to 18% for placebo based on a post-hoc analysis [64]. Complete resolution with vilobelimab compared to placebo was also significantly higher at 40.9% versus 13%. The rates of AEs seen with vilobelimab were similar to those in placebo. Progression of the drug into Phase III trials will further characterize the efficacy and safety.

Avacopan is an oral C5a inhibitor also being considered for use in HS. In its Phase II trial, 398 enrolled patients received either avacopan 10 or 30 mg BID or placebo BID for 12 weeks [65]. At week 12, statistical significance was not met for HiSCR50 scores, but for Hurley stage III patients particularly, there was a significantly greater response in those taking 30 mg of avacopan BID compared to placebo (42.6% vs. 22.2%, $p = 0.0349$). Patients tolerated the medication well with lower rates of AEs and sAEs compared to placebo. A phase III trial is not yet underway.

Tyrosine Kinase Inhibitors

Remibrutinib is a Bruton's tyrosine kinase inhibitor that works by mediating B-cell activation and stimulation involved in the chronic inflammation of HS [66]. Remibrutinib had positive results in its Phase II trial, with 77 patients receiving either 25 mg of remibrutinib BID, 100 mg BID, or placebo for 16 weeks, and 72.7% of patients on 25 mg reached simplified HiSCR compared to 34.7% of those in placebo [67]. Only one sAE was reported, and upper respiratory infections were the most common AE. Phase III trials are underway (NCT06799000, NCT06840392) [68, 69].

Fostamatinib is a spleen tyrosine kinase that also targets B cells and plasma cells involved in HS [70]. A proof-of-concept open-label study with 20 patients with HS administered 100 mg of fostamatinib BID for 4 weeks, and then had participants increase the dosage to 150 mg BID for an additional 8 weeks. At week 4, 85% of participants achieved HiSCR50, and these results were maintained until week 12. The medication was well tolerated, and no grade 2 or 3 adverse events were reported. While the study had a small sample size, the speed and degree of improvement warrant further consideration in a larger scale study. There are no trials of fostamatinib for HS ongoing currently.

OX40-OX40L Inhibitors

Amlitelimab is a monoclonal antibody that inhibits the OX40 ligand (OX40L) and has recently been initiated in a proof-of-concept study for HS [71]. Preliminary data is not yet available for this indication. SAR-442970, a nanobody molecule that inhibits both TNF-α and the OX40L, has shown evidence in animal models of suppressing inflammation similar to that seen in HS skin [72]. A Phase II trial with 86 patients has been completed, but the data are not yet available [73]. Rocatinlimab is a monoclonal antibody that blocks the OX40 receptor, but it does not appear to have been investigated in HS to date.

GLP-1 Receptor Agonists

Glucagon-like peptide-1 receptor agonists (GLP1-RAs) are most well-known for promoting weight loss and improved blood sugar control, and their use in inflammatory diseases has been increasingly explored [74]. HS has a strong association with metabolic dysfunction and suggests that there may be a role for these agents in its treatment, as loss of body weight has been shown to decrease disease severity [75, 76]. A systematic review of the use of GLP1-RAs in HS found that liraglutide and semaglutide have been used effectively to help patients both lose weight and decrease the severity of disease and frequency of flares [76]. Liraglutide and semaglutide were also shown to cause significant improvements in quality of life. Additionally, GLP-1As are thought to have anti-inflammatory properties, suppressing the activity of TNF-α and IL-17 [76]. While sample sizes of the included studies were small and several other GLP-1RAs have not been studied in HS, this class of medications may be beneficial in HS patients with comorbid obesity, particularly in improving quality of life.

Board Review Question Explanation

Which of the following is NOT a key cytokine involved in the pathogenesis of hidradenitis suppurativa?

A. TNF-alpha
B. IL-1
C. IL-13 (Correct)
D. IL-17
E. IL-23
F. IL-36

Answer Explanation

While a number of cytokines have been found to play a role in the pathophysiology of HS, IL-13 is not a key cytokine involved in precipitating disease. As detailed in the introduction above, HS is thought to be mediated primarily by Th1 and Th17 associated cytokines, which are activated inversely to Th2 cytokines such as IL-13. Further investigation is needed to characterize the relationship of IL-13 in HS, but the other cytokines listed have been shown to play a role in the disease process and have been investigated as molecular targets for HS drug development.

Key Takeaway Points

- HS is a complex condition precipitated largely by immune dysregulation, many of the components which are still being discovered.
- The extensive pathophysiologic mechanisms involved in HS provide several cytokines and inflammatory pathways that are potential targets for directed therapies.
- Several existing medications, with indications for other dermatoses, are being explored in their application to HS because of overlap in inflammatory pathways and cytokine activity and/or preliminary evidence supporting clinical efficacy.
- Numerous agents with varying levels of efficacy are currently being developed for use in HS and undergoing clinical trials in mid-to-later stages of development.
- As the treatment armamentarium for HS expands, it is important for clinicians to be aware of the available therapeutic options in order to make the best treatment decision for the patient.
- HS is a difficult condition to treat that frequently displays resistance to monotherapy. Combinations of different medications may be required and need to be considered in patients with particularly severe and/or unresponsive disease.
- Not all clinical manifestations of HS are adequately responsive to medical interventions, especially fibrotic and other fixed sequelae; comprehensive management of HS often requires integration of physical/surgical approaches.

References

1. Ballard K, Shuman VL. Hidradenitis suppurativa. [Updated 2024 May 6]. In: StatPearls [Internet]. Treasure Island (FL): StatPearls Publishing; 2025. Available from: https://www.ncbi.nlm.nih.gov/books/NBK534867/.
2. Melchor J, Prajapati S, Pichardo RO, Feldman SR. Cytokine-mediated molecular pathophysiology of hidradenitis suppurativa: a narrative review. Skin Appendage Disord. 2024;10(3):172–9. https://doi.org/10.1159/000536268.
3. Del Duca E, Morelli P, Bennardo L, Di Raimondo C, Nisticò SP. Cytokine pathways and investigational target therapies in hidradenitis suppurativa. Int J Mol Sci. 2020;21(22):8436. https://doi.org/10.3390/ijms21228436. Published 2020 Nov 10.
4. Kim Y, Lee J, Kim HS, et al. Review of scoring systems for hidradenitis suppurativa [retracted in: Ann Dermatol. 2024 Aug;36(4):255. doi: 10.5021/ad.36.001.]. Ann Dermatol. 2024;36(1):9–17. https://doi.org/10.5021/ad.23.090.
5. Kimball AB, Kerdel F, Adams D, et al. Adalimumab for the treatment of moderate to severe Hidradenitis suppurativa: a parallel randomized trial. Ann Intern Med. 2012;157(12):846–55. https://doi.org/10.7326/0003-4819-157-12-201212180-00004.
6. https://www.accessdata.fda.gov/drugsatfda_docs/label/2008/125057s0110lbl.pdf.
7. Kimball AB, Okun MM, Williams DA, et al. Two phase 3 trials of adalimumab for hidradenitis suppurativa. N Engl J Med. 2016;375(5):422–34. https://doi.org/10.1056/NEJMoa1504370.
8. Zouboulis CC, Okun MM, Prens EP, et al. Long-term adalimumab efficacy in patients with moderate-to-severe hidradenitis suppurativa/acne inversa: 3-year results of a phase 3 open-label extension study. J Am Acad Dermatol. 2019;80(1):60–69.e2. https://doi.org/10.1016/j.jaad.2018.05.040.

9. Kimball AB, Jemec GBE, Alavi A, et al. Secukinumab in moderate-to-severe hidradenitis suppurativa (SUNSHINE and SUNRISE): week 16 and week 52 results of two identical, multicentre, randomised, placebo-controlled, double-blind phase 3 trials [published correction appears in Lancet. 2024 Feb 17;403(10427):618. doi: 10.1016/S0140-6736(24)00266-6.]. Lancet. 2023;401(10378):747–61. https://doi.org/10.1016/S0140-6736(23)00022-3.
10. Casseres RG, Prussick L, Zancanaro P, et al. Secukinumab in the treatment of moderate to severe hidradenitis suppurativa: results of an open-label trial. J Am Acad Dermatol. 2020;82(6):1524–6. https://doi.org/10.1016/j.jaad.2020.02.005.
11. Martora F, Marasca C, Cacciapuoti S, et al. Secukinumab in hidradenitis suppurativa patients who failed adalimumab: a 52-week real-life study. Clin Cosmet Investig Dermatol. 2024;17:159–66. https://doi.org/10.2147/CCID.S449367. Published 2024 Jan 23.
12. Kimball AB, Bechara FG, Badat A, et al. Long-term efficacy and safety of secukinumab in patients with moderate-to-severe hidradenitis suppurativa: week 104 results from the SUNSHINE and SUNRISE extension trial. Br J Dermatol. 2025;192(4):629–40. https://doi.org/10.1093/bjd/ljae469.
13. Kimball AB, Jemec GBE, Sayed CJ, et al. Efficacy and safety of bimekizumab in patients with moderate-to-severe hidradenitis suppurativa (BE HEARD I and BE HEARD II): two 48-week, randomised, double-blind, placebo-controlled, multicentre phase 3 trials. Lancet. 2024;403(10443):2504–19. https://doi.org/10.1016/S0140-6736(24)00101-6.
14. Glatt S, Jemec GBE, Forman S, et al. Efficacy and safety of bimekizumab in moderate to severe hidradenitis suppurativa: a phase 2, double-blind, placebo-controlled randomized clinical trial. JAMA Dermatol. 2021;157(11):1279–88. https://doi.org/10.1001/jamadermatol.2021.2905.
15. https://www.accessdata.fda.gov/drugsatfda_docs/label/2024/761151s005s006s007lbl.pdf.
16. https://www.accessdata.fda.gov/drugsatfda_docs/label/2021/103772s5401lbl.pdf.
17. Shih T, Lee K, Grogan T, De DR, Shi VY, Hsiao JL. Infliximab in hidradenitis suppurativa: a systematic review and meta-analysis. Dermatol Ther. 2022;35(9):e15691. https://doi.org/10.1111/dth.15691.
18. Ghias MH, Johnston AD, Kutner AJ, Micheletti RG, Hosgood HD, Cohen SR. High-dose, high-frequency infliximab: a novel treatment paradigm for hidradenitis suppurativa. J Am Acad Dermatol. 2020;82(5):1094–101. https://doi.org/10.1016/j.jaad.2019.09.071.
19. Pan A, Gerriets V. Etanercept. [Updated 2023 Jul 24]. In: StatPearls [Internet]. Treasure Island (FL): StatPearls Publishing; 2025. Available from: https://www.ncbi.nlm.nih.gov/books/NBK545252/.
20. Adams DR, Yankura JA, Fogelberg AC, Anderson BE. Treatment of hidradenitis suppurativa with etanercept injection. Arch Dermatol. 2010;146(5):501–4. https://doi.org/10.1001/archdermatol.2010.72.
21. Lee RA, Dommasch E, Treat J, et al. A prospective clinical trial of open-label etanercept for the treatment of hidradenitis suppurativa. J Am Acad Dermatol. 2009;60(4):565–73. https://doi.org/10.1016/j.jaad.2008.11.898.
22. Klint S, Feldwisch J, Gudmundsdotter L, et al. Izokibep: preclinical development and first-in-human study of a novel IL-17A neutralizing Affibody molecule in patients with plaque psoriasis. MAbs. 2023;15(1):2209920. https://doi.org/10.1080/19420862.2023.2209920.
23. Manalac T. Acelyrin's lead assetizokibep fails in late-stage hidradenitis suppurativa trial. BioSpace. News release. Accessed 12 Sept 2023. https://www.biospace.com/article/acelyrin-s-lead-asset-izokibep-fails-in-late-stage-hidradenitis-suppurativa-trial/.
24. Papp KA, et al. Efficacy and safety of izokibep, a novel IL-17A inhibitor, in moderate-to-severe hidradenitis suppurativa: week 12 results from a randomized, double-blind, placebo-controlled, multicenter, phase 3 study. Presented at: European Academy of Dermatology and Venereology (EADV) Congress, Amsterdam, Netherlands, 25 Sept 2024. Abstract ID: 7995.
25. Papp KA, Weinberg MA, Morris A, Reich K. IL17A/F nanobody sonelokimab in patients with plaque psoriasis: a multicentre, randomised, placebo-controlled, phase 2b study [published correction appears in Lancet. 2021 Jun 5;397(10290):2150. doi: 10.1016/S0140-6736(21)01068-0.]. Lancet. 2021;397(10284):1564–75. https://doi.org/10.1016/S0140-6736(21)00440-2.

26. Kimball AB, Okun MM, Zouboulis CC, et al. Efficacy and safety of the IL-17A- and IL-17F-inhibiting Nanobody® sonelokimab in patients with active, moderate-to-severe hidradenitis suppurativa: results from the global, randomized, double-blind, placebo-controlled phase 2 MIRA trial. Presented at: 32nd European Academy of Dermatology and Venereology (EADV) Congress, Berlin, Germany, 11–14 Oct 2023.
27. Kimball AB, Kirby B, Bechara FG, et al. Efficacy and safety of the IL-17A- and IL-17F-inhibiting Nanobody® sonelokimab in patients with moderate-to-severe hidradenitis suppurativa (HS); week 24 results from the phase 2 MIRA trial. Presented at: American Academy of Dermatology Annual Meeting, San Diego, California, 8–12 Mar 2024. Abstract 56014.
28. Pinto Salgueiro G, Yilmaz O, Nogueira M, Torres T. Interleukin-17 inhibitors in the treatment of hidradenitis suppurativa. BioDrugs. 2025;39(1):53–74. https://doi.org/10.1007/s40259-024-00687-w.
29. Kimball AB, Prens EP, Bechara FG et al. Hidradenitis suppurativa responds to a novel anti-IL17 antibody (CJM112) in a controlled clinical trial vs placebo. Presented at: 24th World Congress of Dermatology, Milan, Italy, 10–15 June 2019.
30. Kearney N, Hughes R, Kirby B. Treatment of hidradenitis suppurativa with brodalumab in biologic treatment failures: experiences from a specialty clinic. Clin Exp Dermatol. 2023;48(7):790–2. https://doi.org/10.1093/ced/llad130.
31. Esme P, Botsali A, Akoglu G, Caliskan E. An anti-interleukin-17A monoclonal antibody, ixekizumab, in the treatment of resistant hidradenitis suppurativa: a case series. Skin Appendage Disord. 2022;8(4):342–5. https://doi.org/10.1159/000521860.
32. Calabrese L, Malvaso D, Coscarella G, et al. Therapeutic potential of IL-1 antagonism in hidradenitis suppurativa. Biomolecules. 2024;14(2):175. https://doi.org/10.3390/biom14020175. Published 2024 Feb 1.
33. Cvetkovic RS, Keating G. Anakinra. BioDrugs. 2002;16(4):303–14. https://doi.org/10.2165/00063030-200216040-00005.
34. Leslie KS, Tripathi SV, Nguyen TV, Pauli M, Rosenblum MD. An open-label study of anakinra for the treatment of moderate to severe hidradenitis suppurativa. J Am Acad Dermatol. 2014;70(2):243–51. https://doi.org/10.1016/j.jaad.2013.09.044.
35. Tzanetakou V, Kanni T, Giatrakou S, et al. Safety and efficacy of anakinra in severe hidradenitis suppurativa: a randomized clinical trial. JAMA Dermatol. 2016;152(1):52–9. https://doi.org/10.1001/jamadermatol.2015.3903.
36. Gottlieb A, Natsis NE, Kerdel F, et al. A phase II open-label study of bermekimab in patients with hidradenitis suppurativa shows resolution of inflammatory lesions and pain. J Invest Dermatol. 2020;140(8):1538–1545.e2. https://doi.org/10.1016/j.jid.2019.10.024.
37. AbbVie. Lutikizumab showed positive results in a phase 2 trial of adults with moderate to severe hidradenitis suppurativa as program advances to phase 3. AbbVie Newsroom. Published January 8, 2024. Accessed 6 June 2025. https://news.abbvie.com/2024-01-08-Lutikizumab-Showed-Positive-Results-in-a-Phase-2-Trial-of-Adults-with-Moderate-to-Severe-Hidradenitis-Suppurativa-as-Program-Advances-to-Phase-3.
38. Kimball AB, Prens EP, Passeron T, et al. Efficacy and safety of risankizumab for the treatment of hidradenitis suppurativa: a phase 2, randomized, placebo-controlled trial. Dermatol Ther (Heidelb). 2023;13(5):1099–111. https://doi.org/10.1007/s13555-023-00913-3.
39. Kimball AB, Podda M, Alavi A, et al. Guselkumab for the treatment of patients with moderate-to-severe hidradenitis suppurativa: a phase 2 randomized study. J Eur Acad Dermatol Venereol. 2023;37(10):2098–108. https://doi.org/10.1111/jdv.19252.
40. Masson R, Seivright J, Grogan T, et al. Ustekinumab in hidradenitis suppurativa: a systematic review and meta-analysis. Dermatol Ther (Heidelb). 2024;14(7):1901–16. https://doi.org/10.1007/s13555-024-01207-y.
41. Alavi A, Prens EP, Kimball AB, et al. Proof-of-concept study exploring the effect of spesolimab in patients with moderate-to-severe hidradenitis suppurativa: a randomized double-blind placebo-controlled clinical trial. Br J Dermatol. 2024;191(4):508–18. https://doi.org/10.1093/bjd/ljae144.

42. Bader, Kaitlyn. Imsidolimab development for HS discontinued. Dermatology Times. Published May 29, 2024. Accessed 8 June 2025. https://www.dermatologytimes.com/view/imsidolimab-development-for-hs-discontinued.
43. Padda IS, Bhatt R, Parmar M. Tofacitinib. [Updated 2023 Jul 3]. In: StatPearls [Internet]. Treasure Island (FL): StatPearls Publishing; 2025. Available from: https://www.ncbi.nlm.nih.gov/books/NBK572148/.
44. Sadeghzadeh Bazargan A, Pashaei A, Goodarzi A. Successful treatment of hidradenitis suppurativa with tofacitinib: two cases and a review of the literature. Oxf Med Case Rep. 2023;2023(3):omad003. https://doi.org/10.1093/omcr/omad003. Published 2023 Mar 25.
45. Shaharir SS, Jamil A, Chua SH, Arumugam M, Rosli N. A case paradoxical hidradenitis suppurativa with janus kinase inhibitor, literature review and pooled analysis of biological agent-induced HS. Dermatol Ther. 2020;33(6):e14021. https://doi.org/10.1111/dth.14021.
46. Kimball AB, Ackerman L, Schlosser BJ, et al. Efficacy and safety of upadacitinib in moderate-to-severe hidradenitis suppurativa: a phase 2, randomized, placebo-controlled study [43799]. J Am Acad Dermatol. 2023;89(3):AB42. https://doi.org/10.1016/j.jaad.2023.07.172.
47. Ackerman LS, Schlosser BJ, Zhan T, et al. Improvements in moderate-to-severe hidradenitis suppurativa with upadacitinib: results from a phase 2, randomized, placebo-controlled study. J Am Acad Dermatol. 2025;92(6):1252–60. https://doi.org/10.1016/j.jaad.2024.12.046.
48. Kirby JS, Okun MM, Alavi A, et al. Efficacy and safety of the oral Janus kinase 1 inhibitor povorcitinib (INCB054707) in patients with hidradenitis suppurativa in a phase 2, randomized, double-blind, dose-ranging, placebo-controlled study. J Am Acad Dermatol. 2024;90(3):521–9. https://doi.org/10.1016/j.jaad.2023.10.034.
49. Andrus E. Povorcitinib demonstrates promising phase 3 results for hidradenitis suppurativa treatment. Dermatology Times. News Release. Published May 30, 2024. Accessed 11 June 2025. https://www.dermatologytimes.com/view/povorcitinib-demonstrates-promising-phase-3-results-for-hidradenitis-suppurativa-treatment.
50. Jaguan D, Nguyen KT, Goldfarb N. Selective small molecule inhibitors for hidradenitis suppurativa: today and tomorrow. J Am Acad Dermatol. 2024;91(6S):S31–6. https://doi.org/10.1016/j.jaad.2024.09.014.
51. Padda IS, Tripp J. Phosphodiesterase inhibitors. [Updated 2023 Jun 26]. In: StatPearls [Internet]. Treasure Island (FL): StatPearls Publishing; 2025. Available from: https://www.ncbi.nlm.nih.gov/books/NBK559276/.
52. Vossen ARJV, van Doorn MBA, van der Zee HH, Prens EP. Apremilast for moderate hidradenitis suppurativa: results of a randomized controlled trial. J Am Acad Dermatol. 2019;80(1):80–8. https://doi.org/10.1016/j.jaad.2018.06.046.
53. Aarts P, Vossen ARJV, van der Zee HH, Prens EP, van Straalen KR. Long-term treatment with apremilast in hidradenitis suppurativa: a 2-year follow-up of initial responders. J Am Acad Dermatol. 2021;85(1):258–60. https://doi.org/10.1016/j.jaad.2020.08.113.
54. Kerdel FR, Azevedo FA, Kerdel Don C, Don FA, Fabbrocini G, Kerdel FA. Apremilast for the treatment of mild-to-moderate hidradenitis suppurativa in a prospective, open-label, phase 2 study. J Drugs Dermatol. 2019;18(2):170–6.
55. Nielsen VW, Holgersen NK, Ring HC, Egeberg A, Thyssen JP, Gyldenløve M, Thomsen SF. 52267 Effectiveness and safety of oral roflumilast in patients with hidradenitis suppurativa: a prospective single-center study. J Am Acad Dermatol. 2024;91(3):AB192.
56. Frederiksen CG, Sedeh FB, Taudorf EH, Saunte DM, Jemec GBE. Orismilast for the treatment of mild to severe hidradenitis suppurativa: week 16 data from OSIRIS, a phase 2a, open-label, single-centre, single-arm, dose-finding clinical trial. J Eur Acad Dermatol Venereol. 2024;38(5):920–30. https://doi.org/10.1111/jdv.19770.
57. Boyles JS, Beidler CB, Strifler BA, et al. Discovery and characterization of a neutralizing pan-ELR+CXC chemokine monoclonal antibody. MAbs. 2020;12(1):1831880. https://doi.org/10.1080/19420862.2020.1831880.

58. Forman S, Patel D, Kimball AB, et al. Safety and efficacy of LY3041658, a novel septa-specific monoclonal antibody to CXCR1 and CXCR2 ligands, in a phase 2 study in hidradenitis suppurativa. Late-breaking research. Presented at 2023 Annual Meeting of the American Academy of Dermatology, New Orleans, Louisiana, 17–21 Mar 2023.
59. McDonald A, Karnik R, Campbell V, et al. IRAK4 is overexpressed in hidradenitis suppurativa skin and correlates with inflammatory biomarkers. J Invest Dermatol. 2025;145(2):323–333.e10. https://doi.org/10.1016/j.jid.2024.04.035.
60. Ackerman L, Acloque G, Bacchelli S, et al. IRAK4 degrader in hidradenitis suppurativa and atopic dermatitis: a phase 1 trial. Nat Med. 2023;29:3127–36. https://doi.org/10.1038/s41591-023-02635-7.
61. A phase 2 study to evaluate the efficacy and safety of SAR444656 compared with placebo in adult participants with moderate to severe hidradenitis suppurativa (ZEN). ClinicalTrials.gov identifier: NCT06028230. Updated March 4, 2025. Accessed 14 June 2025. https://clinicaltrials.gov/study/NCT06028230.
62. Kanni T, Zenker O, Habel M, Riedemann N, Giamarellos-Bourboulis EJ. Complement activation in hidradenitis suppurativa: a new pathway of pathogenesis? Br J Dermatol. 2018;179(2):413–9. https://doi.org/10.1111/bjd.16428.
63. Giamarellos-Bourboulis EJ, Argyropoulou M, Kanni T, et al. Clinical efficacy of complement C5a inhibition by IFX-1 in hidradenitis suppurativa: an open-label single-arm trial in patients not eligible for adalimumab. Br J Dermatol. 2020;183(1):176–8. https://doi.org/10.1111/bjd.18877.
64. Bosslett M. InflaRx presents efficacy and safety data on vilobelimab at AAD 2025. Dermatology Times. Published March 11, 2025. Accessed 14 June 2025. https://www.dermatologytimes.com/view/inflarx-presents-efficacy-and-safety-data-on-vilobelimab-at-aad-2025.
65. Kirby J, Prens E, Jemec GB, Malathong V, Prasad S, Schall T, Staehr P, et al. LB791 Avacopan, a highly selective small molecule inhibitor of C5a receptor, in patients with hidradenitis suppurativa: initial results from a randomized, double-blind, placebo-controlled, phase 2 study (AURORA). J Invest Dermatol. 2021;141(8):B19. https://doi.org/10.1016/j.jid.2021.07.121.
66. van Straalen KR, Piguet V, Gudjonsson JE. Hidradenitis suppurativa: key insights into treatment success and failure. J Clin Invest. 2024;134(21):e186744. https://doi.org/10.1172/JCI186744. Published 2024 Nov 1.
67. Kimball, A. Efficacy and safety of the oral Bruton's tyrosine kinase inhibitor, remibrutinib, in patients with moderate to severe hidradenitis suppurativa in a randomized, phase 2, double-blind, placebo-controll. Late-breaking research: session 1. Presented at: 2024 American Academy of Dermatology Meeting, San Diego, CA, 8–12 Mar 2024. https://am2024.aad.org/sessions/16895.
68. NCT06799000. A phase 3 study to assess efficacy, safety, and tolerability of remibrutinib in adult patients with moderate to severe hidradenitis suppurativa (RECHARGE 1). ClinicalTrials.gov. Updated June 11, 2025. Accessed 14 June 2025. https://clinicaltrials.gov/study/NCT06799000.
69. NCT06840392. Study to assess efficacy, safety, and tolerability of remibrutinib in adult patients with moderate to severe hidradenitis suppurativa (RECHARGE 2). ClinicalTrials.gov. Updated May 6, 2025. Accessed 14 June 2025. https://clinicaltrials.gov/study/NCT06840392.
70. Jepsen R, Edwards C, Flora A, Kozera E, Frew JW. A proof-of-concept open-label clinical trial of spleen tyrosine kinase antagonism using fostamatinib in moderate-to-severe hidradenitis suppurativa. J Am Acad Dermatol. 2023;89(4):694–702. https://doi.org/10.1016/j.jaad.2023.05.076.
71. NCT06118099. Proof-of-concept study assessing the efficacy and safety of subcutaneous amlitelimab in adult participants with moderate to severe hidradenitis suppurativa. ClinicalTrials.gov. Updated February 26, 2025. Accessed 15 June 2025.
72. Leeuw T, Šimaitė D, Heyninck K, et al. Combined TNF-α and OX40L targeting as a new treatment option for hidradenitis suppurativa. J Allergy Clin Immunol Glob. 2025;4(3):100483. https://doi.org/10.1016/j.jacig.2025.100483. Published 2025 Apr 23.

73. NCT05849922. A study to test the efficacy and safety of SAR442970 in adults with hidradenitis suppurativa (HS OBTAIN). ClinicalTrials.gov. Updated January 23, 2025. Accessed 15 June 2025. https://clinicaltrials.gov/study/NCT05849922.
74. Collins L, Costello RA. Glucagon-like peptide-1 receptor agonists. [Updated 2024 Feb 29]. In: StatPearls [Internet]. Treasure Island (FL): StatPearls Publishing; 2025. Available from: https://www.ncbi.nlm.nih.gov/books/NBK551568/.
75. Phan K, Charlton O, Smith SD. Hidradenitis suppurativa and metabolic syndrome—systematic review and adjusted meta-analysis. Int J Dermatol. 2019;58:1112–7. https://doi.org/10.1111/ijd.14500.
76. Krajewski PK, Złotowska A, Szepietowski JC. The therapeutic potential of GLP-1 receptor agonists in the management of hidradenitis suppurativa: a systematic review of anti-inflammatory and metabolic effects. J Clin Med. 2024;13(21):6292. https://doi.org/10.3390/jcm13216292. Published 2024 Oct 22.

Index

N. Brownstone (ed.), *Clinical Cases in Hidradenitis Suppurativa*, Clinical Cases in Dermatology, https://doi.org/10.1007/978-3-032-15200-8